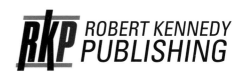
ROBERT KENNEDY
PUBLISHING

ANABOLIC PRIMER

Ergogenic Enhancement for the Hardcore Bodybuilder

By Gerard Thorne

Published by Robert Kennedy Publishing
400 Matheson Boulevard West
Mississauga, ON
L5R 3M1 Canada
Visit us at www.emusclemag.com or www.rkpubs.com

Art Directors: Alex Waddell and Jason Branidis
Copy Editor: Jacqui Hartley
Proofreader: James De Medeiros
Cover Photos: Jason Breeze

Library and Archives Canada Cataloguing in Publication

Thorne, Gerard, 1963-
        Anabolic Primer : ergogenic enhancement for the hardcore
bodybuilder / Gerard Thorne.

Includes index.
ISBN 978-1-55210-066-0

        1. Bodybuilding--Physiological aspects. 2. Bodybuilders--Drug
use. 3. Bodybuilders--Nutrition. 4. Metabolism--Effect of drugs on.
5. Dietary supplements. I. Title.

RC1220.W44T56 2009   615'.739   C2009-902014-9

10 9 8 7 6 5 4 3 2 1

Distributed in Canada by NBN (National Book Network)
67 Mowat Avenue, Suite 241
Toronto, ON
M6K 3E3

Distributed in USA by NBN (National Book Network)
15200 NBN Way
Blue Ridge Summit, PA
17214
Printed in Canada.

Robert Kennedy Publishing Book Department
Art Director: Gabriella Caruso Marques
Senior Production Editor: Wendy Morley

DISCLAIMER

Robert Kennedy Publishing and Gerard
Thorne do not condone the use of anabolic
steroids or any other illegal substances. The
sections in this book pertaining to these topics are for information purposes only. In
countries where certain substances discussed within are illegal, please obey the law.

WARNING

This book is not intended as medical advice,
nor is it offered for use in the diagnosis of
any health condition or as a substitute for
medical treatment and/or counsel. Its purpose is to explore advanced topics on sports
nutrition and exercise. All data are for information only. Use of any of the programs
within this book is at the sole risk and choice
of the reader. Before undertaking any form
of formal exercise or a new nutrition regimen, consult your healthcare professional.
Ask for a physical stress test to ascertain
your tolerance for strenuous exercise.

ACKNOWLEDGMENTS

Brave is the individual who attempts to compile a book of this size on his own. I claim no such bravery, and for this reason I'd like to thank the following individuals.

Special thanks to Jennifer Kelly for all of her painstaking editing and suggestions. An author could not hope for a better editor. Thanks cookie.

Thanks to Bertha Thorne for her continued support and financial counseling. I'm still not retired and out of debt, but that's not her fault!

Thank you to Wendy Morley for her help over the past few years.

Finally to Robert Kennedy, thanks for giving me yet another opportunity to help millions of people around the world improve their physiques and overall health. Bob took a big chance 10 years ago, asking an unknown to write a series of books for him. I hope I've managed to do the *MuscleMag* name proud.

TABLE OF CONTENTS

BOOK ONE
Evolution and Current Perspectives

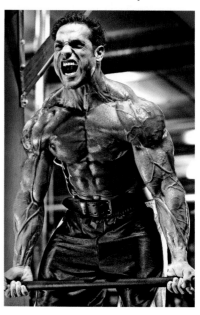

BOOK TWO
Hormone Manipulation

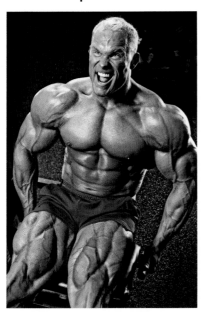

BOOK THREE
Fat Burning

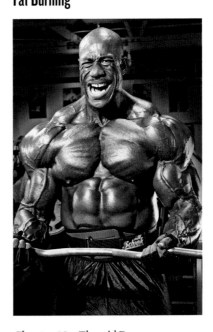

TABLE OF CONTENTS

BOOK FOUR
Stimulants

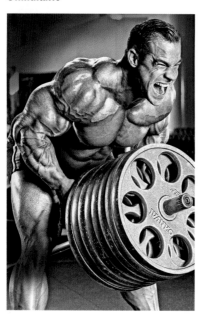

BOOK FIVE
Painkillers

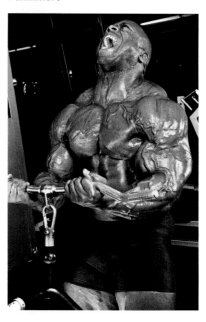

BOOK SIX
Protein and Amino Acids

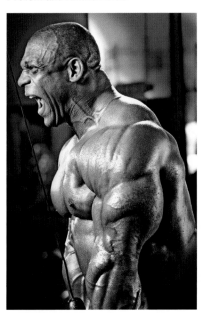

BOOK SEVEN
Ergogenic Nutrients

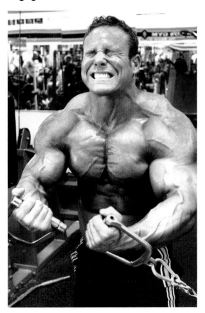

TABLE OF CONTENTS

BOOK EIGHT
Natural Anabolics and Anti-Catabolics

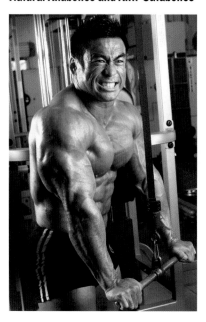

BOOK NINE
Ergogenic Techniques

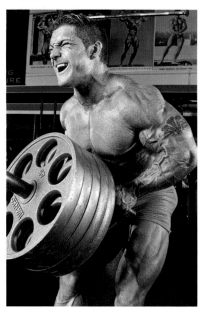

BOOK TEN
Putting It All Together

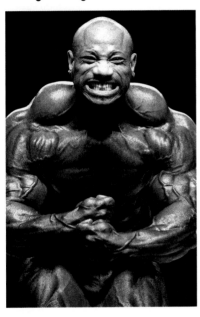

PREFACE

If there's one aspect separating *MuscleMag International* from its magazine competitors it's in the treatment of performance-enhancing drugs and ergogenic aids. Where most other monthly mags either pretend the issue doesn't exist or bombard readers with a plethora of horror stories, *MuscleMag* has always tried to provide readers with an objective look at this controversial topic. In fact, it was such honesty that led to the original publishing of *Anabolic Primer*. No sooner had it hit bookshelves when readers demanded a sequel, and *Anabolic Edge* was born. Nearly 10 years have passed and the murky world of performance enhancement shows no signs of a clear path ahead. Every month sees a new compound on the market that advertisers claim will put "20 pounds of muscle on your body" or "drive your strength levels through the roof."

Despite the popularity of drugs and supplements, many body-builders and athletes are still looking for natural ways to increase their size and strength without having to fork out hundreds of dollars every month on supplements or risk being arrested by the Drug Enforcement Administration (DEA) for illegal use. The growing interest in drug-free muscle building is why we've included totally new chapters informing you how to use diet and exercise to promote anabolic reactions in the body. Of course, we also realize that readers want the latest information on the newest supplements – rest assured we've included a thorough recap of what biochemistry has made available over the last 10 years.

We should point out that many of the supplements fall into two or more categories. For example, ephedrine and caffeine are used both as stimulants and fat-burning supplements. Because compounds such as these carry out dual functions in the body, you'll find descriptions of them in more than one chapter.

We'll also examine in detail the health and safety aspects of the various compounds presented in the pages within. While it's true that law makers and the media industry often inflate the dangers of supplement use, the fact remains that most drugs and over-the-counter supplements can be dangerous if taken in mega doses – a practice that has more recently become all too common.

One comment readers made about the original *Anabolic Primer* and *Anabolic Edge* was that these two books lacked information from star athletes. This rewrite of *Anabolic Primer* suffers no omissions in this regard, and an entire chapter has been devoted to pre-contest training tips from top bodybuilders.

Since the first two publications were released, certain laws and regulations for many of the drugs and supplements discussed in this book have become increasingly strict. For example, supplements such as ephedrine that were once sold over the counter are now banned or highly restricted. So, even if you question the rationale behind such legislation, the fact remains that you could face prison time if you decide to use any of these illegal substances.

Our aim in *Anabolic Primer* is to provide you with the most up-to-date and accurate information on performance enhancement and the associated drugs and compounds. We present the history, the facts and even the controversies, giving you not just a glimpse into this world, but a full and honest perspective on the topic. Knowledge is a powerful tool, and that's the very reason you'll find such vital information within this book.

INTRODUCTION

When the original *Anabolic Primer* was published in 1998, the sports community was still recovering from the fallout 10 years earlier at the 1988 Olympic Games. Canadian sprinter Ben Johnson's positive test for anabolic steroids in Seoul, South Korea, exposed the general public to the seedier side of athletics and the "win-at-any-cost" mentality that had permeated into modern sports. Prior to those Games, steroids and other performance-enhancing drugs were believed to be solely the domain of bodybuilders and weightlifters. But the Johnson scandal set in motion a chain of events that would reveal just how widespread drug use in sports really was.

While Johnson was the first big-name athlete to be caught using performance-enhancing drugs, many others have come under scrutiny since then. Superstar athletes such as Major League Baseball players Mark McGwire, Barry Bonds and Roger Clemens; sprinter Marion Jones; and Tour de France winner Floyd Landis have all been exposed for their drug use – either by their own admission or through independent investigations including drug tests. The banned substance issue has reached a point where the general public assumes most athletes are using drugs. Positive drug tests certainly no longer garner the same degree of shock and surprise as when Ben Johnson filled his urine sample cup back in 1988.

A LONG TRADITION

Contrary to popular opinion, drug use to boost athletic performance is not a modern invention. As early as 776 BC, the Greek Olympians were reported to have used substances such as dried figs, mushrooms and strychnine to gain a competitive edge over their opponents. During the days of the Roman Empire, chariot racers were said to have fed their horses a potent mixture to make the animals run faster, and many gladiators "doped up" to make their fights sufficiently more violent and bloodier for the paying spectators.

Athletes got their first real competitive edge thanks to the help of medical science. Perhaps the most significant occurrence was in 1889 when Dr. Charles Edward Brown-Sequard announced at a scientific meeting in Paris, France, that he had found a compound that eliminated most of his 72-year-old body's ailments. He reported having injected himself with the extract of dog and guinea pig testicles under the assumption these organs had "internal secretions that acted as physiologic regulators." As bold (and foolhardy) as Brown-Sequard's experiment was, the French scientist was on to something – his early investigations eventually led to the discovery of hormones in 1905 and the consequent isolation of testosterone in

1935. Soon thereafter, Russian weightlifters began to outpace American Olympians with their "Eastern Bloc Secrets." Not wanting to be left behind, U.S. coach Dr. John Ziegler did some research of sorts, discovering the "secret" to the Russians' success after having a few drinks with Russian weightlifting coaches. Ziegler then teamed up with chemists to produce an anabolic steroid (now known as Dianabol) for American athletes.

Now, readers should not be misled into thinking that steroids are the only drugs used by athletes. In the 1930s, amphetamines were synthesized and quickly made their way into gym bags. Other chemical goodies such as diuretics, painkillers and growth hormone were also added to the athletic arsenal as soon as they hit pharmacy shelves.

Recognizing the inroads drugs had made into the Games (although not to the full extent) the International Olympic Committee (IOC) began official drug testing at the 1968 Olympics in Mexico City. At first the only tests conducted were for amphetamines and other related performance-enhancing drugs. Anabolic steroids weren't added to the list of banned substances until 1973. Steroid testing became mandatory starting at the Montreal Olympics in 1976.

To get an idea of the modern athlete's mindset, a now well-known survey was conducted in the 1990s in which aspiring Olympians were asked two basic questions: "If you were offered a banned performance-enhancing substance that guaranteed you would win an Olympic medal and you could not be caught, would you take it?" Remarkably, 195 of 198 athletes answered yes. And, "Would you take a banned performance-enhancing drug under a guarantee that you will not be caught, will win every competition for the next five years, but will then die from adverse effects of the substance?" Amazingly, over 50 percent of the athletes answered that they would still take the drug.[1]

The results of this survey sent a clear message about the sporting world: Modern athletes are willing to sacrifice everything – even their lives – for a better chance at achieving Olympic glory.

The crackdown on drugs was what helped spearhead the growth of the "natural" supplement industry. But as we'll see in later chapters, there is a fine line separating the definitions of "drug" and "natural." A large gray area exists within this topic, and some of the supplements touted as safe and natural are potentially even more dangerous than their drug counterparts.

Reference

1) Bamberger M., Yaeger D. Over the edge: special report. *Sports Illustrated*. (1997) 86:64.

EVOLUTION AND CURRENT PERSPECTIVES

B1

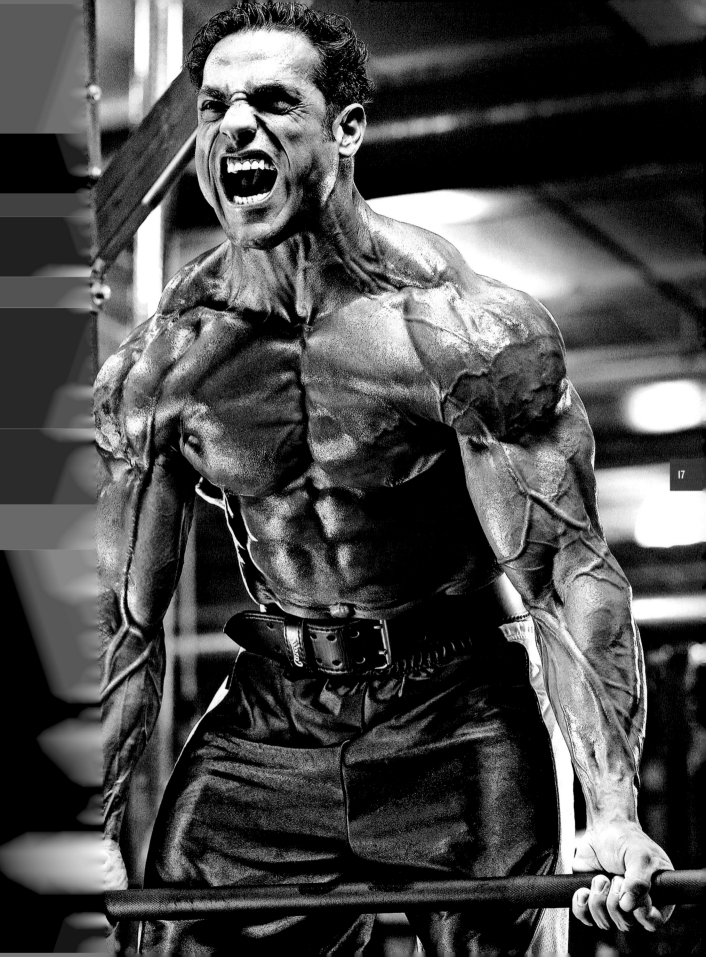

THE EVOLUTION OF THE SUPPLEMENT INDUSTRY

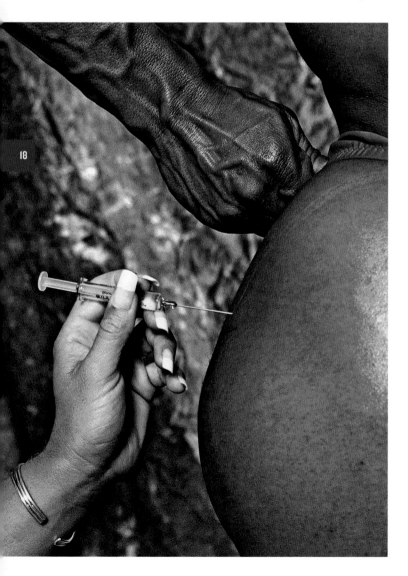

18

In the broadest sense, ergogenic supplements are substances used by bodybuilders and other athletes with the belief that they will improve performance, whether by increasing strength, size or power (strength over time). The term ergogenic comes from the Greek *ergo* – to work, and *genesis* – the beginning. Ergogenic aids exist in many forms including powder, liquid, tablet and capsule, solid, and yes – injection. Most types are taken with meals and snacks, but compounds such as steroids and growth hormone are injected.

Although the prefix words "ergogenic" and "food" are often used interchangeably, there is a difference between the two. For most people a food supplement is merely a way to add extra nutrients to their diets. Increasing athletic performance is not usually a consideration. For a bodybuilder, however, every nutrient entering his body is taken with the sole purpose of increasing muscle strength and size. While food supplements are used by the general population, ergogenic compounds are primarily limited to use among bodybuilders and other athletes.

It should also be made clear that ergogenic supplements can include both legal and illegal compounds. Of course, illegal and legal simply represent moments in time, and many compounds discussed in the first *Anabolic Primer* and *Anabolic Edge* are now banned.

Photo by Jim Amentler

IN THE BEGINNING

Until the early 1990s the most popular name in the supplement industry was Weider. Joe Weider was a former Canadian whose name came to symbolize bodybuilding. Starting with his first magazine *Your Physique* in 1939 (later renamed *Muscle Builder Power* and then *Muscle and Fitness*), Weider built a California-based publishing and supplement empire that cofounded the International Federation of Bodybuilders (IFBB) and brought a young Arnold Schwarzenegger to America in 1968.

Weider was the first publisher and supplement manufacturer to realize that marketing was the most important tool for selling food supplements. By combining photos of the latest bodybuilding stars with persuasive writing, Weider could convince millions of young readers that the key to their bodybuilding success was using his supplements. The fact that most of the featured stars didn't use his products (but did use steroids and other performance-enhancing drugs) was conveniently omitted. By the early 1990s, Weider had a virtual monopoly in the food supplement business and was grossing hundreds of millions of dollars a year. Of course any time that amount of money is being made, sooner or later a challenger will come along to shake up the market. The upstart's name was Bill Phillips, and the industry hasn't been the same since his arrival.

WHO NEEDS CALIFORNIA?

Until 1986, Bill Phillips was just another aspiring bodybuilder who headed to California with the hopes of making it big on the bodybuilding scene. He soon realized he didn't have the genetics to make his mark in bodybuilding and moved back to Colorado. Bill's four years in California was not time wasted, however, as he made a point to learn everything he could about anabolic steroids. With just $185 and a small office in his mother's basement, Bill began to publish a newsletter called *The Anabolic Reference Update*. Word spread quickly about Bill's frank discussions of steroids, and by 1992 his

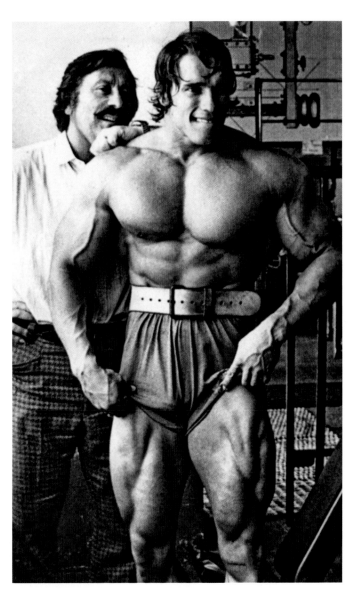

ABOVE: It was bodybuilding legend Joe Weider and his growing empire that attracted Arnold Schwarzenegger to the U.S. in the late 1960s.

LEFT: The vast array of ergogenic supplements include everything from liquids and powders to capsules and tablets, some forms are even injected.

> "It probably wasn't too long after the invention of the barbell that bodybuilders started ingesting various concoctions in an effort to enhance their progress. Probably not long after that, a shrewd businessman thought of selling some exotic elixir that promised to more quickly build bigger and stronger muscles. As athletes became more sophisticated, so did the promotion techniques of the hucksters."
>
> – Nelson Montana, *MuscleMag International* contributor

basement publication had grown into a glossy monthly magazine that rapidly vaulted to the No. 1 position in muscle magazine sales. Called *Muscle Media 2000*, the magazine focused almost entirely on performance enhancement. Bill's next goal was to get into the supplement business by teaming up with Dr. Scott Connelly to promote MET-Rx. At that time, MET-Rx was the world's first hardcore meal-replacement product, and thanks to the popularity of *Muscle Media 2000* and heavy marketing, it became the industry's top-selling supplement. Their partnership was short-lived, though – Phillips wanted to sell the product exclusively through the magazine while Connelly wanted to make it mainstream. After parting ways, Bill acquired the rights to a small company called Experimental and Applied Sciences (EAS), and, as with Met-Rx, brought it to the top of the supplement industry with heavy promotion in *Muscle Media 2000*.

By 1997 EAS was the No. 1 supplement company in the world, ending nearly 50 years of domination by Weider. Realizing nothing lasts forever, Bill decided to go mainstream that year, and he changed the name *Muscle Media 2000* to just *Muscle Media*. Instead of targeting hardcore bodybuilders, the new format was geared more toward overall health and fitness. In theory the mainstream market should have been more lucrative, but it wasn't. A combination of losing longtime, loyal readers and Bill's departing from the supplement business led to the magazine's decline in sales and final shutdown in 2004.

AND ALL THE REST

Lest readers assume the supplement industry has been all EAS since the early 1990s, nothing could be further from the truth. Though displaced from the top of the supplement heap, Joe Weider was still a major force in that world. Aside from publishing his collection of monthly magazines including *Flex*, *Muscle and Fitness*, and *Shape*, Joe and his brother Ben continued to run the IFBB and sponsor its numerous pro contests. There are also the new kids on the block. We say "new," but some have been operating for decades. It's just that these companies finally emerged from Weider's shadow during the 1990s thanks to Bill Phillips' industry shakeup. Some of the more recent heavyweights in the supplement industry include MuscleTech, TwinLab, ProLab and Optimum Nutrition. Every year these businesses (and hundreds of others) fight for their piece of the estimated 20-billion dollar supplement pie.

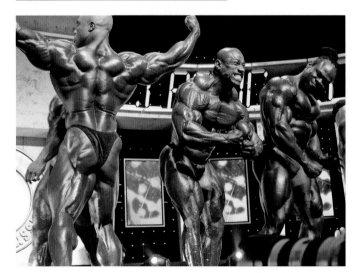

ABOVE: For bodybuilders, choosing the right supplements is a key part of creating a contest-winning physique.

Photo by Gordon Smith
Model Phil Heath, Dexter Jackson and Kai Greene

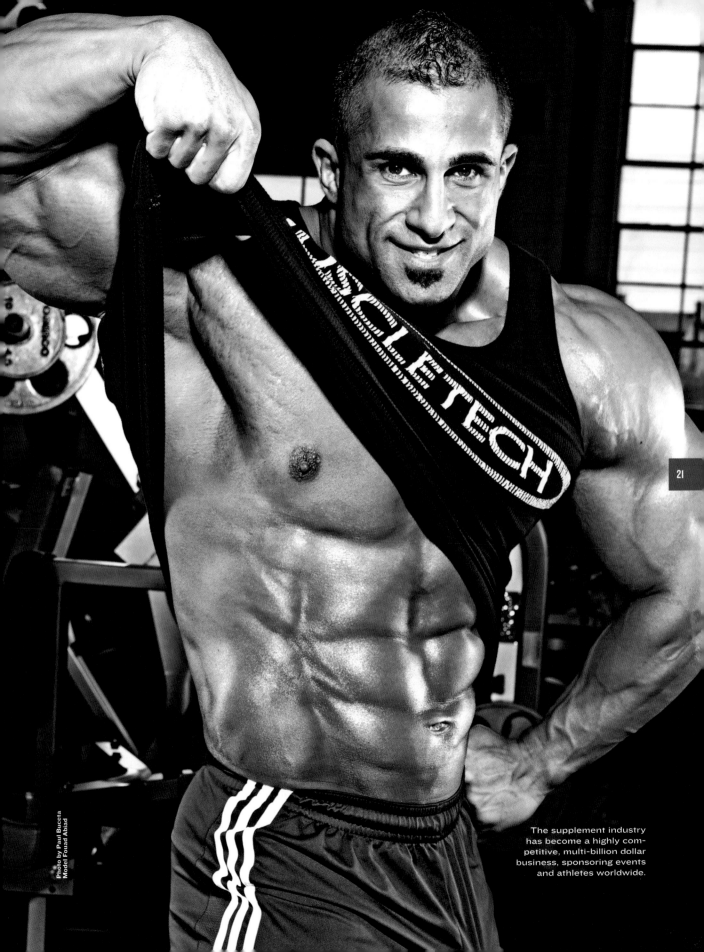

21

The supplement industry has become a highly competitive, multi-billion dollar business, sponsoring events and athletes worldwide.

THE MODERN SUPPLEMENT SCENE

"After the release of *Pumping Iron* in 1976, gym membership numbers soared. This was a mixed blessing for bodybuilding promoters because home gym equipment sales declined. Supplements then became the main sales objective."

– Nelson Montana, *MuscleMag International* contributor

These days a trip to the health-food store carries the same degree of bewilderment and discovery as a trek up the Amazon. It also involves similar risks. While supplement manufacturers are big on claims and advertising, most fall far short when it comes to providing hard scientific data to back up the effectiveness of their products. Circus promoter extraordinaire P.T. Barnum once said, "There's a sucker born every minute." Barnum may be long gone, but his philosophy lives on in the minds of many supplement makers. And the current state of health-food regulations doesn't help the matter. As it stands right now, dietary supplement manufacturers are not required to test their products for purity or effectiveness. Essentially, this means they can take a page right out of Dr. Joseph Goebels' diary (Goebels was Adolf Hitler's minister of propaganda). Much of Hitler's success was based on the premise that if you tell a lie often enough, people will eventually start believing it. The strategy in the supplement industry is no different. Every month *MuscleMag International, Flex* and other popular bodybuilding magazines are filled with full-page, glossy ads telling bodybuilders how just "three pills per day" or "two scoops" can turn 140-pound weaklings into 280-pound pillars of muscularity. The pro bodybuilders in the ads realize the difference, but the naive 16-year-old staring wide-eyed at the image of his hero assumes what the ad is saying is true.

Perhaps the most sobering aspect of the supplement effectiveness debate is their ease of availability. If over-the-counter (OTC) supplements were as effective as claimed, by definition they'd be drugs and would require a prescription. These products would also be heavily regulated. But go into any health-food store and you'll see row upon row of eye-catching bottles and containers all readily available for the "manufacturer's retail price."

Now does this mean all OTC supplements are worthless and potentially dangerous? Of course not. Bodybuilders can thank Bill Phillips for making quality and safety important to more supplement companies. During his EAS days, Bill made a point to base much of his claims on results from scientific studies. Granted researchers can easily find ways to "influence" and "misinterpret" study results if the manufacturer is providing the grant money. Nevertheless, Bill changed the way supplement companies designed and marketed their products. The bigger, more reputable manufacturers in the current industry try to cite medical studies to back some of the claims in their ads. They also run quality control tests to ensure their products are pure and free of contaminants. The same, however, cannot be said of some of the smaller, get-rich-quick companies. Because the supplement industry is poorly regulated, and given its worth, it tends to attract some unsavory characters. Before popping a pill or swallowing some liquid, ask yourself a few basic questions: Why am I taking this? What do I expect to achieve by using this supplement? Just how much do I know about this company? Are they new to the scene or well-known and established? Remember it's your body and you only have one copy.

BELOW: Buying supplements has become a bit like piecing a puzzle together – a combination of research, science and promotional marketing has led to an influx of products to choose from.

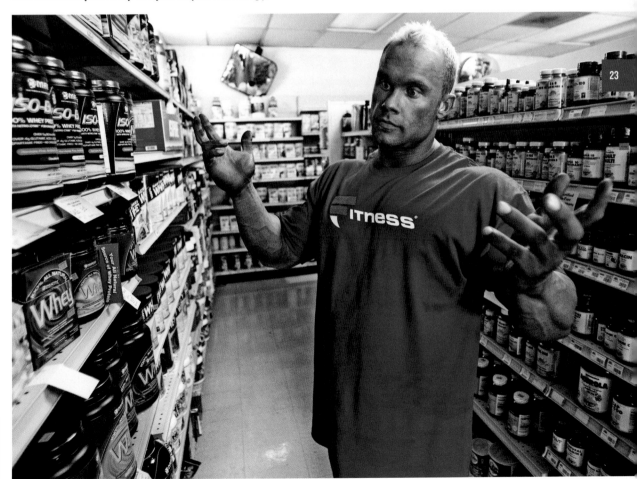

Photo by Robert Reiff
Model Ben Pakulski

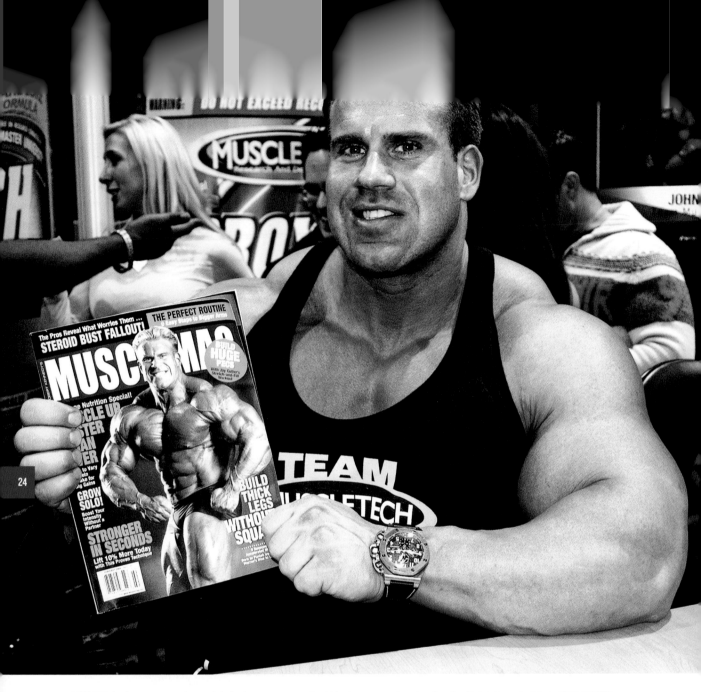

ABOVE: A close connection exists between bodybuilding, magazine publishing and supplement sales – magazines promote the bodybuilders, athletes promote the mags and supplement companies drive the entire sport with marketing and sponsorship.

BODYBUILDING & SUPPLEMENTS — THE ETERNAL PARTNERSHIP

Of all the sports associated with supplements, none play a bigger role than bodybuilding. In fact the two are so heavily interdependent it's doubtful one could survive without the other. Bodybuilders rely on supplements as a means to increase their muscle size and strength, and decrease their recovery time between workouts. Pro bodybuilders also depend on the industry itself as a source of income. Most of the leading manufacturers pay top bodybuilders big bucks to promote their products at contests, conferences and seminars. Companies also pay bodybuilders for the rights to use their photos in ads. Supplement manufacturers support the sport as a whole by

Photo by Garry Bartlett
Model Jay Cutler

sponsoring contests. The monthly bodybuilding magazines similarly serve a crucial role, both promoting the sport and serving as the primary marketing platform for the hundreds of supplement lines. Contrary to popular belief, most of the operating revenue generated by these magazines comes from supplement ads, not OTC sales. To give you an idea of the amount of money involved, a full-page, glossy ad in *MuscleMag International*, *Flex*, or *Iron Man* costs thousands of dollars per month. One quick flip through any recent copy and you'll see dozens of such ads. Some of the bigger supplement companies may have eight to 10 ad pages. We're talking top dollars here, most of which gets recouped from supplement manufacturer's best friends: bodybuilders!

BODYBUILDERS – THE MOST LUCRATIVE MARKET

Though athletes in virtually every sport use supplements these days, by far the biggest users (in all respects) are bodybuilders. The relationship between the two dates back to the late 1940s and early 1950s when the first protein supplements came on the scene. Initial ads were tame by today's standards – usually a good-looking bodybuilder standing on a beach, holding a tin of protein in one hand and a beautiful blonde in the other. The message to teenaged males was obvious: use this product and you'll build a muscular physique and be swarmed by beautiful women.

As the supplement industry and products evolved, so too did the ads. Nowadays supplement manufacturers capitalize by using the latest computer graphics and professional photography. Companies also spend millions of dollars on the packaging of their products. Those plain, boring-looking tins with block lettering from the '60s and '70s have been replaced by attractive, eye-catching bottles and boxes that rival the top pharmaceutical products.

THE LONG ARM OF THE LAW

Some consider it the most progressive piece of legislation in athletic history. Others view it as nothing short of Draconian and the biggest boost to the illegal drug trade since

BELOW: Early strategic marketing techniques enticed young athletes with the promise that supplementing would bring muscle ... and the ladies.

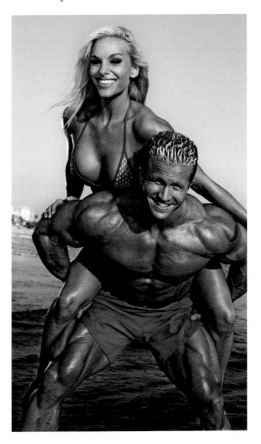

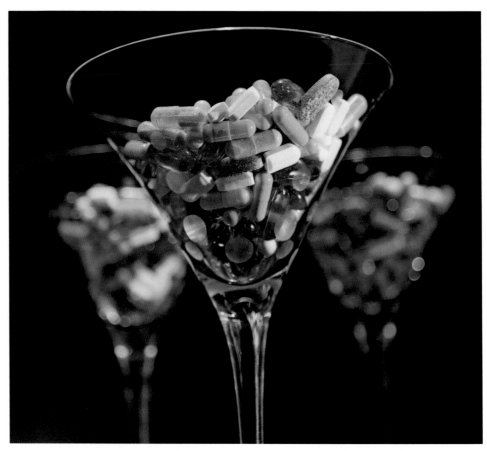

ABOVE: The effects of certain drugs and substances are amplified when combined. "Synergism," as it's called, has led to a growing popularity of drug cocktails in the sport.

prohibition. We're talking about the Anabolic Control Act of 1990. We'll be discussing the legal aspects of steroids and other performance drugs much more in a later chapter, so suffice it to say here that the Anabolic Control Act of 1990 was a boon to supplement manufacturers. When steroids were classified as controlled substances in 1990, the supplement industry knew bodybuilders and other athletes would be looking for alternative options. In response the manufacturers cleverly started marketing their products using catch terms such as "Anabolic," "Steroid replacer," "Hormonal," "Testosterone" and "Metabolic." The old, simple lettering was replaced with detailed biochemical assays, tables and charts. You'd almost need a PhD to decipher the ads, given the copious use of scientific language. Many ads are now disguised as articles complete with references. Such advertising has helped the evolution of bodybuilding as well. A careful balancing of amino acids, creatine reserves and training tempos have replaced the days when "all you can eat, all you can lift" were words to live by.

Photo by Paul Buceta

26

COSTS AND DANGERS

If there's one thing bodybuilders have inherited from the steroid industry with regards to supplements it's the issue of mega-dosing. As bodybuilders gradually upped their steroid dosages over the years, so too was there a dramatic increase in the amount of supplement consumption. Many bodybuilders spend hundreds, and in some cases thousands, of dollars a month on dietary products. If an individual wanted to consume at least one pill or scoop from all of the major supplement groups (i.e., protein, creatine, glutamine, etc.), his monthly expenditure would easily exceed $1,000. We then need to ask the question, is it worth it? Are bodybuilders achieving the strength and size gains they're paying for?

We should start by asserting that no OTC food supplement is anywhere near as effective as any anabolic steroid when it comes to increasing muscle size, strength and recovery abilities. And while the potential dangers of steroids far outweigh the dangers of most supplements, the bottom line is that on a dollar-per-dollar cost basis, steroids are far more effective.

That being said, we'll now look at the issue from an opposing viewpoint. When taken separately, no OTC supplement produces near the same degree of effects that anabolic steroids do. There is evidence, however – both scientific and anecdotal – to suggest that when some of the best supplements are combined, they do produce moderate degrees of anabolism. In some individuals the results may be similar to that of small doses of steroids, and it's believed they arise from what pharmacologists call a "synergistic effect." Synergism occurs when two or more compounds produce added effects that are greater than the sum total of those produced when the compounds are taken separately. Put more simply, this means that instead of 2+2 = 4, you may have 2+2 = 6, 8, 10 or more.

Now while the performance-enhancing outcome of such supplement cocktailing may be clear, the safety aspects are still a mixed bag. Until the early 1990s, bodybuilders really had only a few categories of supplements to choose from. The most popular were protein products and vitamin and mineral derivatives. However, starting with creatine in 1992–'93, the modern bodybuilder was afforded more choice, with now literally hundreds of different compounds to choose from. No one knows what the long-term consequences of such multi-compound mega-dosing might be. Granted most of the top sellers such as creatine, protein, glutamine, nitric oxide and the like are naturally occurring compounds. The key point, however, is that these substances don't exist naturally in the human body in the amounts ingested by bodybuilders. No long-term studies investigating the effects of these compounds have been published yet. A four-week experiment looking at performance-enhancing

"When I'm sponsored by a company I try out their entire line and settle on a few products I like to use, but do I go out of my way to spend my own money on every product that comes out? No, definitely not."

– Lee Priest, professional bodybuilder

effects cannot be used to sufficiently predict the health outcomes of taking a compound for 10 or 20 years – a time span of use many of today's bodybuilders have surpassed or will eventually reach.

We must also be cautious of the purity of many supplements. As mentioned earlier, the amount of money to be made in the supplement industry is enormous. While most of the larger manufacturers have reputable quality-control practices, the same cannot be said for some of the smaller fly-by-night operations. Regulatory agencies usually become interested in supplements only when a particular manufacturer goes too far with advertising claims. Healthcare professionals take notice only when a specific health issue can be traced back to a certain supplement. Unfortunately this type of reactionary response can backfire, as was illustrated when the amino acid tryptophan came under scrutiny.

During the late 1980s, the amino acid tryptophan (commonly used as a sleeping aid) was linked to a painful muscle disorder called Eosinophil-Myalgia Syndrome (EMS). In 1991, after 1,500 cases were diagnosed and 38 deaths were reported, the U.S. FDA banned all sales of tryptophan. It was later determined, however, that the amino acid wasn't at fault but rather a contaminated batch of product from one Japanese manufacturing plant. It took 10 years before the FDA recognized their mistake and allowed tryptophan to again be put on store shelves for sale.

THE PLACEBO EFFECT

No discussion of supplements would be complete without a brief mention of the placebo effect. Physicians – particularly those who work in combat situations – have long known about the power of the mind when it comes to influencing a drug's effect. It was discovered during times of war (and portrayed in at least one episode of the popular TV show "M.A.S.H.") that by giving a soldier an inert sugar or salt injection and telling him it was morphine, the soldier's perception of pain disappeared. Despite the fact that the pill or injection had no pain-killing properties, the soldier's belief that it did caused the pain to lessen or disappear. In simple terms, a placebo is an inert (non-active) compound that produces the same results as a drug, based on the individual's belief in the compound. The OTC cold-medication industry relies heavily on the placebo effect. Most cold and flu remedies contain very small amounts of active ingredients, but a majority of people have their favorites and will swear by their effectiveness.

Placebos also play a major role in scientific studies and research. Before a new prescription drug is released to the general public it must undergo a battery of tests called trials. Most trials involve dividing test subjects into two groups: experimental and control. The experimental group is given the new drug while the control group is

"The key point is that these substances don't exist naturally in the human body in the amounts ingested by bodybuilders. A four-week study looking at performance-enhancing effects cannot be used to sufficiently predict the health outcomes of taking a compound for 10 or 20 years."

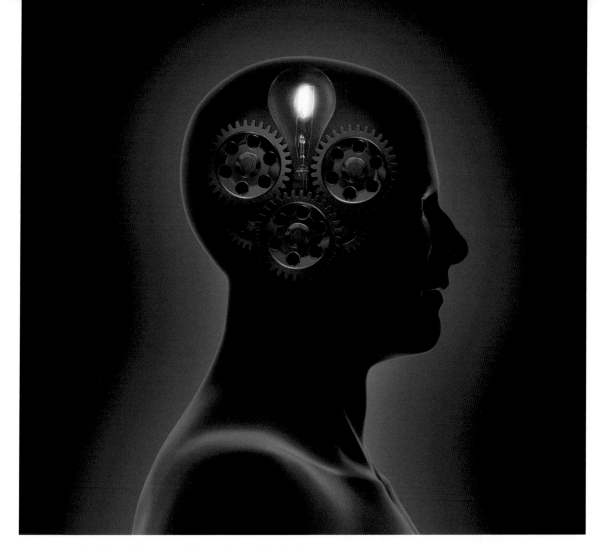

given a placebo (though they are told it is the real drug). The experiment is run and the data is then collected and analyzed. The purpose of such tests is to determine if the new drug does what the manufacturer is claiming or if most of the results can be explained by the placebo effect.

So what does all this have to do with performance enhancement? Many nutritional experts are convinced that most of the effects derived from supplements are related to the placebo effect. Nothing convinces young, naive bodybuilders of a supplement's effectiveness like a full-page, glossy ad complete with tables, charts and testimonials from pro bodybuilders. The ads are so professional in their appearances that readers are left with but one conclusion – these products will have a pronounced effect on muscle size and strength. And you know what? Chances are that when people do use the product, they will get results. The fact that the placebo effect may be the biggest contributing factor never comes into play. And even those who admit it could be more mind over matter don't really care, as long as they are seeing the outcomes they desire. This way of thinking is fine if your bottom line is strictly results, but ask yourself whether you want to continue paying big bucks for a product that is primarily a psychological bluff.

ABOVE: The mind is a powerful tool – so much so that many experts in the field of nutrition argue that supplement efficacy has more to do with the placebo effect than biochemistry.

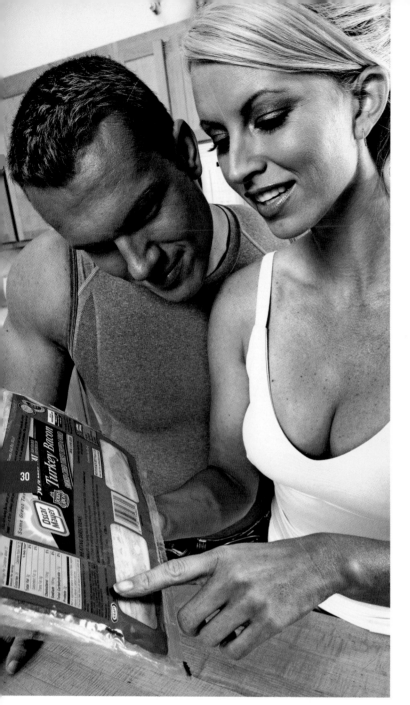

ABOVE: Being knowledgeable and conscious of the nutrients and ingredients in the foods you eat will help you stay on track with your nutritional goals.

WHEN NUTRIENT SUPPLEMENTATION MAY BE NEEDED

It's amazing the number of nutritionists who still maintain that you can get all the nutrients you need from a healthy diet. In theory they're correct, but unfortunately food-processing techniques, outdated measuring methods and busy lifestyles have created a large gray area when it comes to nutrients and individual needs.

Much of the food we eat – especially anything canned – is cooked at least three times before it arrives on store shelves for us to buy. Cooking the food at home then brings the total to four. Granted, cooking is necessary in order to kill any harmful microorganisms, but it also destroys much of the nutrient value, particularly vitamins (minerals are more resistant to heat). And fruit sources are not immune either, as a combination of chemicals and light may decrease their vitamin content by 50 percent.

Even food that holds its nutrient value may not be adequate. It used to be that you couldn't turn on a TV show or read a magazine article without coming across some reference to RDAs – Recommended Daily Allowances. RDAs are values and amounts for each of the known nutrients that were developed by the government in response to both the Great Depression and the negative effects of food-processing techniques. Recognizing that the U.S. population was at risk for developing nutrition-related diseases, the U.S. government established nutrient minimums as a means to guide the general public's food choices and eating. Also enacted was the Enrichment Act of 1942, which required food-processing companies to fortify foods with extra nutrients to help offset what was lost through manufacturing techniques.

THAT'S ALL FINE, BUT ...

You'd think that something as official and important as government-established nutritional guidelines would be the end-all to nutrient consumption, but unfortunately the RDAs have their own flaws.

Photo by Robert Reiff
Models Tom Voss and Aubrie Lemon

For starters, the RDA values were originally calculated from sedentary (non-exercising) individuals. Nowadays it's generally accepted that athletes have higher nutrient demands than the non-exercising population. So, those outdated 50- or 60-year-old RDAs probably just don't cut it. Many people have also questioned why the RDAs were even calculated in the first place. Initially the purpose of the guidelines was to suggest nutrient levels necessary to sustain life. During the 1930s and into the 1940s, sicknesses and deaths from malnutrition were tragically all-too-common occurrences. Today, however, the incidence of starvation (at least in Western societies) has declined substantially.

Yet another reason to question the RDAs is the population base that was used to calculate the values. The primary sample groups were young and healthy people. The numbers derived from such samples didn't take into account individuals with metabolic deficiencies or diseases. Furthermore, the nutrient minimums may not be adequate amounts for older individuals. It's generally understood that as we age our digestion and absorption abilities decrease. As such, common sense should dictate that the older population would benefit from ingesting nutrient values above those of the RDAs.

31

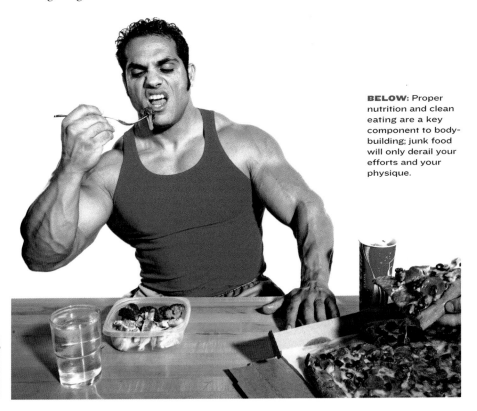

BELOW: Proper nutrition and clean eating are a key component to body-building; junk food will only derail your efforts and your physique.

These days the outdated RDAs aren't commonly used as a base point to determine nutrient needs. Two main dietary recommendation systems have since been established to replace the previous RDAs. The RDI (Reference Daily Intake or Recommended Daily Intake) values were the first of the two, set by the FDA for use in nutrition labeling – RDIs are still used to determine the "Daily Values" printed on food labels in the U.S. and Canada. Based initially on the upper limit of each RDA, the RDIs were calculated to meet the requirements of nearly all healthy individuals, and were aimed to assure needs were met for all age groups of each sex.

The most recent set of nutrient recommendations are the DRI (Dietary Reference Intake) guidelines. These values were formulated by the Food and Nutrition Board of the Institute of Medicine in 1997. Essentially, the RDAs were revised and updated, and they became one part of a broader set of guidelines – the DRIs. And it's the DRIs that may eventually be the basis for updating the RDI values.

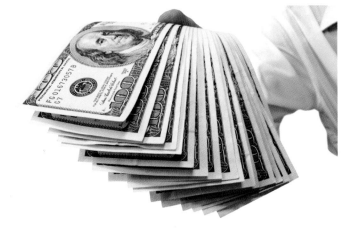

ABOVE: Using supplements is a major investment. Do your research to ensure your money is well spent.

RIGHT: Paul Demayo lost his life at the age of 37 in June 2005 – his death was the result of recreational drug abuse.

A FEW FINAL WORDS

For those readers who are ready to fork out their hard-earned cash on the latest supplements, we offer a few words of caution. First and foremost, research is very limited on the long-term side effects of mega-dosing with multiple supplements. They may be "natural" substances and may come from respectable supplement companies. This, however, doesn't erase the fact that little to nothing is known about the synergistic effects and health problems that a cocktail of 10 or 20 compounds may cause 20 or 30 years from now.

Another point of concern is legitimacy. Most readers have no doubt heard the phrase "If it sounds too good to be true it probably is." No truer words have been spoken with regards to the supplement business. If an ad claims that "studies have shown ...," take the time to check out the actual studies. A majority of large colleges and universities carry such major journals as *JAMA* (the *Journal of the American Medical Association*) and *The New England Journal of Medicine*, and most journals are also online now. Before a study is published it has to be reviewed by a number of peers (experts in the same field) and scrutinized to make sure the researchers have followed proper scientific methods. The results and conclusions are also verified. Once you've established that a study actually exists, you should then check to see if the supplement manufacturer is portraying it accurately. The best example to illustrate this point involves the amino acid arginine. In the 1980s, supplement manufacturers made millions of dollars selling arginine as an "anabolic" compound. The study they kept flouting indeed showed that arginine could cause muscular gains (by increasing levels of growth hormone), but a couple of key points were conveniently omitted. For starters, the test subjects were not bodybuilders but rather individuals with various debilitating diseases. Dosages were another factor to consider. Instead of milligram amounts in the hundreds range, the researchers were administering multiple gram-sized dosages. Through creative advertising, bodybuilders were left with the impression that a couple of 500-milligram tablets could turn skinny, 150-pound individuals into 250-pound, rock-hard Mr. Olympias.

Aside from safety and legitimacy issues, another point to take into account is cost. The $20 tins of protein from the '70s are long gone. Nowadays supplements can cost hundreds of dollars for only a month's supply. Likewise, buying three or four of the top-selling products will take a huge chunk out of your wallet each month. This expense is fine if you have the expendable cash and are seeing some decent results from your investment. You should question the practice, though, if all you end up with is the most colorful (and expensive) urine in town!

A final comment (and one that should now be second nature to you) concerns knowledge, or more correctly, the acquisition of it. Just as you continue reading muscle magazines every month to find out the latest training tips, so too should you keep up with the latest supplement information. Under no circumstances do you want to put anything in your body that you're not familiar with. Before consuming any pill, powder or oil, do some investigating. At the very least you may save yourself a heap of cash – but you could also save your own health. We'd like to think this book is a fantastic starting point.

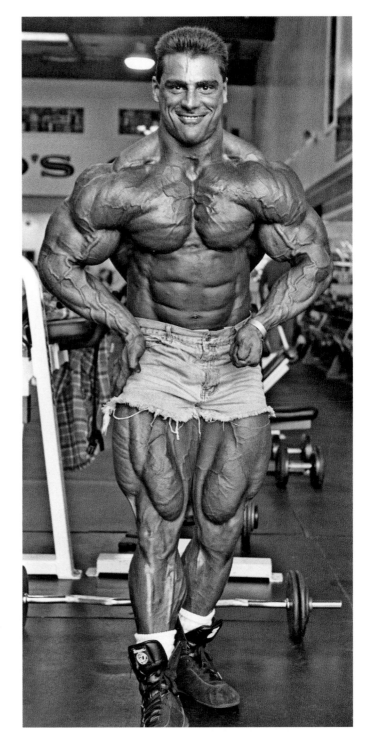

Photo by Jason Mathas
Model Paul DeMayo

33

HORMONE
MANIPULATION

B2

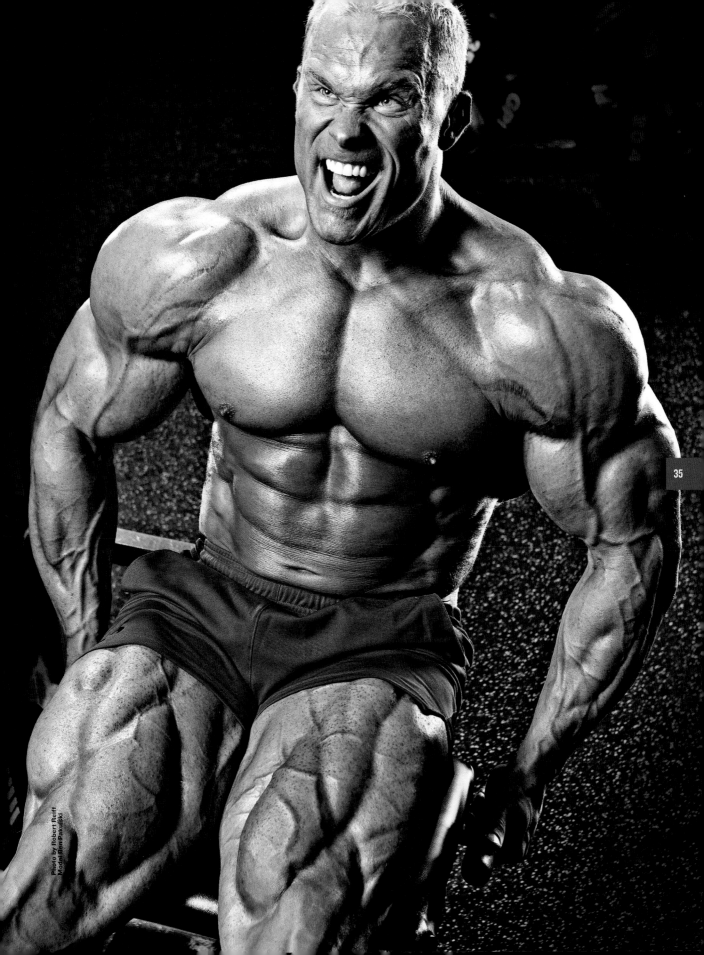

HORMONAL CONTROL

While bodybuilders and other athletes employ various strategies to boost performance, by far the most common (and effective) is modifying biochemistry – particularly the body's various hormone systems. The reason is quite simple: Under normal circumstances your body has a fixed rate at which it can utilize nutrients. Adding extra nutrients to your diet will not speed up the rate at which they are converted into new muscle tissue. Think of it like a bricklayer who's building a wall. Giving him 200 bricks makes no sense if he can only lay a maximum of 100 bricks per hour. The extra bricks will simply pile up. The same holds true for the human body – surplus nutrients and calories will only get stored as fat if they are not used. Once scientists discovered that various compounds could speed up the rate at which additional nutrients are utilized by the body, it wasn't long before bodybuilders started including the substances as part of their training regimens.

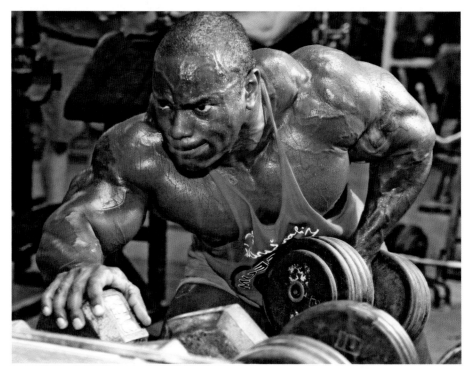

RIGHT: Many bodybuilders use substances specifically geared to modify their hormone systems, all to amplify training and growth.

Photo by Jason Breeze
Model Johnnie Jackson

36

THE ENDOCRINE SYSTEM

The human body contains two main control systems: nervous and endocrine. While the nervous system plays a role in performance enhancement, it's the endocrine system that bodybuilders and other athletes devote the most attention to when it comes to modification.

The primary units or messengers of the endocrine system are hormones. They can be peptide (protein) or steroid in nature. Peptide hormones are made from amino acids, and steroid hormones are synthesized from cholesterol. Unlike the nervous system, which has its own highway (i.e., nerves) the endocrine system relies on the vast network of blood vessels in the cardiovascular system to carry hormones throughout the body.

Hormones are similar to enzymes in that they rarely start chemical reactions but instead speed up the rate of existing reactions, and they do so in a number of ways. Hormones can

- speed up the production of enzymes, which in turn modify chemical reactions.
- increase or decrease the amount of reactants available for a reaction.
- increase the permeability of cell membranes to allow reactants easier access to cell interiors.

Like most bodily systems the brain controls the endocrine system. The brain's primary command center for most endocrine functions is the hypothalamus – a small structure located toward the front of the brain. The hypothalamus is responsible for such behaviors as hunger, thirst, anger, and yes – sex drive!

Another small structure closely related to the hypothalamus is the pituitary gland. This gland is divided into two sections: posterior and anterior. The posterior pituitary releases such peptide hormones as vasopressin (a water-conserving hormone) and oxytocin (the hormone responsible for inducing labor).

Despite the posterior pituitary's importance in hormone release, the anterior pituitary is the most crucial to bodybuilders because it controls the various sex hormone-producing structures (i.e., testes and ovaries). For both of these structures to function properly they must be stimulated by hormones produced by the anterior pituitary – luteinizing hormone (LH) and follicle-stimulating hormone (FSH). Once released LH and FSH literally tell the testes or ovaries to start synthesizing testosterone or estrogen.

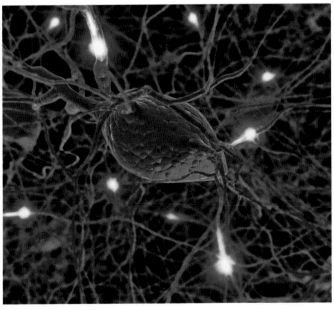

ABOVE: The endocrine system transports hormones in the body using the intricate network of blood vessels.

37

Testosterone and estrogen are the two sex hormones that differentiate males from females – it's the relative concentrations that have led to each being gender specific.

38

Photo by Robert Kennedy
Models Frank Sepe and Stacey Lynn

FEEDBACK CONTROL

Over the course of human evolution the body has developed a mechanism whereby the endocrine system regulates itself. That is, two sets of hormones each constantly influence the manufacture and release of the other through a process called feedback control.

The best analogy to explain this mechanism is the common household thermostat and furnace. When you set the thermostat at 20 degrees, for example, the furnace will kick in and produce heat until the thermostat reads a temperature of 20 degrees. It then tells the furnace to turn off. If the temperature drops below 20, the thermostat once again signals the furnace to start up and produce heat. This interplay is called feedback control, and once set (i.e., the thermostat is set at the desired temperature), it's independent from outside forces.

The human body has systems that function in a similar way. In males, the anterior pituitary releases LH to stimulate the testes to produce testosterone. Once testosterone reaches a given level, it signals the anterior pituitary to shut down LH production. When testosterone levels fall, LH production resumes and again triggers the testes to boost testosterone. Later in the book we'll focus on how anabolic steroids can interfere with this feedback loop.

THE SEX HORMONES

When it comes to separating the "boys" from the "girls," no hormones have a more central function than the sex hormones – testosterone and estrogen. They are the primary reason for the major physical differences between males and females. We should point out that males and females each have both hormones, but males have far more testosterone while estrogen is dominant in females. It's the relative concentrations that have led to testosterone being called a male hormone and estrogen a female hormone. Estrogen may have a small role in performance enhancement (there is some evidence to suggest it can make testosterone receptors more sensitive to testosterone), but testosterone (and its offspring – anabolic steroids) is the main contributor to increasing muscular size and strength.

TESTOSTERONE — THE MOST POWERFUL ANABOLIC STEROID

Testosterone serves two primary functions in males – sperm production and the development of secondary sex characteristics. As sperm production has little to do with performance enhancement, suffice it to say sperm cells are the male reproductive cells that contain half the human chromosome number (23). During sex, one sperm cell combines with a female egg to form the complete human chromosome number (46). And nine months later you can look forward to 3 a.m. feedings, frequent diaper changing, and then, "Are we there yet?"

"When it comes to separating the 'boys' from the 'girls,' no hormones have a more central function than the sex hormones. Males and females each have both hormones, but males have far more testosterone while estrogen is dominant in females."

39

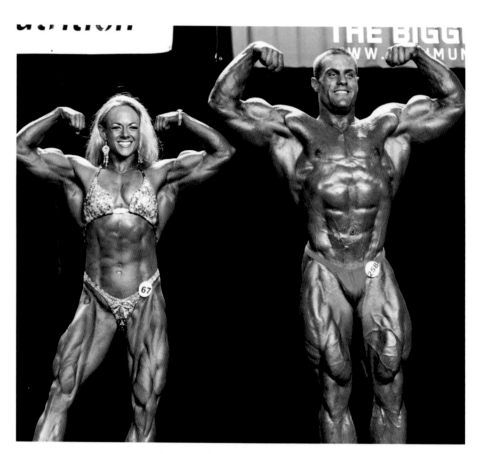

ABOVE: Because men have greater amounts of testosterone circulating in their systems, they are naturally bigger and stronger than women.

The second major function of testosterone is to produce and maintain the male secondary sex characteristics. These traits can be subdivided into anabolic and androgenic. Anabolism itself makes up one half of all the body's chemical reactions, called metabolism. Anabolic reactions are those in which small compounds combine to form larger units. Conversely catabolic reactions involve large molecules breaking down into smaller compounds. The key to building muscle strength and size is to maximize anabolic reactions and minimize catabolic reactions.

Testosterone is primarily anabolic in nature and chief among its effects is promoting increases in muscle size and strength. One of the main reasons males are, on average, bigger and stronger than females is because males have higher circulating levels of testosterone.

Testosterone also produces androgenic effects. These include growth of the reproductive organs, deepening of the voice, hair growth and acne. As you may have guessed by now, these bodily processes are most pronounced at puberty when circulating levels of testosterone are at their highest.

Photo by Ralph DeHaan
Models Kristy Hawkins and Evan Centopani

AND THERE'S MORE ...

Aside from testosterone, there are other hormones subject to body-builder tinkering in their quest for ultimate size and strength. Closely related to testosterone (at least in anabolic effects) is Human Growth Hormone (HGH or GH). This peptide hormone is one of the most powerful anabolic compounds in the human body, and GH use in athletics is widespread because it's undetectable (as of the writing of this book). Another hormone used and abused by many bodybuilders is insulin. Long known for regulating sugar levels, insulin also speeds up the rate at which amino acids are converted into protein and ultimately new muscle tissue. Unfortunately insulin can induce a life-threatening coma in mere minutes – hardly a worthwhile tradeoff for a few extra pounds of muscle mass.

Some bodybuilders also take synthetic versions of thyroid hormones as a means to drop their bodyfat percentages. The thyroid gland is largely responsible for regulating metabolism. By artificially speeding up metabolic rate, you can drop your bodyfat level to a low, single-digit percentage. However, you can also damage your metabolism to the point where you'll ultimately gain hundreds of pounds of fat.

Before looking at some of the various drugs and compounds bodybuilders use to modify their hormonal systems, a few points are worth repeating. Many of the drugs discussed in the next few chapters are illegal in many countries including the United States. Anabolic steroids, for example, are treated no different in the legal system than cocaine and heroin in many states. Unless you want to share a cell with some butt-loving Neanderthal, we suggest you obey the law.

You can't overlook the safety issues either. Insulin can quickly lead to coma or death. Thyroid abuse can screw up your metabolism. And while anabolic steroids might not kill you, they can cause severe side effects if abused. For these reasons (among others) we suggest teenagers never use any of these drugs, and adults should only do so under strict medical supervision.

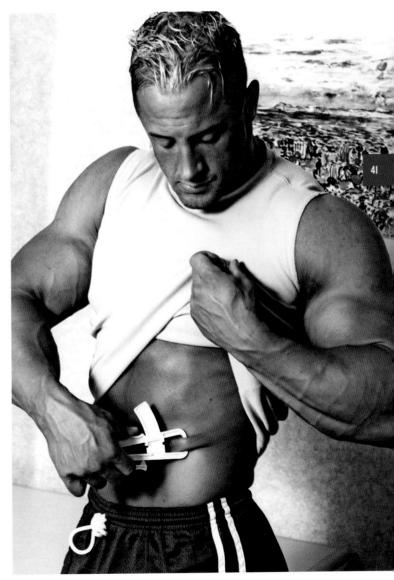

BELOW: Low bodyfat percentages are a key goal for many bodybuilders, so they use artificial means to speed up their metabolisms.

Photo by Irvin Gelb
Model Erick Seng

41

ANABOLIC STEROIDS

Of all the drugs linked to bodybuilding and other sports, none have captured public imagination like anabolic steroids. If you ask virtually anyone on the street to name a performance-enhancing drug, you can almost be guaranteed they'll say "steroids." Although steroids really only made it to the front pages of the world's newspapers after Canada's Ben Johnson tested positive at the 1988 Summer Olympics, these compounds have been part of bodybuilding (and many other sports we might add) since the 1950s. Virtually every sport that requires short bursts of strength and speed has had its fair share of "steroid scandals." In recent years Major League Baseball has been the torch carrier for the steroid set, and such superstars as Barry Bonds, Mark McGwire and José Canseco (by his own admission) have been linked to the powerful muscle builders.

HISTORICAL PERSPECTIVES

Despite the media attention given to today's top athletes, steroids as a class of drugs were not developed specifically for athletic enhancement. They were originally designed for legitimate medical reasons. Early researchers were not trying to bench press 500 pounds or knock a record number of baseballs out of ballparks; they were instead looking for a pharmaceutical equivalent of the Fountain of Youth – particularly as it related to male sexuality. For thousands of years it was known that "something" in the male testes gave men their physical strength and secondary sex characteristics. Proof of this "something" was easily demonstrated by removing the testes. The unfortunate male subjects quickly lost their strength and sex drive, and gained bodyfat. For hundreds of years singing choirs of eunuchs (males whose testes were removed before puberty) were considered the finest in the world because their voices did not deepen and retained a childlike flexibility.

The first scientist to investigate the relationship between the testes and masculinity was Dr. Charles-Édouard Brown-Séquard who in 1889 injected himself with a solution made from dog testes. Despite claims of increased sexual performance and vitality, few of his colleagues took him seriously. Whatever effect the compound might have had in his bedroom, however, it didn't extend his life as he died within five years.

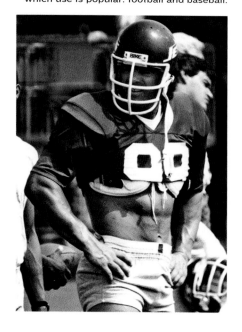

BELOW & RIGHT: Steroid use infiltrated many sports, as athletes were and still are focused on being stronger and faster. Lou Ferrigno, shown here, played two sports in which use is popular: football and baseball.

42

The next big step in hormone research took place at the turn of the 20th century when researchers tried to implant monkey testes in humans. Again the "rejuvenating" results were probably more related to the placebo effect than any real increase in hormone levels. And even if some meaningful science was occurring, it was offset by the unfortunate fact many of the recipients received monkey syphilis.

The first legitimate discovery in testosterone chemistry took place in Germany during the 1930s when scientists isolated crystals from bull testicles. Dutch scientists later named the new compound testosterone. Once biochemists discovered testosterone had a steroid molecule as its nucleus, it wasn't long before the hormone was being synthesized from such common steroid-based molecules as cholesterol.

SYNTHESIS

A detailed description of testosterone synthesis is unnecessary, but a brief discussion of testosterone biochemistry is warranted to fully understand the relationship between the hormone and anabolic steroids.

Given the amount of negative press surrounding cholesterol, it may shock readers to learn that this much-mangled molecule has numerous benefits in the human body including testosterone production. There are many steps involved, but at a basic level cholesterol is converted into four intermediate compounds before finally becoming testosterone. The entire process takes place in the male testes with an average of 2.5 to 10 milligrams being secreted each day.

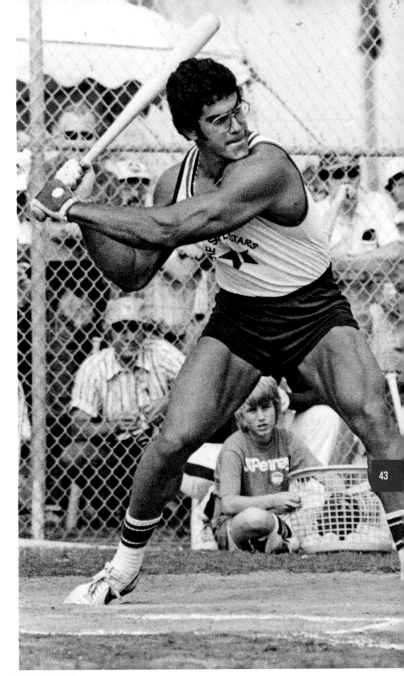

SYNTHESIS PATHWAY

Cholesterol → Pregnenolone →
17-hydroxypregnenolone →
Dehydroepiandrosterone →
Androstenediol → Testosterone

"I think steroid use is at an all-time high. Most users are just young guys who want to have big arms and a big chest to fill out their strap shirts."

– Lee Priest, professional bodybuilder

THE ORIGIN OF ANABOLIC STEROIDS

Once testosterone could be naturally synthesized in quantities, it soon began being used for medical purposes. At first this hormone was used to treat individuals with endocrine problems. Later, those recovering from surgery or starvation were added to the list. One of the most important applications was treating the victims of concentration camps following World War II. Testosterone became one of the drugs of choice because of its ability to cause rapid increases in muscle size and strength – two characteristics that were desperately needed by post-war victims recovering from starvation and trauma.

On the surface testosterone seems perfect for drug therapy, but unfortunately there are limits to its benefits. For starters, testosterone produces the androgenic effects discussed earlier. While treatment with this hormone may be fine among males, most females are not keen on developing facial hair and masculine voices. The hormone's short half-life (the amount of time necessary for one half of a given drug to degrade in the body) must also be considered. In the case of testosterone this timeframe is only 10 to 20 minutes.

These limiting aspects of testosterone are what led researchers to look for derivatives that would maximize its anabolic effects and minimize its androgenic effects. Biochemists started with testosterone's steroid nucleus, and, through a series of chemical steps, modified it so the resulting compound would mimic the positive qualities while reducing or eliminating the hormone's undesirable attributes.

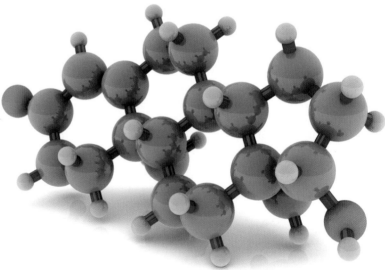

Because the new compounds were anabolic in nature (i.e., muscle building) and possessed a steroid molecule as their nucleus, they were named "anabolic steroids."

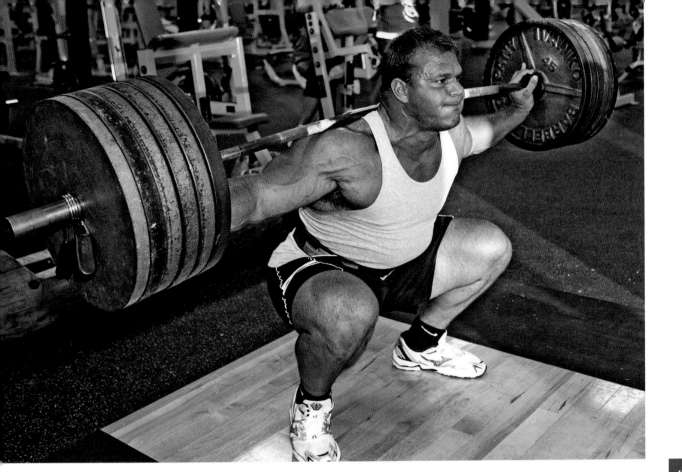

GREEK IDEALS

Brave is the individual who tries to pinpoint the exact moment in time when steroids made their debut in sports. The first credible report involves four Swedish athletes who admitted to using Rejuven, a German-made drug, in 1931.[1] While not an anabolic steroid (the class of drugs didn't exist until the late 1940s and early 1950s), Rejuven did contain small amounts of testosterone. Whether such a small dose of testosterone made a notable impact is unclear, but at that point the genie was let out of the bottle, and modern athletics haven't been the same since.

ZIEGLER'S FOLLIES

The next defining moment in anabolic steroid history occurred in 1954 when Dr. John Ziegler accompanied the U.S. weightlifting team to Vienna, Austria. After years of U.S. domination in weightlifting, the Soviet athletes suddenly vaulted to the top of the podium. Ziegler even noticed that many of the Soviet's female athletes had a degree of masculinity that could only come from artificial means. But what was the source? Finding the answer would involve the age-old Russian tradition: vodka drinking!

Not one to sit back and accept defeat, Ziegler, as the story goes, managed to corner some of the Russian doctors and coaches over a few glasses of vodka. A few glasses apparently became a few bottles and before long their secret was out – the Soviet athletes were using testosterone.

ABOVE: A big turn in steroid history came when after years of U.S. domination, Soviet weightlifters began winning with relative ease. The reason? Testosterone.

Photo by Ralph DeHaan
Model Derek Poundstone

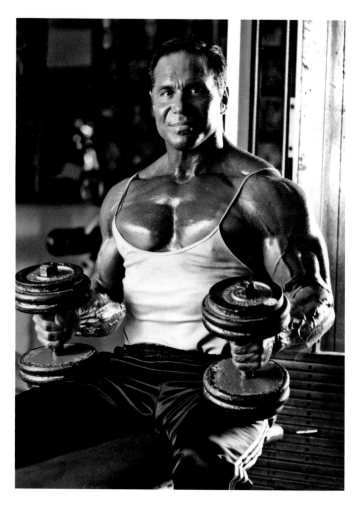

At the time Dr. Ziegler was working as a researcher with the Ciba pharmaceutical company. He was also a dedicated iron-pumper himself, closely associated with the York Barbell Company. At first he tried the Russian route by using testosterone, but the limited results left him searching for something better. Through his contacts at Ciba, Ziegler was able to develop a far more effective compound called methandrostenelone. Ciba marketed the drug under the name Dianabol, and within a few short years the York Barbell Club became famous for its supersized weightlifters.

Ziegler attributed the success of his athletes to new training techniques (sound familiar?), but the truth soon came out and other anabolic steroids were being developed. Throughout the '60s Ziegler kept a close association with both Ciba and the York Barbell Club. He quickly developed a disdain for the whole situation, however, when he discovered some of his charges were ingesting over 20 times the dosage he was prescribing. In 1967 he'd finally had enough and parted company with York. Ziegler died in 1983 of heart disease, having attributed his own medical problems to steroid use 20 years before.

ABOVE: A pioneer of sorts, Bill Pearl was the first documented champion bodybuilder to use steroids.

RIGHT: Many of the big players in our sport, including Tom Platz and Larry Scott, have admitted to using steroids.

FAR RIGHT: Mike Mentzer was a top competitor during the '70s, when steroids became the most popular drug for performance enhancement.

BODYBUILDING GEARS UP

If Olympic weightlifters were the first group of athletes to experiment with anabolic steroids, bodybuilders were a close second. This is no surprise considering both groups often trained side by side in the same gyms. While the use of steroids by a few champion bodybuilders during the late '50s and early '60s is probably lost to the ages, the first documented use is by multi-Mr. Universe winner Bill Pearl. In an interview published in the June 1987 issue of *Muscle and Fitness*, Pearl tells of being passed information about the Soviet steroid use from Dr. Arthur Jones (who later achieved fame by inventing the Nautilus line of exercise equipment). Unlike some of the carefree types Ziegler was working with, Pearl placed great value on his health. He did not want to start blindly ingesting a substance he was unfamiliar with, so Pearl went to the University of California to do some research. Around the same time, a veterinarian told him about the dramatic effects the new steroid Nilivar was having on cattle. His curiosity was aroused, and Pearl did a low-dose, three-month cycle – he gained over 20 pounds of solid muscle mass and experienced a dramatic increase in strength.

THE RACE WAS ON

Given the closeness within the bodybuilding community, it wasn't long before most other top bodybuilders of the 1960s had jumped on the steroid bandwagon. Despite claims by certain individuals that they were "totally natural," no less of an authority than *MuscleMag International* founder Robert Kennedy has stated that, in his opinion, about 95 percent of the "old timers" were on steroids.

At the end of the 1960s and into the early 1970s, anabolic steroids became by far the most popular performance-enhancing drugs. Stories are told of steroids literally being available over California gym counters. And the results were obvious – each new generation of bodybuilding superstars were bigger and harder than their predecessors. Because steroids were not classified as illegal drugs until the early 1990s, many top stars from the '60s, '70s and '80s later admitted to using the substance. Some of the big names who confessed outright to taking steroids (or at least alluded to it) include Larry Scott, Mike Mentzer, Mike Matarazzo, Tom Platz and yes, even the Governator himself Arnold Schwarzenegger.

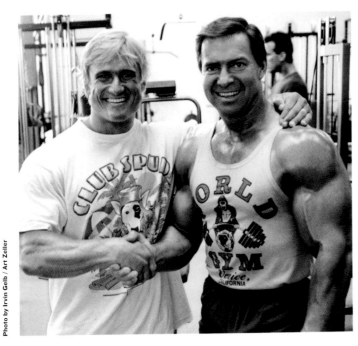

Photo by Irvin Gelb / Art Zeller

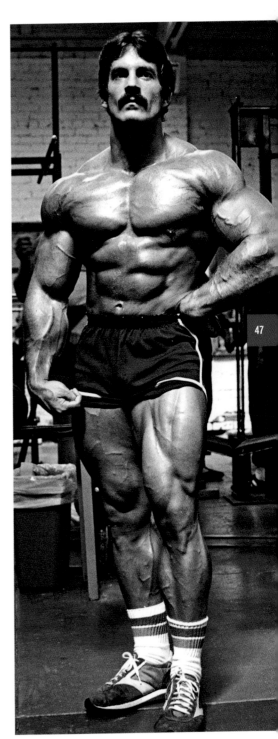

47

OUR LITTLE SECRET

Before Canadian sprinter Ben Johnson tested positive for Stanozolol at the 1988 Summer Olympics, the vast majority of the general public had no idea the extent to which steroids were used in mainstream sports. Most assumed steroids were limited to bodybuilding and weightlifting, or used by the occasional East German shot-putter. All that changed, thanks to Johnson. Within a few years of his suspension, current and former athletes from many popular sports began talking – some out of guilt, others out of necessity. It seemed the scientists developing the drug tests had become somewhat successful at catching drug-using athletes, and during the 1990s just about every sport had its own "steroid scandal."

From the testimonies of retired athletes, it appears as though football was probably the first mainstream sport where steroids made serious inroads. Most football players were training at the same gyms as bodybuilders and Olympic lifters, which was likely an influencing factor. Furthermore, football is a sport where size and strength are virtual requirements. If you're not convinced simply by the word of ex-football players, look at the average weight increase of players. Since the NFL-AFL merger in 1970, the average player is nearly 25 pounds heavier, weighing 245.

48

BELOW: Although drug and steroid use is common in a wide spectrum of sports, football players were the first mainstream athletes to experiment with steroids.

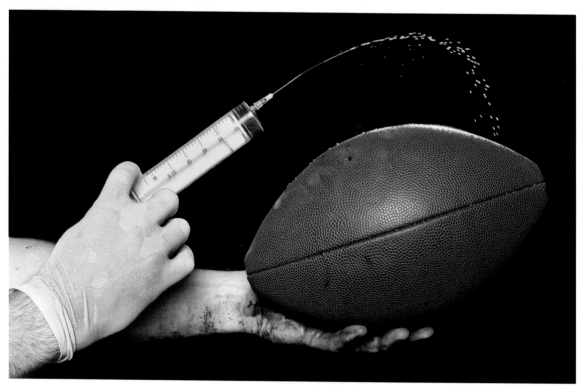

Over the same time period the average weight of an offensive lineman has increased by 62 pounds and the defensive lineman tips the scale 34 pounds heavier. Even the fleet-footed running backs and quarterbacks are not immune to the higher weights – they average an additional 17 and 26 pounds, respectively. Given that the human body takes hundreds of thousands, if not millions, of years to evolve, something other than natural selection must have occurred here. Weight training can of course account for part of the increases, but not 62 pounds!

Once steroids had become entrenched in football and other professional power sports, amateur and Olympic athletes were quick to follow the trend. The 1970s are considered the decade in which drug use in sports really exploded. Without restarting the Cold War, it's probably safe to say that Russian and East German athletes took the practice to new levels. There were always suspicions about East German swimmers and numerous Russian track athletes, but it took the fall of the Berlin Wall to confirm such accusations. The governments of the old Soviet Bloc countries kept very detailed records on their drug agendas. These records became public in the 1990s at which time it became obvious just how organized their drug program really was. Instead of the North American practice, where drug use was run at the coach level, the Eastern Bloc program was organized at the state level with everyone from coaches, sports directors and government officials working together to ensure their athletes dominated international sports. Ironically, the individuals who knew the least about what was going on were the athletes themselves!

Since the first edition of this book, the general public has seen an explosion in the number of competitive athletes who have tested positive for steroids or voluntarily confessed to using them. As this edition goes to print the fallout from the Mitchell Report is still working its way through the courts. In December 2007, Senator George Mitchell released the 409-page report summarizing his investigation into the use of performance-enhancing drugs by Major League Baseball players. In gathering evidence Mitchell interviewed over 700 people including 68 baseball players. In all, there were 89 current or former players identified including such big names as Jason Giambi, Roger Clemens, Barry Bonds and José Canseco. The fact that Canseco was pinpointed came as no surprise considering his past association with drugs. In 2005 he admitted to using steroids in a tell-all book, *Juiced: Wild Times, Rampant 'Roids, Smash Hits & How Baseball Got Big*. Canseco also claimed that up to 85 percent of Major League players took steroids, a figure disputed by many in the game. In the book Canseco specifically identified former teammates Jason Giambi, Mark McGwire, Rafael Palmeiro and Iván Rodriguez as steroid users. He even admitted to having injected most of them. As expected, most of the players named denied their drug use.

"All I can say is that recreational drugs have never seemed to be as big a problem as they are today in the sport. But it's rampant in our society, not just bodybuilding. Bush lost my vote when he emphasized how dangerous steroids were in his 2004 State of the Union Address. For him to come out against steroids while so many people's lives are being destroyed – more every year – by drug and alcohol abuse and addiction, was just irresponsible."

– Ed Connors, former owner of Gold's Gym

49

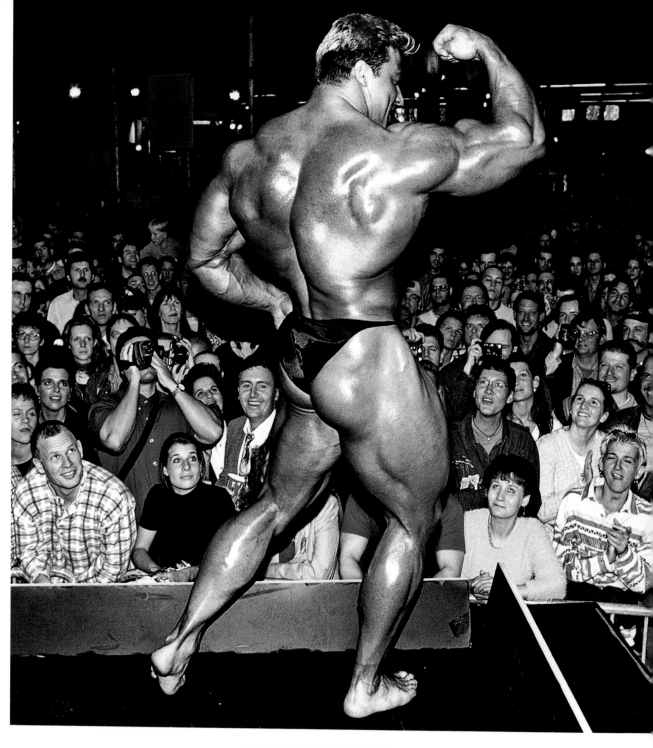

ABOVE: When a professional athlete takes drugs, he impacts more than his own body – young athletes are more likely to start using steroids knowing their "role models" use them.

TEENAGER SEE – TEENAGER DO

Considering the amount of media attention centered on professional athletes, rampant steroid use at the teen level doesn't come as a shock. The pressure on teen athletes to excel and make the "big leagues" is enormous. When you combine the stress on young athletes from parents and coaches, and the knowledge that many of their heroes are on drugs, it's understandable that many teenagers would hit the juice. A lot of parents even jump the gun and actually introduce the drugs to their sons or

Photo by Irvin Gelb
Model Gunter Schlierkamp

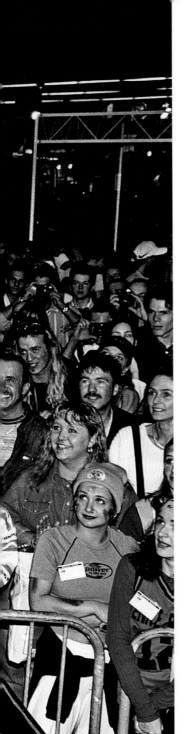

daughters. In one noteable case, a federal judge gave James Gahan a six-year sentence after he admitted to giving his son synthetic testosterone and human growth hormone. Consequently, Corey Gahan, a champion inline skater, was banned from the sport for at least two years. The father confessed that he provided the drugs to his son starting when the boy was 13. However, James Gahan later denied his involvement, instead accusing his son's trainer and a clinic operator of giving Corey the drugs without his knowledge, according to Gahan's plea agreement.

Many pro athletes readily point fingers at their coaches for encouraging them to hit the juice when they were younger. While a few actually specified the drugs by name and bluntly told the athletes which to use, most coaches simply said unless athletes packed on 15 or 20 pounds – and quick – they had no hope of ever making it to the college or pro ranks. It was obvious what those coaches were talking about, and many young, impressionable athletes with dreams of Olympic gold medals or million-dollar contracts quickly took the hint.

AN ONGOING STRUGGLE

Despite the best efforts of sports officials and drug testers, the use of performance-enhancing drugs is still rampant in the world of sports. Similar to the workings of terrorism and counterterrorism, the athletes are usually one step ahead. When a test for steroids was developed in the 1970s, athletes simply started using other drugs to mask the presence of steroids. When those drugs were added to the list of banned substances, athletes began switching urine samples. As testing procedures became more scrutinized, athletes turned to undetectable drugs such as growth hormone and "designer" steroids.

Reference

1) Reuters, Nurmi won with drugs in Olympics, Swede says, *The Globe and Mail*, December 14, 1990, A-19.

51

"I don't follow baseball at all, and 10 years ago I knew half the players, both amateur and professional, were juiced up. Even when I graduated high school in 1989 I knew many players were on the stuff. Now the powers that be are making it out to be such a new, shocking discovery. Everyone is juiced up, even at the almighty Olympic Games. They are the worst of the worst. Take away the drugs and the entire sporting world will suffer. I'm just keeping it real."

– King Kamali, professional bodybuilder and *MuscleMag International* columnist

STEROID PHARMACOLOGY

Like most drugs and compounds, the effects of steroids and testosterone are produced at the cellular level. The primary site for action is called a receptor. Most steroid receptors are located in the center (nucleus) of the cell. Each receptor is specific for one particular type of drug compound, and molecular biologists and biochemists use the "lock-and-key hypothesis" to describe the unique affinity of one drug and receptor pair. Just as one key will only fit a certain lock, a receptor can only be "turned on" by a compound with one specific molecular arrangement. Once the drug binds to the receptor we have what biochemists call a drug-receptor complex. This system then initiates a series of chemical reactions that produce a biological response. In the case of steroids, the biological feedback is an increase in RNA and protein synthesis.

BELOW: When steroids enter the body's system, they bind to a specific receptor and become active through a sequence of chemical reactions.

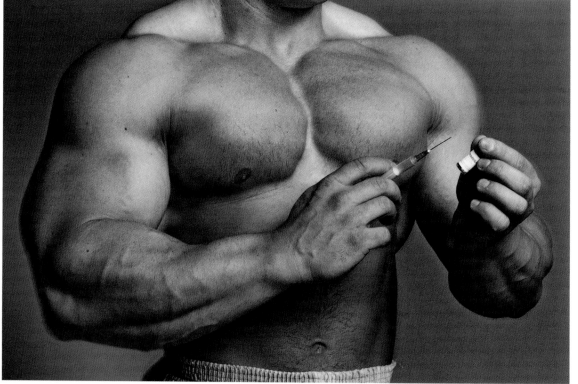

Photo by Alex Ardenti

One of the interesting points about biological responses is that there may be considerable variation among individuals. For example, one user may gain 20 pounds of muscle mass on a four-week cycle of a given steroid while another may gain just five. There are also those unfortunate users who make virtually no strength or size gains. Numerous factors may impact the differences in results, but the most logical explanation is that the individual who makes no gains may have few receptors appropriate for that particular steroid. A simple switch to another steroid will often produce the desired strength and size gains.

ROUTES OF ADMINISTRATION

A drug is useless unless it somehow gets inside the body and reaches the receptors. There are numerous ways steroids can be delivered into the human body (called routes of administration), and the following are the more popular methods.

Oral

Not counting pure testosterone, oral steroids were the first to be developed. As the name suggests, the drug exists in pill or tablet form and is taken by mouth. In terms of safety (as it applies to the route of administration), oral steroids are the easiest and simplest to use. Individuals who take them just swallow one or two with a glass of water or other beverage. Unfortunately, no steroid comes without a price and orals are probably the harshest on the liver. The reason lies within biochemistry: To help them survive passing through the digestive tract, oral steroids have been chemically modified. If you refer back to the steroid molecule pictured earlier (page 44), you'll see they are three-ring structures joined together. Though not shown, each corner contains a carbon atom. To simplify the naming process of different compounds biochemists numbered the carbons. In the case of oral steroids the chemical modification takes place at the 17th carbon position. The modification is called 17-alkylation and while it allows more of the steroid to enter the bloodstream, it can also wreak havoc on the liver. Long-term, heavy usage of orals has been linked to abnormal liver enzymes, peliosis (characterized by randomly distributed, multiple blood-filled cavities throughout the liver) and possibly cancer.

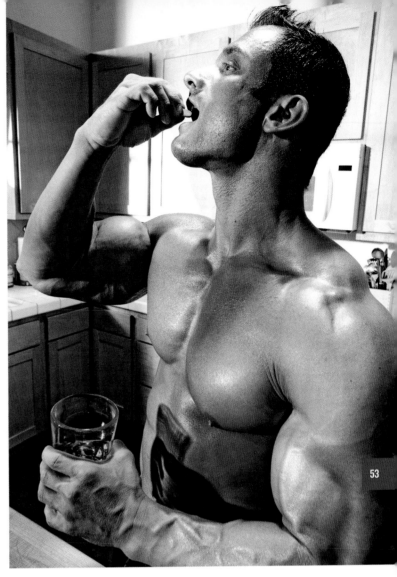

53

ABOVE: While oral steroids are the easiest to use because of the convenience of tablets and pills, this form is the most detrimental to the liver.

Photo by Robert Reiff
Model Dan Decker

Injectable

Steroids administered by injection are introduced into the bloodstream by way of a long (usually 1- to 1½-inch) hypodermic needle.
Although the method sounds more dangerous, injectable drugs are
safer than orals as they don't possess the same degree of chemical
modification, making them less harsh on the liver. Many anti-steroid
advocates cite the dangers of injectable drugs as reasons to avoid
steroids. And while there are risks, virtually all can be eliminated if
proper hygienic measures are followed. Let's face it – millions of
children safely inject themselves with insulin and other medicines
every day without problems.

BELOW: Either the glutes or quads are the
most common steroid injection sites – because the injection is intramuscular, these
areas are ideal.

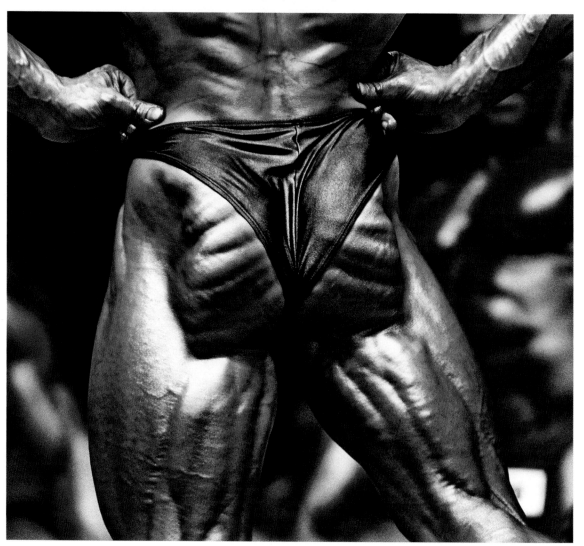

Photo by Robert Kennedy

54

IM, NOT IV!

One of the myths about injectable steroids is that they're injected directly into veins. This is simply not true. The injection is intramuscular (IM – into a muscle), not intravenous (IV – into a vein). Most bodybuilders prefer to inject into either their quads or glutes. The quads are easy to reach but have slightly more nerve endings than the glutes and are thus a little more painful. Conversely, the glutes have less nerve endings but are awkward to reach. For this reason most bodybuilders have a friend do the injection if they opt for the glutes.

TYPES OF INJECTABLE STEROIDS

There are two basic subcategories of injectable steroids: oil-based and water-based. The terms oil- and water-based refer to the medium the steroid is mixed or suspended in. The oils used are primarily sesame or cottonseed. Many water-based types are called suspensions because the steroid floats around in the mixture. When left sitting for extended periods of time, the steroid crystals fall to the bottom of the vial (much like the sugar you find at the bottom of your coffee mug). This occurrence is not a big deal – the vial just needs to be shaken to re-suspend the crystals before use.

RISKS OF INJECTABLE STEROIDS

Much like orals, injectables are not a free ride and carry their own associated risks. For starters, you have to understand that injecting a drug into the body is a minor medical procedure. Nurses and doctors spend years perfecting their techniques. One lesson from Danny Deltoid at the local gym will in no way prepare you for open heart surgery. Before stabbing your thigh with a long, sharp needle, you need to be familiar with the basic blood vessel layout of the quads. If you rupture your femoral artery you'll bleed to death within minutes. Even puncturing some of the lesser blood vessels in the upper leg can leave you in a precarious situation. If you experience an injection mishap, at the first sign of major blood vessel damage apply pressure, elevate your leg and seek medical attention. It's far better to be embarrassed and safe than dead!

Aside from the blood vessels you also have to be aware of the body's vast network of nerves. If you strike one of the main nerves, you'll experience an instantaneous jolt of excruciating pain. Nerve damage can also lead to paralysis or atrophy of the muscle.

Yet another issue to consider is infection. The skin is the body's primary outer defense against invading organisms. As soon as you break or puncture it, you are opening the door for dastardly little pathogens to enter. Always wipe the area with alcohol before and after injecting. And under no circumstances should you ever share needles – we don't care how close you and your buddy are. You may

> "A study published in *The New England Journal of Medicine*, considered one of the most prestigious medical and scientific journals in the world, found that healthy men who were given 600 milligrams of testosterone enanthate per week did not suffer any side effects, negative effects in lipid profiles, increases in prostate-specific antigens or increased aggression."
>
> – Will Brink, bodybuilding and nutrition writer

think you know his complete sexual history, but don't risk finding out differently five or 10 years down the road when you develop AIDS or hepatitis.

There is also a risk of poisoning associated with injectables, as many steroids on the black market are counterfeit. While some are of the same quality as the legitimate brands, others have been produced in basement labs where hygiene is virtually nonexistent. If you inject a "dirty" drug into your body you could start experiencing chills, muscle cramps and nausea. In some cases the infection may become so severe that gangrene may set in. If the thought of developing gangrene isn't enough to frighten you, understand that the only cure for this condition is partial or full amputation of the leg. You'd be hard-pressed to win the "Best Legs" category at the next bodybuilding contest with just one leg.

OTHER ROUTES OF DELIVERY

Although orals and injectables make up the vast majority of steroid types used by bodybuilders, there are other routes of administration available.

Spray

After the fall of the Berlin Wall, numerous Eastern Bloc athletes began opening up about their steroid use behind the Iron Curtain. One of the most intriguing accounts concerned a steroid-based nasal spray that was used like a common cold medication. The lining of the nasal passage is very thin, so absorption of the spray is very fast. Furthermore, the reports suggested that the drug leaves the body's system in as little as three days. The benefits of such a fast clearance time for drug-tested athletes should be obvious. They could continue using the drug right up until week of the event, maximizing on the performance-enhancing benefits while still passing any drug tests.

Transdermal

Another route of administration that holds promise is transdermal. With this type the active drug is dissolved in an alcohol or alcohol-related compound and placed on a patch, which then gets placed on the skin. Upon contact the drug is absorbed by the skin and passed into general circulation. Although great success has been achieved with transdermal delivery for smokers (the nicotine patch) and heart patients (the nitroglycerine patch), the results for testosterone and anabolic steroids remain limited. The chief issue with transdermals is the very small amount of drug that actually gets absorbed. AIDS researchers are continuously looking for ways to increase the dosage delivered by transdermal patches in an attempt

"Not long after the invention of different types of steroids, bodybuilders started combining or 'stacking' two or more in the same cycle. Stacking reached a new level of insanity in the 1990s with the practice of 'shotgunning' – the addition of GH, insulin, diuretics and just about every other performance-enhancing drug to stacks."

to slow down the degree of muscle wasting brought on by the disease. ALZA Pharmaceuticals has released a patch called Testoderm that is showing promise in regards to absorption, and no doubt future advancements will see this delivery form become much more popular with bodybuilders.

Sublingual

Further to sprays and transdermals, an additional method of taking steroids is by sublingual absorption. The area under the tongue has a very high density of blood vessels and the skin in this region is very thin. Cardio patients have been using nitroglycerine tablets via sublingual absorption for decades to ward off heart attacks – it's not surprising that researchers began experimenting with this method of delivery using testosterone. Similar to transdermals, the success of sublingual absorption with AIDS patients shows promise, and males with low sex drive seem to benefit from sublingual testosterone. The technique, however, has limited value for bodybuilding purposes. With each tablet only supplying a small dosage for a short period of time, a large 220- to 230-pound bodybuilder would need to consume 20 or 30 tablets per day just to get the same dosage as a couple of oral steroid tablets or one injection.

TERMINOLOGY

Anabolic steroid use, like many other practices, has its own distinct language and vocabulary. Bodybuilders refer to the drugs by a number of different names including "roids," "juice" and "gear." You are most likely familiar with the first term as media outlets frequently include references to "roid rage" in their discussions of steroids.

Most bodybuilders – at least the smarter ones – don't stay on steroids continuously, but instead alternate periods of use with nonuse. This practice is called cycling, and it's believed to produce less side effects and better strength and size gains. Of course many bodybuilders throw caution to the wind and base cycles more on their finances than time. As long as they have available cash they're on the juice. As we'll explain later, this approach is dangerous as the risk of side effects is proportionate to the duration of use – the longer the time period the greater the risk.

Another common gym term within the realm of anabolic steroids is "stacking." Not long after the invention of different types of steroids, bodybuilders started combining or "stacking" two or more in the same cycle. As expected, strength and size gains increased, but so too did the risks and side effects. Stacking reached a new level of insanity in the 1990s with the practice of "shotgunning" – the addition of growth hormone, insulin, diuretics and just about every other performance-enhancing drug to stacks. This type of

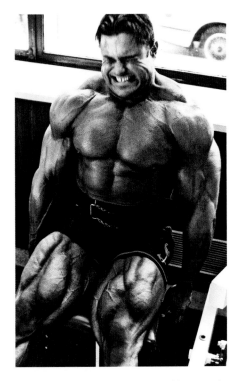

ABOVE: Steroids may help you add size and strength to your legs, but if you inject a bogus or fake drug, you could end up with an infection so severe that amputation is necessary.

57

Photo by Irvin Gelb
Model Tommi Thorvildsen

> "As crazy as this may sound, there are wannabe chemists out there who try to set up steroid-producing labs in their basements. The problem is only complicated by the fact that literature is still circulating both in print and online, telling readers how to cook up their own anabolics. This is reckless and dangerous if you don't have the necessary skills (at minimum, a degree in chemistry) to follow such technical chemical synthesis."

approach is one of the reasons today's pro bodybuilders are tipping the scales at 280 to 300 pounds. It's also believed this form of stacking may be why so many pro bodybuilders are suffering from numerous health issues. The human body was not meant to endure such an intense chemical cocktail.

MAKING YOUR OWN STEROIDS

As crazy as this may sound, there are wannabe chemists out there who try to set up steroid-producing labs in their basements. The problem is only complicated by the fact that literature is still circulating both in print and online, telling readers how to cook up their own anabolics. A few sources even advise readers to pick up the latest copy of the Merck Index (a pharmacology book that outlines the manufacturing procedures for most of the world's drugs). This is reckless and dangerous if you don't have the necessary skills (at minimum, a degree in chemistry) to follow such technical chemical synthesis.

Before you decide to bypass chemistry 101, there are numerous reasons why you should steer clear of basement chemistry. The first involves the preciseness at which chemical reactions must take place. Following a recipe written on a few scraps of paper is a sure way to produce products that could be downright lethal. Such variables as temperature, pressure, ingredient amounts and solvents used must be exact. If even one of them is skewed, you could end up with a host of toxic byproducts.

Equipment is another area of consideration – Mom's cupboard in no way compares to the million-dollar labs at Upjohn or Dow Chemical Company. A few kitchen pots and pans are no substitute for sterile glassware, test tubes and centrifuges. And even if by some remote chance you had access to some of this expensive equipment – do you know how to use it? Like any profession – particularly the sciences – laboratory pharmacology requires many years of specialized training.

A final issue of concern is the consequences of a chemical explosion. Even with the best safeguards in place, the major chemical companies have experienced mishaps. This is why they have labs specifically designed to contain and control such explosions. The walls are often on hinges to absorb the shock, fire suppression systems are in place to help put out any fires and sophisticated gas extraction units help reduce the risk of inhaling toxic fumes. Compare this to the battery-powered smoke detector on your ceiling and the hand-held fire extinguisher on your wall.

Hopefully you're convinced enough to avoid trying to make your own steroids. A few writers try to make it sound like a safe and profitable process, but they won't be the ones at your funeral after a chemical accident has scattered your remains all over the neighborhood.

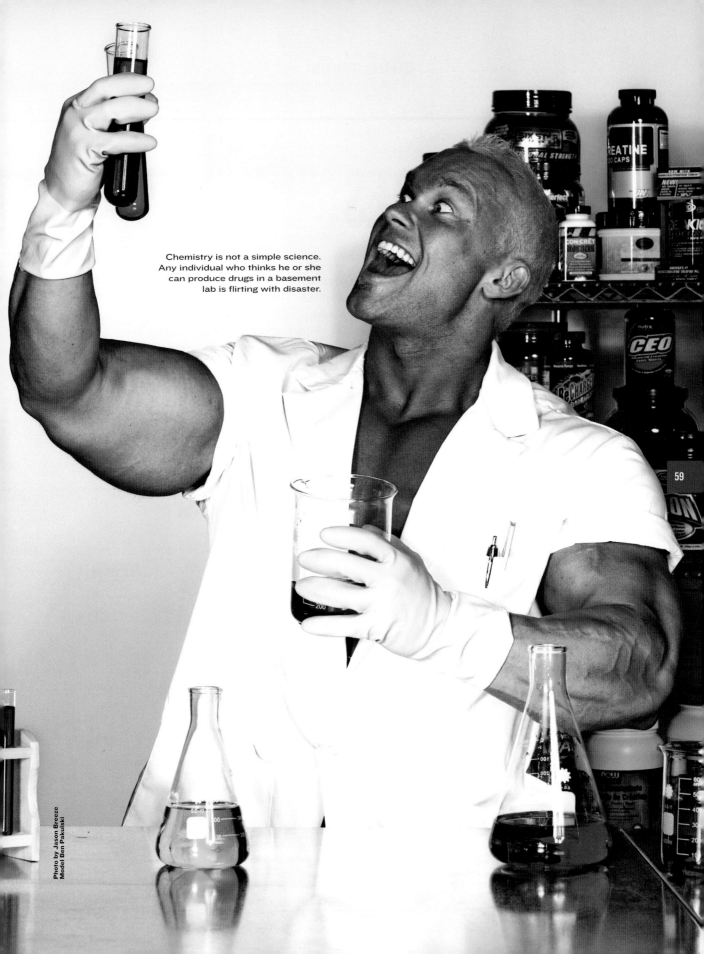

Chemistry is not a simple science. Any individual who thinks he or she can produce drugs in a basement lab is flirting with disaster.

59

STEROID CYCLES

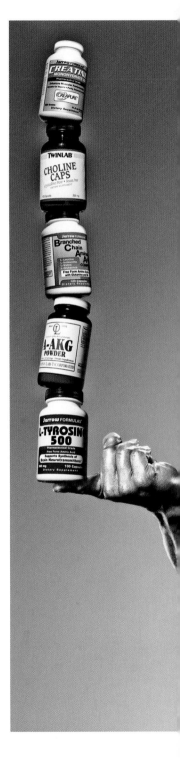

The issue of steroid cycling is quite complex, and understanding it requires more than a mere definition. Most bodybuilders divide their training into two phases: off-season and pre-contest. During the off-season, their primary goal is developing maximum size and strength. Workouts tend to be shorter with heavier weights, and calorie consumption is much higher. About three to four months out from a contest bodybuilders then switch to the pre-contest phase of their training, which is characterized by longer workouts using lighter weights for higher reps. They also follow a much stricter nutrition plan, cutting down on fats and simple sugars (although they don't eat huge amounts of these types of foods during the off-season either).

Because of the two styles of training from off-season to pre-contest and the different goals involved, bodybuilders tailor their steroid cycles accordingly. As expected, during the off-season they primarily use mass- and strength-building drugs, then switch to steroids that increase fat loss and don't cause water retention during the pre-contest phase. Athletes must also take into account whether they are competing in drug-tested events, as sufficient time will be needed for the drug and drug metabolites (breakdown products) to clear their systems.

When they're about two weeks out from a contest, the majority of bodybuilders eliminate most, if not all, drugs to allow for as much water and salt to clear their bodies as possible. Shedding the water weight and flushing out the salt helps them appear vascular and ripped on contest day.

RIGHT: Over the course of a year, bodybuilders will adjust their stacks and cycles based on off-season and pre-contest goals.

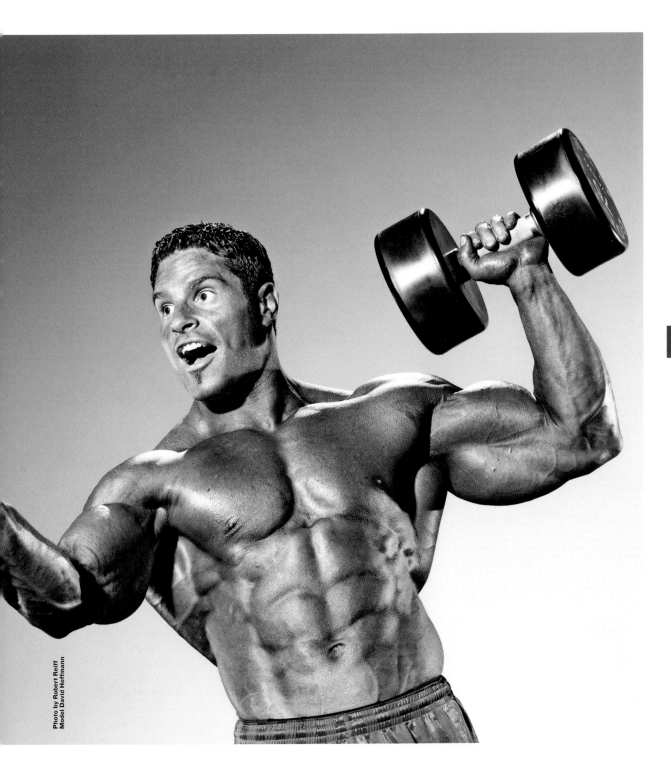

Photo by Robert Reiff
Model David Hoffmann

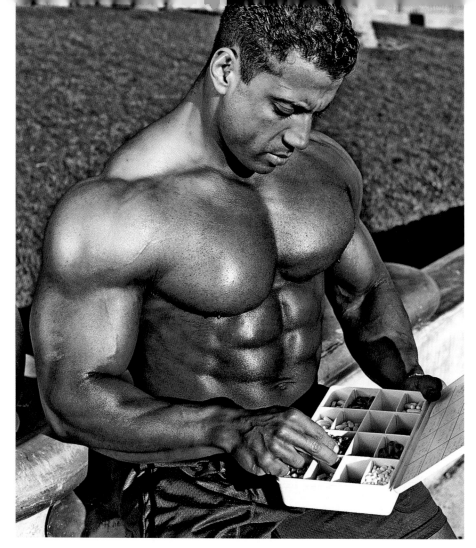

Photo by Irvin Gelb
Model Jamo Nezzar

ABOVE: Jamo Nezzar shows that supplements and cycling aren't basic. Choosing the right ones for your individual needs requires research and planning.

These training factors and contest considerations have influenced bodybuilders over the years to come up with a number of steroid patterns and cycles to suit their competitive needs. The following are the five most popular.

STRAIGHT ARROW

The "straight arrow" consists of a steroid stack in which the dose of each drug taken by the athlete remains constant during the cycle. The addition of any drugs after the start of the cycle does not change this designation, provided the dosage of the steroid added also remains the same throughout the cycle.

CLIFFHANGER

The "cliffhanger" is one of the most abrupt patterns of anabolic steroid cycles. It involves an overall increase in dosage during the cycle, but there is no tapering off at the end. This approach would only be used during the off-season, as an athlete would not pass a drug test with such a high concentration of steroids in his or her system. The cliffhanger's major disadvantage is that the body's hormonal system is not given a chance to normalize at the end of the cycle. As a result, the athlete often experiences problems with low sex drive, impotence and a general lack of motivation. These symptoms, however, are transitory and will disappear once the body's own hormonal system kicks back in or the athlete begins another cycle.

SKI SLOPE

Of all the different types of anabolic steroid cycles the "ski slope" is probably the safest and most popular pattern among athletes. In this stack the steroid dosages decrease over the duration of the cycle. From a health perspective the ski slope has an advantage over the other approaches because decreasing dose amounts limit the risks of taking the drugs. This method is used by many athletes during the pre-competition phase of their training – the rationale being that it will result in very low drug levels in their systems near or at the time of drug testing.

PYRAMID

The "pyramid" pattern is probably the most complex steroid cycle. It is characterized by three distinct, consecutive phases. The first phase involves an increasing dosage, the second marks the peak where the highest dosage is reached, and the third is defined by a decreasing dosage. As with the ski slope, the pyramid is favored as a pre-competition cycle. The plateau during the third phase leaves low drug levels in the body, and the athlete thus has a better chance of passing a drug test.

NON-CYCLIC

Although considered the five most popular patterns among body-builders, the vast majority of steroid users do not follow any of the previous four types of cycling. They instead take as much as they can afford for as long as possible. If the cash is available, they stay on the cycle and never come off. This type of approach is crazy, not to mention dangerous – even the most diehard steroid users readily admit that the risk of side effects is directly proportionate to the length of the cycle and the dosages of steroids used. Perhaps the most frightening aspect of these never-ending cycles is that a high percent-age of those who follow the non-cyclic pattern are teenagers. The extensive media attention these days on steroid use among baseball players and pro wrestlers has impacted thousands of teenage males (and numerous teenage females, we might add) to the point where they've turned to the juice. Many of these teens hold down lucrative part-time jobs and use their earnings to buy cycles that rival those of professional bodybuilders. Teens should not be using these drugs – as we'll discuss in more detail in a later chapter – the risks and side effects are just too great.

"I nearly keel over when they tell me how much shit they're on. In most cases it's more than I have ever used for a cycle, and it's even more than most of the pros I know use. But these guys don't look anything like what you'd expect them to. This reality again proves drugs aren't the be-all and end-all that so many make them out to be."

– Lee Priest, professional bodybuilder

63

ANABOLIC EFFECTS

The effectiveness of steroids is one of the great debates between users and the medical establishment. Body-builders swear by them for building strength and size while anti-steroid groups argue the results are primarily linked to the placebo effect or are exaggerated. While medical literature on the topic is inconclusive, it's generally accepted that an individual using steroids will produce faster and far greater gains in muscle size and strength than a non-user.

Current published medical findings are so sadly lacking in "proof" about steroid efficacy because ethics and legalities prevent researchers from using the same dosages that bodybuilders regularly use. Where a medical researcher may use one or two times the recommended dosage for a particular drug study, a typical bodybuilder will take anywhere from five to 10 times the dosage of the same steroid. Bodybuilders also combine three or four (or more) drugs in a stack and will stay on the cycle for months at a time. Conversely, medical studies generally involve just one steroid and last for a period of maybe four to six weeks. Drawing a comparison of the results between these two groups would be like comparing apples and oranges.

Aside from increasing muscle size and strength, steroids have other physiological effects. No less an authority than NASA has looked at the potential of steroids to offset the loss of bone minerals during long space flights.[1] NASA's investigations concluded that steroids counteract mineral loss by increasing the absorption of calcium by bones.

And calcium isn't the only element in the body influenced by anabolic steroids: they also increase the retention rate of other minerals and ions (electrically charged atoms or molecules) including potassium, chloride and nitrogen. Both potassium and chloride play a role in nerve conduction and muscle contraction, and a positive nitrogen balance is the most desirable environment for new muscle-tissue synthesis – by impacting the levels of potassium, chloride and nitrogen within the body, steroids also affect the functions of which these minerals and ions control.

Another function of steroids is their ability to counteract the negative effects of catabolic hormones such as cortisol. As we discussed in Chapter 3, catabolic hormones are those in which larger compounds are broken down into smaller subunits. The best example of

"What the medical experts don't know about steroid use may be even more important than what they do know, so let us cut to the chase."

– Dr. George H. Elder, *MuscleMag International* contributor

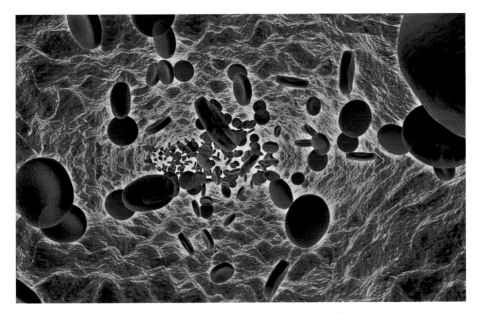

LEFT: The more red blood cells in the bloodstream, the greater muscle stamina will be, as higher amounts of oxygen can be carried in the blood.

this in bodybuilding terms is when protein is broken down into individual amino acids, the end result of which is muscle wasting. One of the reasons individuals who are under stress lose weight is because their bodies are flooded with catabolic stress hormones. Under normal circumstances, healthy individuals produce enough anabolic hormones to counteract the catabolic hormones. There's a continuous tug of war taking place where amino acids are being moved into and out of the muscles. And while not fully understood, it is believed that anabolic steroids compete with catabolic hormones for receptor sites, and the anabolics usually win. These anti-catabolic effects are so pronounced that many biochemists suggest a more appropriate name for the drugs might be anti-catabolic steroids.

A final effect associated with anabolic steroid use is increased production of a hormone in the body called erythropoietin. Erythropoietin is generated by the kidneys and stimulates bone marrow to speed up formulation of red blood cells (RBCs). More RBCs mean a higher oxygen-carrying capacity in the blood and hence greater muscle stamina. One of the side effects of a heightened RBC count is an elevated number of blood vessels. This is one of the reasons steroid-using bodybuilders have increased vascularity when they drop their bodyfat levels.

Reference

1) Stepaniak P., Furst J., Woodward D. Anabolic steroids as a countermeasure against bone demineralization during space flight. *Aviation, Space and Environmental Medicine*. Feb. 1986.

PHYSIOLOGICAL SIDE EFFECTS

If the issue of whether steroids cause increased muscle size and strength is hotly debated, then the topic of side effects creates nothing short of nuclear war. Every day seemingly brings forth some new proclamation about the horrors of anabolic steroids. Various media outlets and anti-steroid groups almost trip over themselves in their condemnation of drug-using athletes. Many health problems, from brain cancer and liver disease to psychosis and depression, are blamed on steroids. The fact that little or no credible medical evidence exists to back these claims seems to be conveniently ignored.

We've broken this topic into two sections: This chapter will address the physiological side effects of steroid use, and Chapter 9 will focus on the psychological side effects.

BELOW: Anti-steroid groups go to many lengths, including public protests, to convey their opposition to drug use and the "claimed" side effects.

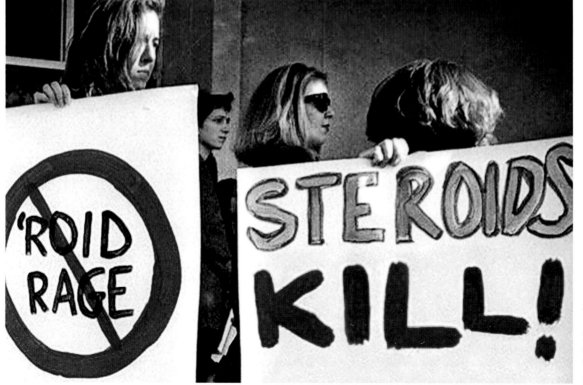

Photo by Mark Costantini

CANCER

Next to "roid rage" (which will be discussed in Chapter 9) cancer is probably the most commonly talked about side effect of anabolic steroids by groups who oppose the drugs. There is not one shred of medical proof, however, that links cancer with steroid use.

In North America, cancer ranks second only to heart disease as the primary cause of death. The term cancer does not apply to one disease but rather collectively represents a group of conditions all sharing a common denominator: the uncontrollable growth of body cells. Such growth causes the formation of masses called tumors, which often ultimately lead to death. In some cases, even when treatment takes place the diseased cells cannot be destroyed and the outcome for those affected is fatal.

Researchers currently do not have a definitive answer as to what initiates and promotes the growth of cancerous cells. Numerous theories exist about such factors as environmental toxins, diet and genetics, but the exact underlying source is not known. Now please re-read the last two sentences carefully – if the origin has not been discovered, how can anti-steroid groups say steroids cause cancer? By doing so, these groups are either suggesting they're far more knowledgeable than the world's top cancer researchers or are simply spreading propaganda.

To prove conclusively that a drug or compound is cancer-causing takes years of research and millions of dollars for studies and analyses. Researchers need to conduct long-term comparison studies involving drug-using and non-using groups. If after five or 10 years it could be shown that the steroid-using group had a higher incidence of developing cancer, only then could claims be made that a relationship exists between steroid use and cancer. To date there are no such long-term comparison studies – the only "evidence" in medical literature linking the two is from case studies.

For those not familiar, case studies are individual in nature – each focuses on one person who is dying or has died from cancer and just happened to have taken steroids. Groups who oppose steroids generalize the details in these case studies in order to draw a connection between the drugs and the disease. But such logic has no merit. Consider, for example, the analogy of the blue car we've used in previous writings. Someone with an axe to grind could find examples of 50

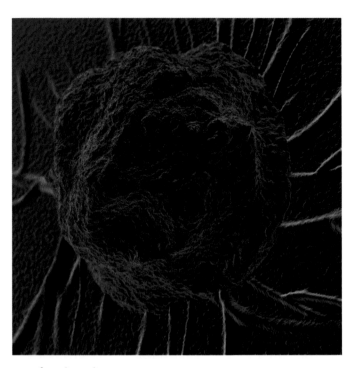

ABOVE: There is currently no science to back the claim that steroids cause cancer. Cancerous cell growth afflicts many seemingly healthy, non-drug users.

67

> "In 1996 the *Canadian Journal of Applied Physiology* published an extensive meta-analysis of the available research on the side effects of steroids called 'Androgen use by athletes: a re-evaluation of the health risks.' Because of this study, a great deal of fear about steroids was put to rest. The authors did an exhaustive search and evaluation of the studies to date that really looked at the use of anabolic steroids by athletes and the associated side effects. The researchers' conclusion: 'Side effects resulting in serious harm or death to athletes from androgen self-administration are exceedingly rare.' Not exactly what the media wants us to believe is it?"
>
> – Will Brink, bodybuilding and nutrition writer

or 100 individuals who had died of cancer and who also just happened to have driven blue-colored cars. With a bit of creative writing and the right media connections, this person could make it sound as if there is a relationship between driving a blue car and developing cancer. Carried to the extreme, automobile manufacturers would likely have to stop painting cars blue. As far-fetched as this scenario may sound, it mirrors what anti-steroid groups are doing by quoting case studies as evidence to establish a cancer-steroid connection. But the relationship just doesn't exist.

Not wanting to concede this debate, some anti-steroid groups argue that while evidence may be limited right now, users will probably develop some form of cancer in the future. There is no proof, however, to back that statement; steroids have been used since the 1960s with the first generation of users now in their 60s and 70s. If steroids were cancer generators we'd expect an epidemic among bodybuilders and other athletes of that age range – this type of mass affliction hasn't yet happened and it remains to be seen whether it ever will.

LIVER DISEASE

While it's true that steroids cause liver abnormalities, most occurrences are transitory and disappear with cessation of the drug. An elevation of liver enzymes is the primary side effect, which is logical because the liver is the body's primary detoxifying organ. Blood gets filtered as it passes through, and compounds such as drugs and toxins are removed and deactivated. Therefore, common sense should tell you the more drugs sent through the liver the harder it has to work. Over time, this added exertion will take its toll and sooner or later the organ will start wearing out. The best example of this process in the liver is long-term consumption of alcohol. The ingredients in alcohol negatively affect the liver and eventually cause the organ to no longer function properly. Heavy drinkers often develop a condition called cirrhosis characterized by severe liver damage.

With respect to liver effects, steroids are no different than other drugs – any individual who's using heavy dosages of multiple drugs for extended periods of time is risking damage to this organ. The first symptom is usually elevated liver enzymes followed by jaundice (yellowing of the skin, tissues and body fluids). While the presence of jaundice will be obvious, enzyme irregularities can only be detected in a blood test. This type of "silent" symptom is why readers who are using or contemplating steroids should do so only under medical supervision.

We should add that virtually all instances of liver side effects documented in medical literature involve orally active C-17 alkyl derivatives. As we discussed earlier, such steroids have been chemically modified to survive the harsh environment in the digestive

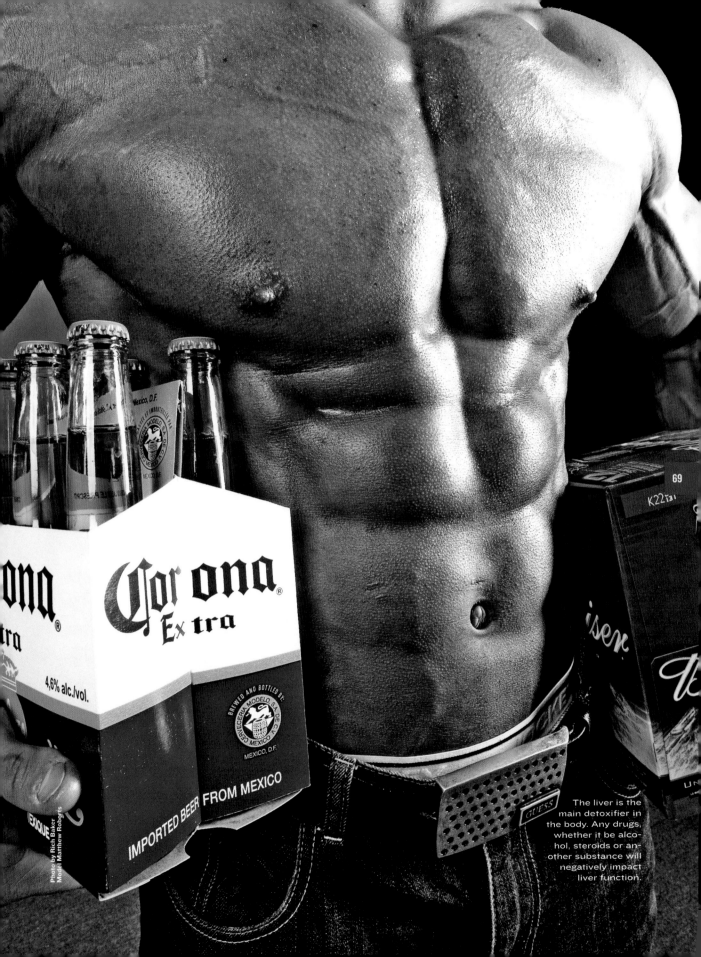

The liver is the main detoxifier in the body. Any drugs, whether it be alcohol, steroids or another substance will negatively impact liver function.

system. Unfortunately, while this modification guarantees that more steroid will reach the bloodstream, it may also result in damage to the liver. This result is why most regular steroid users only stay on orals for short, six- to eight-week cycles.

HYPERTENSION – HIGH BLOOD PRESSURE

Most individuals who take steroids will experience an elevation in their blood pressure during a steroid cycle. The condition, however, is transitory and blood pressure will normalize after steroid use is stopped. Hypertension occurs during a cycle because steroids pro-

BELOW: Blood pressure is a health aspect affected by steroids, because the drugs promote fluid retention. This elevation only occurs during a cycle, though.

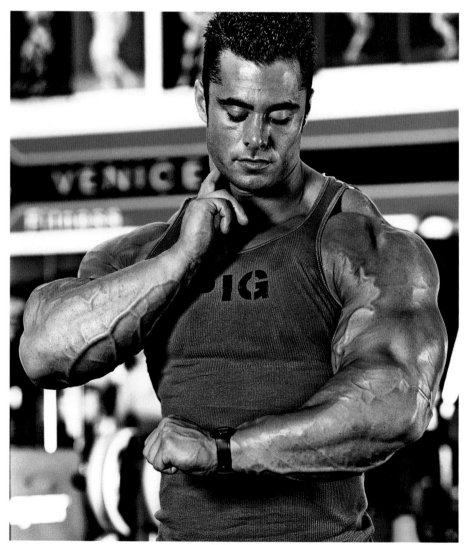

70

mote fluid retention in the body. Most bodybuilders control the state by reducing their salt intake. A few go even further by opting for the diuretic route, but as we'll discuss later, diuretics come with their own set of risks. While short-term hypertension is not serious in healthy individuals (notice we said "short-term" and "healthy"), those who already suffer from cardiovascular or kidney disease or have a family history of stroke should avoid anabolic steroids. Hypertension can aggravate any of those health issues with lethal consequences.

ELEVATED CHOLESTEROL

While medical knowledge on certain effects of steroid consumption is limited, it is known that steroids can change the ratio of LDL cholesterol (bad) to HDL (good) cholesterol.[1] Unfortunately, the change is not a beneficial one – steroids cause an increase in LDL and a decrease in HDL. The LDL:HDL ratio is one of the best predictors as to whether an individual will develop cardiovascular disease later in life. Those with a genetic history of heart disease should limit the length of their steroid cycles, or better yet, avoid steroids altogether.

GYNECOMASTIA

It's ironic that a drug taken by males to increase masculinity may also give them breast development that would rival a Playboy playmate! Through an interesting twist in the evolution of the human body, one of the breakdown products of testosterone is estrogen – a female or feminizing hormone. In some males the conversion (endocrinologists use the term aromatization) may be excessive. Increased estrogen on its own is not a problem, but unfortunately the male body also has estrogen receptors, which are largely concentrated in the breast region. Once stimulated these receptors may cause the appearance of female breasts. Bodybuilders use the term "bitch tits" to describe the condition. In most instances the breast development is not permanent – the swelling will subside and disappear when steroids are no longer present in the body. In some individuals, however, an anti-estrogen drug is needed to reverse the condition (many bodybuilders get a head start on this step by including anti-estrogen drugs in their steroid stacks). For a few unfortunate individuals though, the reversal doesn't occur naturally or with medication and surgery may be required to remove the breast tissue, as growing cells could become cancerous if left unchecked.

Gynecomastia is not a health issue limited only to bodybuilders on steroids. Newborn babies can often exhibit the condition if their mothers leaked estrogen into the placenta during pregnancy. Teenage males can also develop gynecomastia because their bodies are flooded with testosterone during puberty. Older males may experience this same breast tissue growth as a result of having higher

"Remember I know nothing about your medical history such as how much alcohol you drink, if you use oral steroids, whether you take pain killers. So I am making some generalizations. When your doctor sees elevated liver enzymes, he simply looks to remove the possible variables by a process of elimination and tries to figure out what's causing the elevation. That's why he wants you to stop taking supplements and take time off from the gym, because 99 percent of the time, taking a week or two off brings enzymes back to normal, thus satisfying the doc. What should you do? Do exactly what your doc wants you to do. There is really nothing to freak out over."

– Will Brink, bodybuilding and nutrition writer

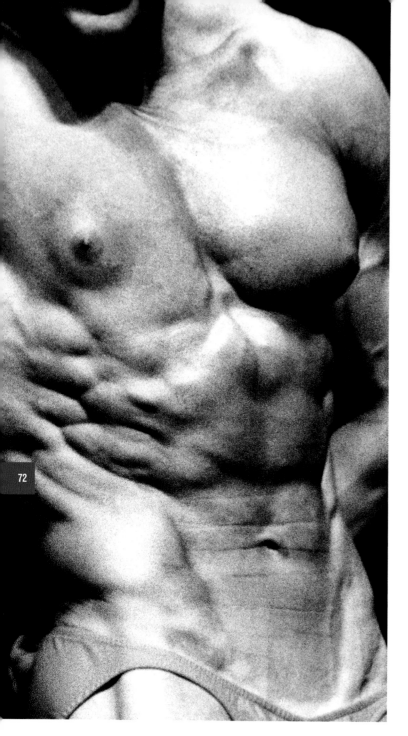

concentrations of a plasma hormone called sex hormone-binding globulin (SHBG) in their bodies. This hormone binds to testosterone and decreases the amount necessary for masculinizing reactions. Increased fat deposits are also a contributing factor because they elevate levels of aromatase – the enzyme that converts testosterone to estrogen.

There is no definitive way to predict who is susceptible to gynecomastia, but similar to acne, males who encounter the condition naturally at puberty are at greater risk. This is one of the reasons teenagers should under no circumstances use anabolic steroids.

The type of steroid an individual chooses to take may also be a determining factor for gynecomastia. Generally speaking, steroids with high androgenic properties are the most likely to cause breast development in males. Most of the common testosterone drugs such as cypionate, propionate and enanthate also note breast tissue growth as a common side effect. Other drugs that seem to influence the estrogen receptors are GH (growth hormone), thyroid drugs, Valium and yes, even marijuana.

At the first sign of gynecomastia, affected individuals should seek medical help. Granted the effect was most likely brought on by steroids (or one of the natural means discussed earlier), but growth in the breast region can also be a symptom of testicular cancer. While seeing a doctor may be a bit embarrassing, erring on the side of caution is better than risking cancer.

ABOVE: Gynecomastia, or "bitch tits," as those in the sport call them, are a clear visual sign that an athlete is using steroids.

GENITALIA
Men

Although the topic may make good media copy and be the center of much locker room banter, steroids do not cause penis enlargement. This myth probably originated from a combination of factors. First, steroids do in fact cause fluid retention – a slight swelling in the penis from additional fluid being held in the body may create the illusion of a bigger penis. But by no means are we talking about actual size increases here.

Photo by Doris Barrilleaux

Second is a condition called priapism, which is a persistent and painful erection that is not relieved by any type of sexual release including through intercourse. Now before you start wishing for such a long-lasting erection, understand that most sufferers report intense pain and discomfort. Furthermore, the penis was not designed to be under such prolonged pressure. After a certain time period with a severe case of priapism the tissues and blood cavities in your penis will simply give out. Finally, just try to visualize attempting to carry out your day-to-day activities with a constant woody! Being "happy to see someone" is one thing, but your intentions might be embarrassingly misinterpreted!

Steroids do cause an actual size change in a part of the male reproductive system, but this effect is definitely not for the better. Virtually all steroid users will experience mild to moderate shrinkage of their testes. The reason is based on the hormonal feedback loop discussed in Chapter 3. The body treats steroids like testosterone and responds by shutting down production of the male hormone. Because the testes are the primary production centers, they in turn begin to atrophy (shrink) from lack of usage – the process is very much like the "use it or lose it" principle. The extent of an individual's shrinkage depends on numerous factors including his genetics; dosages, type and number of steroids; and perhaps most important, duration of use. In general, the longer a cycle is the greater degree of atrophy that will occur.

Shrinkage will most often stop and the testes will return to their normal size after the steroids are no longer in the body, with rebound time being dependent on the cycle duration (i.e., longer cycle equals more time required for the testes to return to their pre-steroid size). Many bodybuilders opt for a proactive approach by taking a drug such as human chorionic gonadotropin (hCG) to kick-start the testes. This strategy is used for two primary reasons: to increase sex drive and to enable the user to retain most of the gains he made while on the steroid cycle.

Now for those who think steroids may offer some form of birth control, think again. Sperm count will be greatly reduced for those who use the drugs, but the key word is "reduced," not "eliminated." Sperm production does continue during steroid use, and it only takes one of these swimmers reaching and fertilizing an egg to totally alter the next 18 or so years of your life.

Females

While men need to be concerned about shrinkage during a steroid cycle, growth is of paramount importance to women. Many women who use steroids experience a certain degree of clitoral enlargement. In a few cases the size increase may be as much one to two inches in

> "I know one guy at school who has severe gynecomastia, two months after his last cycle. The guy's too embarrassed to take his shirt off in gym class. He's got better breast development than half the girls. He won't even see a doctor about it."
>
> – Anonymous bodybuilding teen

> "Also after a while 200 milligrams didn't have the same kick so I went back to the doc and asked if he could up the dosage, but he wouldn't go for it. It's just as well because eventually even 1,000 milligrams wouldn't be enough."
>
> – "Joe," professional bodybuilder

length, giving the clitoris the appearance similar to that of a small penis. The biological basis for this type of growth goes back to when a fetus is growing in the womb. During fetal development the genital tissue will masculinize with the presence of testosterone. If the hormone is not present at the crucial time during gestation, the tissue becomes female. But, and this is the important point to remember, the female genitalia still contains androgen receptors that will start masculinizing the tissue if testosterone reaches a certain level. As this rarely happens under natural circumstances, the genitalia remain feminine in appearance. As soon as a female starts taking steroids, however, she runs the risk of kick starting the androgen receptors and developing masculine-like genitalia. This condition usually reverses itself after cessation of steroid use, but in a few instances women may need surgery to "demasculinize" their genitalia.

AIDS

While there is no direct physiological link between AIDS and steroid use, anti-steroid groups continue to argue that a connection exists. Given the speculation surrounding this topic, the facts (and fictions) need to be addressed.

AIDS or Acquired Immuno-Deficiency Syndrome is a disease caused by the spreading of a rhinovirus. Although there are exceptions, the primary methods of transmission are unprotected sex with or receiving blood from infected individuals. Once inside the body the virus begins destroying the immune system, leaving the affected individual susceptible to other diseases such as cancer and pneumonia. Contrary to popular belief, the actual AIDS virus is not what causes death, but rather it's the inability of the immune system to fight off other pathogens.

Despite the conclusive knowledge from medical research and studies on this topic, anti-steroid groups continue to support the fallacy that steroids cause AIDS. The incidence of AIDS among bodybuilders, however, is no greater than among the general population. If a bodybuilder engages in unprotected sex with an infected partner, then yes, he's at greater risk for developing the disease. The presence or absence of steroids in the body has zero impact on the situation.

Groups who oppose steroids built much of their argument from a few case studies documenting a group of bodybuilders who all developed AIDS. However, what the anti-steroid groups conveniently omitted from their position was that the bodybuilders were sharing needles and one had contracted AIDS through unprotected sex. Therefore, every time the group all used the same needle they transmitted the infected blood to one another. The contents – whether it was steroids or a different drug – had no influence whatsoever on the AIDS virus being spread. This exact scenario of needle passing among

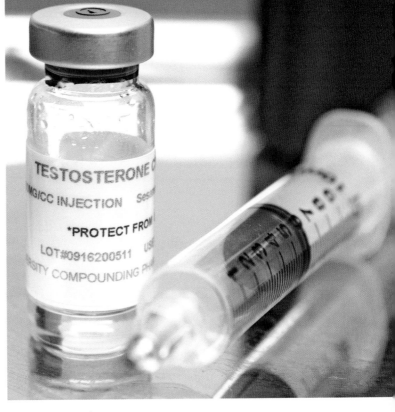

multiple people was what caused AIDS to run rampant through the drug-using community during the 1980s. Anyone who shares injections, regardless of the drug of choice, is putting themselves at risk for contracting AIDS and a host of other deadly diseases.

The irony of this so-called relationship is that steroids not only don't cause AIDS, but they may in fact be one of the best treatments for the virus. (Now how often do you hear anti-steroid groups passing this information along?) Similar to cancer, one symptom of AIDS is the wasting of lean muscle mass. Many steroids such as Deca-Durabolin and Oxandrolone show great promise in their ability to reverse the muscle-wasting effect. No one can dispute that steroids build muscle mass and strength – two important needs of AIDS sufferers. And while steroids are not a cure, their positive impact on muscle tissue will help prolong the lives of those afflicted with the virus.

ABOVE: Regardless of the contents in a vial, it's the sharing of needles that leads to dangerous viruses such as AIDS.

When steroids were classified as illegal in 1990, the political climate became such that no great strides were made to treat AIDS with the drugs; this aversion from using the drugs for medicinal purposes is still largely the case. Researchers and doctors are hesitant to prescribe steroids to AIDS patients because they fear losing their medical licenses or being charged with drug trafficking. It's sad to think a drug that shows such great promise in prolonging the lives of thousands of people is not available simply because some power-hungry politicians are more concerned about getting votes than helping affected individuals.

COSMETIC SIDE EFFECTS

Although cosmetic effects associated with steroid use are the least significant in terms of health, they are by far the most visually obvious. A face covered with acne, after all, will draw more stares and comments than elevated liver enzymes.

One of the main cosmetic side effects for both men and women on steroids is a drastic growth of body and facial hair. Many of the female competitors in bodybuilding contests sport "five-o'clock shadows" most guys would be proud of. Users experience an increase in amount of hair, and there is also a tendency for the strands to be much coarser. For guys, this growth is not as big a deal because they're used to having body hair and it just means extra shaving or waxing at contest time. For women, however, such an increase in body hair can be psychologically traumatic.

Photo by Robert Reiff

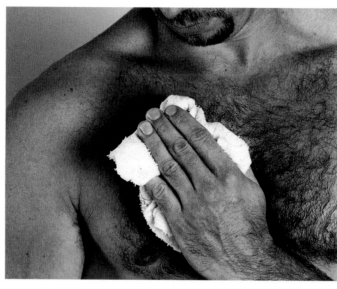

RIGHT: The increased growth of body hair is a fairly common side effect of steroids. Competitors can easily remedy this with shaving and waxing.

76

Interestingly, while steroids cause body hair growth to increase, the effect seems to be opposite on scalp hair. Many bodybuilders in their teens and early 20s have receding hairlines similar to that of a senior citizen. Scientific research has not determined why this occurs, but one theory is that hair loss is influenced by the conversion of testosterone into dihydrotestosterone (DHT), a process mediated by the enzyme 5-alpha reductase. DHT is then believed to attack hair follicles causing them to degenerate. Generally speaking those who have a genetic history of male-pattern baldness are at the greatest risk for steroid-induced hair loss.

One of the most obvious side effects experienced by many steroid-using women is a deepening of the voice. Steroids cause the vocal chords to masculinize leaving many female bodybuilders with deeper voices than their male counterparts. While this condition is in itself embarrassing, more important is that the voice change is permanent and won't be reversed when the user stops taking steroids.

SKELETAL BONES

Steroids cause numerous side effects in teen users, but there is one major outcome that may have huge implications on their social lives and career goals. Steroids have been proven to cause a premature closing or fusing of the epiphyseal plates in human bones. These growth areas at the end of long bones are what give the body its ultimate height. Once fused, these plates cannot be "re-opened" and the individual will not get any taller. Teenagers who use steroids run the risk of stunting their growth, which can often lead to dramatic psychological and social problems.

Photo by John Butler

From a psychological point of view, many teenage males wish they were taller. As superficial as it may sound, height can often be a determining factor of social acceptance during the school years. The most popular guys quite regularly tend to be the athletes who tower over their peers. Being naturally short does not automatically relegate a teen to the doghouse, but those who are of average height or taller commonly have an easier time "fitting in." As such, if a teen starts using steroids he may stunt his growth and as a result suffer severe mental stress.

The social implications associated with stunted growth go beyond school and the teenage years. Height, and its implied power, is also evident in the corporate world. It is a fact that taller individuals have more proven success than shorter individuals when it comes to career advancement. Numerous surveys have reported that the average height of corporate executives is 6'2". So if teenagers whose bones are not fully grown decide to use steroids, they may even be limiting their future career success just for a few extra pounds of muscle mass.

THE GREAT TENDON SCARE

While the primary effects of steroids are on muscle tissue, there are also minor impacts on strength within the tendons. This secondary outcome, however, is directly opposite to what anti-steroid groups would have you believe. Every now and then the media or sporting community focuses attention on some bodybuilder or power athlete who's suffered a tendon tear. Anti-steroid groups are among the first to seize this opportunity to further their crusade against the evils of steroids, their argument being that steroids somehow weaken tendon tissue. But once again, they are jumping to conclusions without the medical evidence to back their claims. There is no credible medical proof that anabolic steroids cause degeneration in tendon tissue strength. Although not conclusive, the generally accepted theory as to why some bodybuilders tear tendons is because steroid use has made their muscles gain strength at a much faster rate than their tendons. A non-user's natural tendon strength tends to keep pace with muscular strength, but a steroid user's muscles often leap way ahead, causing an imbalance – their muscles are capable of generating more power than their tendons can handle. Although the steroids are not directly impacting tendon strength, bodybuilders and other steroid users should still be aware of these risks.

Reference

1) Cohen J.C., et al. "Hypercholesterolemia in male powerlifters using anabolic androgenic steroids," *The Physician and Sports Medicine.* 10:8 (1988), 49–56.

> "One of the most obvious side effects experienced by steroid-using women is deepening of the voice. While the condition itself is embarrassing, more important is that the voice change is permanent."

77

PSYCHOLOGICAL SIDE EFFECTS

Steroids can impact the human body in a variety of ways and many of the effects experienced are psychological in nature. The media and anti-steroid groups address the psychological effects in much the same way as they do the physiological effects — by ignoring medical evidence and exaggerating isolated cases to further their argument.

ROID RAGE

The most well-known (and publicized) psychological side effect of steroid use is roid rage. Many newspaper articles and TV news reports on sports, health or performance-enhancing drugs these days paint a dark picture that all steroid users become homicidal psychotics who are a threat to society.

The term "roid" is a slang that comes from steroid, and "rage" refers to the alleged bouts of intense anger brought on by consuming the drugs. The theory behind roid rage is that steroids cause individuals to exhibit episodes of extreme and uncontrollable anger – sometimes to the point of criminal violence. As with many of the supposed physiological side effects, however, there is no conclusive medical evidence to support this theory. In fact, roid rage owes its existence to the legal field and not the medical profession.

The origins of roid rage go back to the late 1980s when a couple of creative defense attorneys attempted to reason that their clients' criminal behavior was the result of steroid use. One of the accused was a construction worker who had beaten a hitchhiker to death for trying to rob him. Another was an angry motorist who had smashed the windows out of someone else's car after being cut off in traffic. Despite the best efforts of the attorneys, the jurors didn't buy in to the notion of roid rage and both clients were found guilty. The court's decision should have been the end of the issue, case closed, but two groups of individuals – the media and the psychiatric community – saw an opportunity and took action.

THE MEDIA ROLE

During the late 1980s to early 1990s there was an almost endless parade of criminal cases involving flipped-out bodybuilders. The media jumped all over such stories, as they were new and exclusive and far juicier than the mundane court news most reporters typically

Photo by Robert Reiff

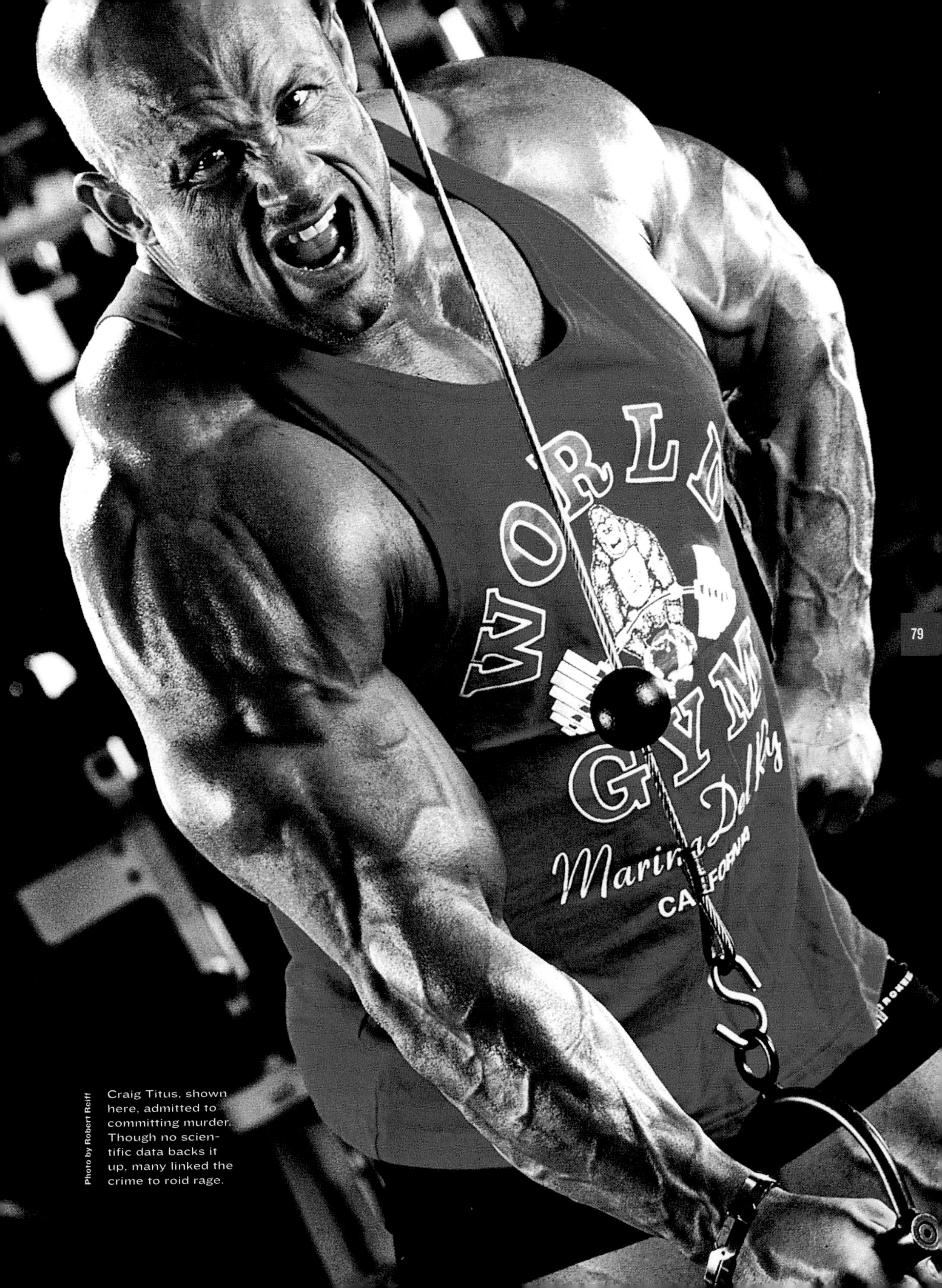

Craig Titus, shown here, admitted to committing murder. Though no scientific data backs it up, many linked the crime to roid rage.

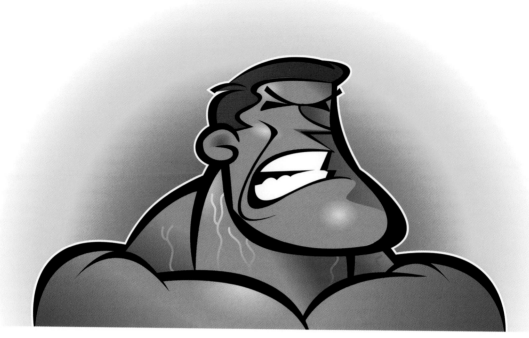

ABOVE: Given that U.S. Congress used roid rage as one of the primary reasons to re-classify steroids as illegal, one would believe the condition has a proven biological basis. But there is no such proof to date.

covered. Headlines tended to be the same: "Mild and meek individual goes on rampage after starting a steroid cycle." On the surface the evidence seemed convincing – especially when the media sensational-ized the story in an attempt to sway listeners into believing that roid rage was a real psychological condition – but the truth was far from what was actually presented.

In virtually all the cases, the individual had a pre-existing his-tory of violent behavior before being charged with the offense. Furthermore, alcohol was also a factor in most of the cases. Does this scenario sound familiar to you as a reader? "Aggressive alcohol user snaps and murders his wife." It's sad that this type of crime has become all too familiar in North American society. Unfortunately, such stories of alcohol abuse have lost their appeal among the gen-eral public, and the media has had to seek out a new hot issue. By raising questions about a link between steroids and psychological problems, regardless of the truth, the media effectively generates excitement around the topic. The issue has become so "popular" that even a few TV show and movie plots have been based on roid rage.

WHAT WOULD FREUD THINK?

The media's sidekicks in spreading the roid rage myth were the psy-chiatrists who made reputations for themselves by becoming "experts" on the condition. Their specific names aren't important, but during the 1990s two relatively unknown psychiatrists at the time used a couple of prominent criminal cases and wrote them up in a few medical journals. Even though these were individual cases (and not the more credible large-sample, long-term comparison studies), they were unexampled at the time, and medical journal editors are

Illustration by Mark Collins

no different than TV and newspaper reporters when it comes to generating interest – they like new twists on issues. The sad part about this situation is that once an article appears in one of these "bibles" in the medical field, the information within is generally accepted as truth. The two psychiatrists were able to get additional articles published and they quickly established themselves as the experts on roid rage. Their "expert" status was quite the accomplishment given their "evidence" came only from isolated case studies not supported by medical proof.

IS ROID RAGE REAL?

Given that U.S. Congress used roid rage as one of the primary reasons for reclassifying steroids as illegal substances in the early 1990s, one would be inclined to believe the condition indeed has a proven biological basis. But there is simply no such proof to date. The sense of realness around the issue comes from the fact that it gets so much attention – the media continues to put these stories in the spotlight because they create more of a buzz than other criminal trials. Take, for example, all the media hype surrounding WWE wrestler Chris Benoit after he killed his wife and young son before taking his own life in 2007. What should have been a domestic violence case of murder-suicide instead became a media circus after testosterone derivatives were found in Benoit's home. At the time of this book's publication, evidence suggests that Benoit suffered brain damage from the years of falls and other heavy-impact wrestling moves he endured in the sport. Numerous medical professionals have indicated that such damage in the brain could lead to a wide spectrum of behaviors including aggression. But somehow Benoit's steroid use is still the central focus of most of the news stories related to the crime.

When you consider that there isn't any conclusive scientific or medical information to prove steroids cause roid rage, it's fairly safe to say steroids users are no more prone to aggressive criminal activity than non-users. As one online writer said, "If you're an aggressive asshole before you use steroids you'll still be an aggressive asshole after you go on a cycle."

AGGRESSION

While the firm evidence for roid rage is insufficient, most users (and their friends) readily admit they get a little "edgy" while on a cycle. This, however, does not mean they are all on the verge of snapping and committing a violent crime at the drop of a hat. What it does mean is aggression levels elevate slightly for most users during a cycle. The degree of increase is usually related to the user's pre-steroid personality. A meek and mild-mannered individual may not notice any

"Thousands upon thousands of men and women have said 'I want to do just one cycle.' But once you've dipped into that bag of tricks, resisting its allure is difficult, and subsequent cycles are almost sure to follow. The better the gains are, the greater the temptation to push the envelope further. Once you get used to feeling like Superman, it's tough to go back to being Mr. Normal. That's when you've got a problem, whether you're willing to admit it or not."

– Nelson Montana, *MuscleMag International* contributor

81

> "Aggression levels elevate slightly for most users during a cycle. The degree of increase is usually related to the user's pre-steroid personality. If someone is 'quick on the trigger' to begin with, steroid use may simply exaggerate the condition."

change in his or her aggression level. Conversely the non-using hot-headed individual may become an aggressive steroid user. If someone is "quick on the trigger" to begin with, steroid use may simply exaggerate the condition. Anti-steroid groups jump on this steroids-cause-aggression bandwagon and make it sound as if using the drugs is a shortcut to criminal activity.

Situational factors are an extremely important aspect in the discussion of aggression and steroids. It's very common for steroid users – especially physically larger individuals – to take jobs in the security field. These jobs such as bouncing, event security, etc. involve dealing with a lot of idiots, many of whom are drunk, on a regular basis. All it takes is for some drunken bar patron to call the bouncer a "juicehead" or "gorilla" and you can likely guess the rest – thrown punches and a bouncer charged with assault. Now this is not to suggest bodybuilders don't initiate any fights or sometimes go too far. Some do. In many cases, however, the aggression is a reaction to the situation and not a side effect of the individual's steroid use.

ANABOLIC ADDICTION

Like most drugs, there is potential for addiction with steroid use. The addiction can be both physical and psychological in nature. A physical addiction occurs when the drug alters the body's chemistry in such a way that it can't function properly without the substance. The normal state becomes the drug state. A psychological addiction is often called "dependence" and refers to the intense craving the individual experiences for the drug. While the body does not physically need the drug, the individual perceives that he or she can't survive without it.

Another closely related issue is tolerance – as the body becomes accustomed to a given drug dosage, gradually the desired effect is no longer produced. The individual then needs to take ever-increasing dosages to achieve the same effect. This issue is further complicated by the fact that once the body becomes accustomed to functioning with a certain level of a drug, a number of potentially severe physical and psychological side effects will be exhibited if usage is stopped. Some of these withdrawal symptoms include depression, agitation, sleep disorders, hallucinations and fatigue.

Among the limited medical evidence to suggest that steroids may cause addiction was one case in which a 24-year-old male weightlifter was admitted as a psychiatric emergency after complaining of bouts of depression and anger outbursts. He admitted to having suicidal thoughts of crashing his car the night before, and had voluntarily sought medical help because he felt controlled by the steroids he was taking. An in-depth assessment of the individual's history showed no sign of any symptoms prior to or for the first three months of his steroid use. The symptoms only started after he switched from cycling only one drug to using five different drugs continuously.[1]

Upon evaluation the admitting psychiatrists found that the individual met six criteria in the DSM-III – the main diagnostic manual at that time for mental illness and drug dependence. The symptoms included:

- Continued use of the drugs for longer than planned.
- Unsuccessful in attempts to cut down on drug use.
- Continued use of the drugs despite their effect on social life.
- Developed tolerance to the drugs.
- Withdrawal symptoms after cessation of drug use.
- Continued use of drugs to avoid withdrawal symptoms.

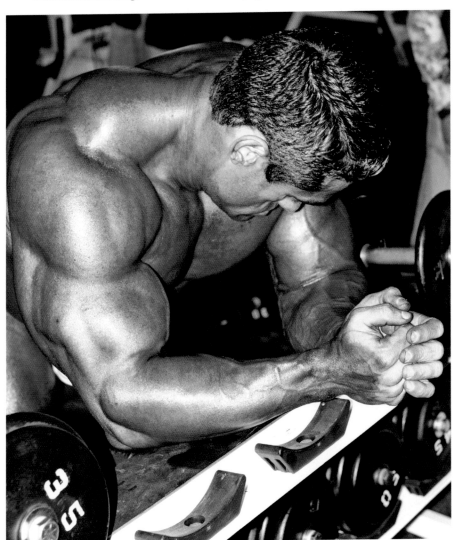

LEFT: When an athlete becomes addicted to a drug, the body's chemistry changes and can't function normally without it. So when the drug is stopped, the body is incapable of working at the same intensity level.

83

Photo by Irvin Gelb
Model Gustavo Badell

You'll notice in the previous list the word "continued" is used in multiple criteria. Many bodybuilders who gain 20 or 30 pounds while on a steroid cycle become so accustomed to this newfound weight that they simply can't handle the thought (or reality) of losing it. Not only are their recovery abilities through the roof, but they're also probably doing reps with weight they couldn't even manage a single lift with before the cycle. Add in the compliments from friends, other gym members and even strangers, and coming off the cycle only to return to pre-steroid strength and weight becomes that much harder.

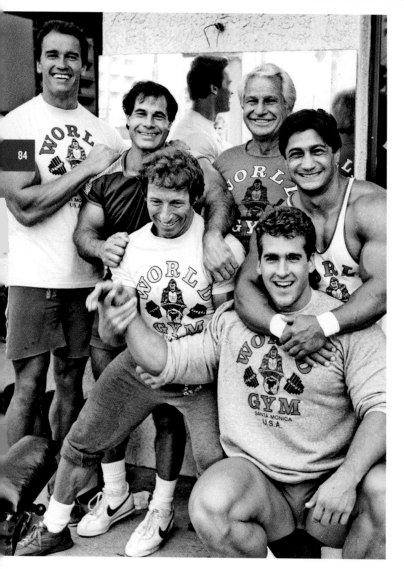

BELOW: A camaraderie exists among bodybuilders, as Arnold Schwarzenegger, Franco Columbu, Joe Gold, Danny Padilla, Eddie Giuliani and Bob Paris prove in this photo. Gym members fuel each other's training fires and serve as key influential factors to do whatever necessary to build the best physique.

DEPRESSION

Although this condition is a rare effect, a few individuals have been diagnosed with depression as a result of their steroid use. Definitions of what constitutes depression differ slightly within the medical field, but most include such symptoms as low self-esteem, loss of appetite, insomnia, low libido, poor personal hygiene and a general lack of interest in social contact.

Similar to addiction, depression can present itself either physically or psychologically. Physical depression is when changes occur to an individual's cellular chemistry, particularly the neurotransmitters (the brain's chemical messengers). Psychological depression is more often triggered by external forces such as the death of a loved one or an ended relationship, whereby the emotions are internalized and begin to affect the individual's ability to carry out regular day-to-day activities.

Steroid use can lead to both types of depression. On a physical level the drugs may alter a user's system to such an extent that it takes weeks if not months to readjust after the drug is stopped. During this "normalizing" process an individual could be more susceptible to experiencing bouts of mild to severe depression.

While steroid users may occasionally suffer from depression due to physical effects, more often the depressed state has a psychological basis. The lives of many

Photo by Art Zeller

bodybuilders revolve completely around their physiques – their whole identity centers on the satisfaction they get from such comments as, "you're as big as a house," or, "you're ripped man, ripped." These types of compliments will usually come fast and furious while a guy is on a cycle, but as soon as the juice is stopped, some amount of weight loss is inevitable. All it takes is a couple of negative comments like, "are you losing weight?" or, "where's the rest of you?," and the individual may get down on himself and slip into a state of depression.

There are numerous factors that contribute to the degree of depression a person experiences. First is the manner in which the steroids were stopped. If the user quits "cold turkey," his or her system is left in a state of shock because of the sudden absence of the compound. They go from one extreme to the other – from drug to non-drug state virtually overnight. Users who stop taking steroids via this approach are more likely to suffer increasingly pronounced depression than those who gradually come off the drugs by tapering down the dosages.

A second variable is the amount of drugs that were being used. Those on high dosages of multiple drugs usually experience more severe symptoms of depression than those who use one or two drugs for short cycles.

A third factor is an individual's post-steroid behavior. If they go off steroids, give up training and don't take anything to boost their natural testosterone levels back to normal, odds are they'll experience a certain degree of depression. In an effort to avoid these symptoms, many bodybuilders start adding human chorionic gonadotropin (hCG) toward the end of their steroid cycle. They also continue to train but at a slightly reduced intensity. While there will still be some loss of muscle mass, most bodybuilders manage to maintain a high proportion of bodyweight. The satisfaction of holding on to most of their weight is in itself usually enough to prevent an individual from becoming depressed.

A final contributing factor to the degree of depression experienced by steroid users is personality. Individual personality types will make individuals more or less prone to encounter a depressive state. Those who have upbeat lives and outgoing personalities tend to suffer less than those with fewer social safety nets. Your personality type is not a fail-proof determinant of whether you'll experience depression, but those who have previously experienced the condition or have poor support networks may want to think twice before using steroids. Depression is a very serious issue and unfortunately many cases lead to numerous health problems, with some even becoming so severe that an individual sees no hope for recovery and takes his or her own life.

> "The lives of many bodybuilders revolve completely around their physiques. [When coming off the juice] all it takes is a couple of negative comments like, 'where's the rest of you?,' and the individual may get down on himself and slip into a state of depression."

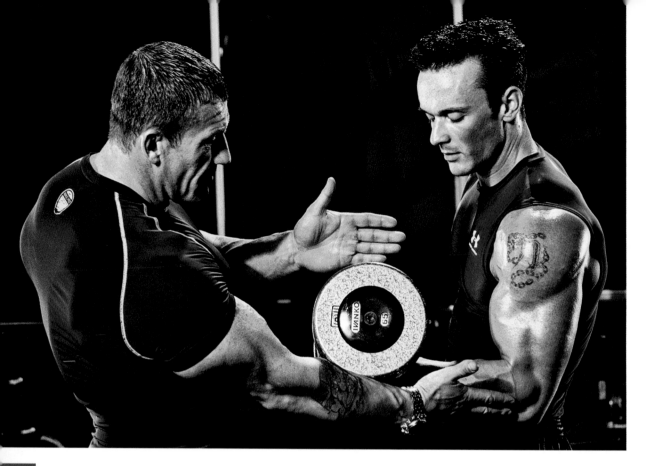

ABOVE: Dorian Yates shows a young trainer the proper lift mechanics – unfortunately, there are some coaches out there who do more harm than good, pressuring young athletes into using drugs.

SUICIDE

It is difficult to prove conclusively that a link exists between steroid use and suicide, but there have been a small number of cases where the drugs were thought to be related to the individual's death. Unfortunately, when left untreated depression can influence some individuals to believe taking their own life is a better option than trying to endure the intense feelings of despair. Some users who go off steroids will struggle with the loss of muscle mass and strength, and they may start to spiral downward emotionally. The decrease in weight and size can be perceived as a loss of identity, and the physical changes associated with stopping the steroids may become overwhelming. Without professional help and support to realize that muscle and strength didn't wholly define them, some of these individuals risk losing all sense of value for life and view suicide as the only way out.

Teenagers are especially at risk for developing symptoms of depression and suicidal thoughts and behaviors. This age group, because of puberty, hormones and biochemical changes in the body, commonly experiences emotional and behavioral swings under normal circumstances – the introduction of steroids into the equation could magnify the problem. It's an unfortunate fact that there have been reported cases of teens who have committed suicide after performing sexual services with adults in exchange for steroids. The teenage mind is a complex entity, still largely misunderstood even by medical professionals. Given that some teens have even committed suicide over such superficial issues (from an adult's perspective) as acne or a relationship break-up, the potential for steroids to cause severe psychological effects is compounded, and use of the drugs among this age group is extremely dangerous.

Although the incidence of steroid-related suicide is medically unproven and largely speculated, users should pay particular attention to any negative psychological symptoms they experience. At the slightest indication of change in mood, inability to sleep, loss of appetite, lethargy or general loss of interest in social life, stop steroid use and seek medical help immediately.

CONCLUSION

Anabolic steroid use, like most other drugs, comes at a cost. There will be side effects. But to say, however, that steroid users are at greater risk for negative side effects than users of other drugs is not supported by research, nor medically credible. In any group or population there will be individuals who experience adverse effects to certain drugs. For example, the vast majority of individuals can safely use the antibiotic penicillin without any problems. For a very small percentage of individuals though, penicillin could cause them to go into allergic shock and die. The same is true for perhaps the most common steroid-based drug in society – birth control pills. Yes, they are steroids but just not the anabolic kind. If you were to look them up in the PDR (Physician's Desk Reference), you'll see a long list of potential side effects – some of which are quite serious. But birth control pills are considered "safe" because the vast majority of women who use them don't experience such side effects. The PDR list is simply a precautionary method to protect the drug manufacturers against legal action should an individual suffer a severe adverse reaction from taking the pills.

Anabolic steroids are no different. Despite what anti-steroid groups, sports officials and media sources continue to preach, the fact remains that most steroid users don't experience the range or degree of side effects commonly linked to the drugs. Indeed, there are risks associated with steroids – we aren't trying to deny that reality. Every drug becomes dangerous if it's abused. To boldly state that steroids are cancer-causing, psychotic-inducing agents, however, is a gross misrepresentation of the facts and medical research. And while there is evidence to support that teens and females should never use the drugs, from a physiological and psychological standpoint, males in their 20s or older can do so in relative safety, under close medical supervision ... though the legal issues are another matter entirely.

Reference

1) Cowart V., Natural Institute on Drug Abuse may join anabolic steroid research, *JAMA*, 261:13 (April 7, 1989).

87

"The teenage mind is a complex entity, still largely misunderstood even by medical professionals. This age group commonly experiences emotional and behavioral swings under normal circumstances – the introduction of steroids into the equation could magnify the problem."

LEGAL ISSUES

The general public's perception is that anabolic steroids are profoundly dangerous and deadly drugs deserving of vilification at every opportunity. Steroid use by adults to enhance physical appearance or athletic ability is labeled by the average American as "abuse," regardless of the amounts, and consequently those who take the drugs are lumped into the same degenerate category as cocaine or heroin users. Law enforcement agents and prosecutors gladly arrest and charge steroid users as part of America's so called "War on Drugs." Only the most progressive physicians accept the legitimacy of anabolic steroids for medicinal use. Most doctors are reluctant or refuse to prescribe the drugs for fear of being labeled a "dealer" and losing their medical licenses.

While rarely reported by the media, there are actually very strong reasons to question current legislation on steroids. Considerable evidence suggests that for healthy individuals, the actual dangers associated with anabolic steroids are significantly less than what were presented to the U.S. Congress in the 1980s. Such laws have ultimately only served to limit research, undermine beneficial applications and, perhaps most importantly, severed any positive association between users and physicians. An argument could even be made that the laws have actually increased the very issues they were created to combat.

THE GOVERNMENT SPEAKS

During the mid 1980s, two steroid-related problems were brought to the attention of Congress: the increasing use of anabolic steroids in professional and amateur sports, and the growing use among high school students. During a two-year period (1988 to 1990), Congressional hearings were held in an attempt to determine the extent of these problems and whether the Controlled Substances Act needed to be modified to include anabolic steroids alongside more serious drugs such as heroin and cocaine.

Numerous witnesses testified at the hearings, including medical professionals and representatives of regulatory agencies like the FDA, DEA and the National Institute on Drug Abuse. All agencies recommended against the proposed changes to the laws, although there was little coverage of this decision by the media. Even the

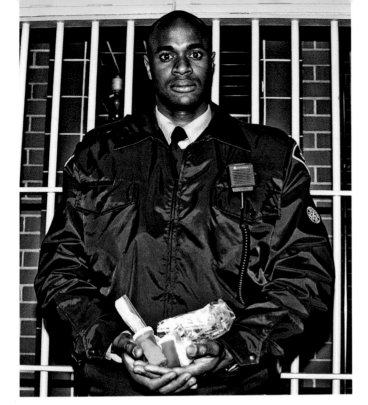

LEFT: Because of the government's decision to clean up sports, law enforcement personnel are quick to arrest and charge steroid users as part of the "War on Drugs."

highly respected AMA (American Medical Association) opposed any modifications, maintaining that abuse of these drugs did not lead to physical or psychological dependence required for scheduling under the Controlled Substances Act.

Unfortunately, it was later revealed that the lack of serious side effects associated with steroids were of secondary importance to Congress. The majority of witnesses called to testify at the hearings were representatives from various athletic organizations. Their testimonies combined with Congress's decision to "clean up" sports seemed to carry the most influence in the courts, and steroids were reclassified as Schedule III controlled drugs in the Anabolic Steroid Control Act of 1990.

ANABOLIC STEROID CONTROL ACT

In some respects this law is one of the most Draconian pieces of legislation ever enacted by Congress. When deconstructed it's certainly one of the most irrational – the core of the Act places steroids in the same legal class as barbiturates, ketamines and LSD precursors. Here are a few main points highlighted within the Anabolic Steroid Control Act:

- Those caught illegally possessing anabolic steroids, even purely for personal use, face arrest and prosecution.
- Under the Control Act, it is unlawful for any person knowingly or intentionally to possess an anabolic steroid unless it was obtained directly, or pursuant to a valid prescription or order, from a practitioner, while acting in the course of his professional practice (or except as otherwise authorized).
- A first offense, simple possession conviction is punishable by a term of imprisonment of up to one year and/or a minimum fine of $1,000.

- Simple possession by a person with a previous conviction for certain offenses, including any drug or narcotic crimes, must get imprisonment of at least 15 days and up to two years, and a minimum fine of $2,500.
- Individuals with two or more such previous convictions face imprisonment of not less than 90 days, but not more than three years, and a minimum fine of $5,000.
- Distributing anabolic steroids, or possessing them with intent to distribute, is a federal felony.
- An individual who distributes or dispenses steroids, or possesses them with intent to distribute or dispense, is punishable by up to five years in prison (with at least two additional years of supervised release) and/or a $250,000 fine ($1,000,000 if the defendant is other than an individual). Penalties are higher for repeat offenders.

These criteria essentially meant that being in possession of even one bottle of Winstrol could land someone in prison next to dealers of crack, heroin and cocaine. As a result of the 1990 Act, a once recreational practice among the bodybuilding and athletic fraternity had become a one-way ticket to lengthy prison terms.

CAREERS MADE

Much like the ambitious psychiatrists who sought to make names for themselves through their "discovery" of roid rage, numerous law enforcement agents viewed the new regulations as a great opportunity to vault up the legal career ladder. The early 1990s were a booming time for many in the law enforcement field who

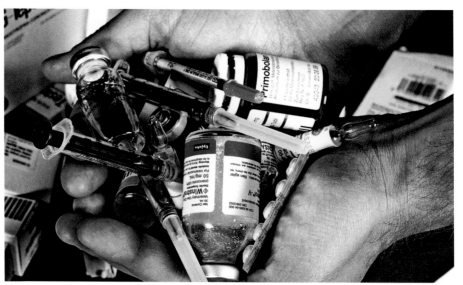

RIGHT: After the Anabolic Control Act was put into effect, anyone possessing steroids, even for personal use, could be faced with jail time.

Photo by Robert Kennedy

sought out steroid users en masse. A criminal "catch" was essentially just a gym bag or locker room away. Drug enforcement agents considered steroid users easy targets because the vast majority were decent, law-abiding citizens. Most users at the time didn't even know steroids had been reclassified as illegal. And having not been part of any prior criminal activity meant they had no experience trying to escape the law. Arrests came quick and easily, and so too did the promotions for those within the enforcement and prosecution fields.

A FAMILIAR PRECEDENT

Despite Congress's rationale for criminalizing steroids, the new legislation only compounded problems. Prior to the crackdown, the average person wouldn't be able to differentiate a steroid from any other drug. But thanks to the steady stream of bodybuilders being tried in court, steroids were thrown into the spotlight and almost everyone and their brother were walking into gyms looking for vials and needles. Forget the standard eating and training programs – people wanted Winstrol and Dianabol. Dealers reported a notable jump during the early 1990s in the steroid business. Many said some shipments were sold before the drugs had even arrived. Despite being aimed at curtailing use, the laws instead gave steroids a Super Bowl-like amount of advertising and publicity.

The drug laws also radically transformed the black market. Prior to 1990 the average steroid "dealer" was often an otherwise law-abiding citizen who was selling steroids to his gym buddies only to cover his own costs. Making millions from a large client portfolio was not the goal of most guys who were dealing. But as soon as steroids became illegal and the increased publicity drove demand through the roof, most of these small-time gym dealers got out of the business. The problem with this situation, however, was that demand was greater than ever.

THE BLACK MARKET

Prohibition in the 1920s; America's "War on Drugs" in the 1980s; the criminalizing of anabolic steroids in 1990. What do these three points in history have in common? They are all instances of when government laws failed to curtail specific drug use despite making the substance illegal to possess. When alcohol was banned in the 1920s, people responded by taking the practice underground. Selling alcohol became a big business and even contributed to establishing the modern Mafia. The same situation happened during the 1980s when the U.S. launched a major crackdown on cocaine. Within months of the legal decision, the term "crime lord" entered into English vocabulary and a few "unknown" Colombians became billionaires selling the drug en masse to the U.S. black market.

"So you've won Mr. Fallopian Tubes, Iowa, and you have a three-foot trophy to prove it. But it cost you $2,000 to $3,000 for steroids and who knows how much in terms of your health and longevity. You want to win the Mr. Olympia and that will take you 10 to 20 years, plus probably 10 more contests that'll cost you about $50,000 for steroids. Is the prize worth the cost?"

– Preston Rendell, bodybuilding writer

91

"The drug laws radically transformed the black market. As soon as steroids became illegal and the increased publicity drove demand through the roof, most of the small-time gym dealers got out of the business."

When a popular drug is or becomes illegal, there will always be someone who's willing to sacrifice the associated risks to sell it. The profits to be made from such sales are just too tempting. The steroid black market was a perfect example. When the Anabolic Steroid Control Act was put into effect, most dealers and suppliers at the time were either arrested or escaped the business. Since demand was at its highest, however, dealers of other street drugs such as heroin and cocaine moved in to fill the void. And as expected, prices of steroids shot through the roof. A bottle of Dianabol that would have sold for $20 or $30 before 1990 instead cost $100 or more. The first generation of steroid dealers never really had profit in mind, but street dealers on the other hand were trying to maximize their gains.

Yet another domino effect of the legislation was that new drugs were introduced to steroid users because the street dealers also sold just about every form of illegal drug available. Teenage males represented the biggest group of users, and seeing the opportunity to drive business, dealers preyed on the aspiring Schwarzeneggers, swaying them to get into hardcore street drugs or worse – sell them. This corrupt drug environment caught the attention of law enforcement agencies and caused a new wave of arrests, a trend that is still ongoing.

BUYER BEWARE

With most doctors now being so opposed to prescribing steroids, because of the potential legal risks to their ability to practice medicine, those in the market have had to seek out other sources. The result is ironic: instead of pure drugs being dispensed and regulated through medical monitoring, individuals are left to test their luck in the black market, risking potential health and legal consequences of one bad roll of the dice.

The trusty gym buddy, who also used to be a popular source for acquiring steroids, is no longer a common go-to option. The majority of bodybuilders nowadays have been put in a position where getting their gear requires illegal measures. Unfortunately, with so many new players on the scene, bodybuilders can never be 100 percent sure where their drugs are coming from. The safest, at least in terms of purity, are those stolen from pharmaceutical labs. And with the potential for profit being so high, not much effort is required on the part of a drug dealer in convincing an employee to divert a few hundred bottles from the stock room before the drugs are logged, catalogued and inventoried. The legal ramifications are still on the forefront, but this scenario at least affords users assurance that what they're buying is real and safe.

Another method to secure illegal steroids is from other countries. In many nations steroids are not classified as illegal drugs. Individuals can literally walk in and buy them from the local drugstore. If a pre-

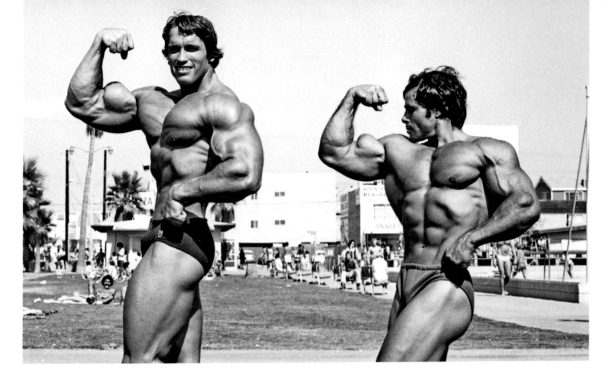

scription is specifically required, the pharmacy often conveniently has a nearby doctor who's qualified to write one on demand. From there, courier services manage to transport the drugs across the U.S. border. Drug smugglers use a number of techniques to bring the drugs into the States, the ins and outs of which could fill an entire book. From rigged hidden storage compartments in cars and trucks to cleverly disguised aerosol containers, smugglers use any means necessary to get the drugs to their given destinations.

The nucleus of North America's current anabolic steroid business is the counterfeit black market. Two main categories of steroids are bought and sold via this source: semi-bogus and bogus. Semi-bogus products are real in the sense that they do contain steroids. However, they are not manufactured in a legitimate pharmaceutical lab and may not contain what's advertised on the label. In most cases, semi-bogus compounds are not a true anabolic steroid, but rather one of the cheaper (but just as potent) testosterone forms. Users usually aren't concerned with these details as long as the drug works without any unexpected side effects. Some of the semi-bogus steroids, however, are just as safe and potent as what's made in big pharmaceutical labs, and in fact may have been produced in facilities outfitted with the latest equipment. Such are the profits to be made on the steroid black market.

Bogus drugs are exactly what they sound like – completely fake. Not a steroid or testosterone derivative can be found in these concoctions. While the vials and labels may look real, the contents contain no anabolic properties whatsoever. Numerous accounts exist of individuals who injected cooking oil into their butts or ingested flour pills under the assumption they were taking steroids. If the person is lucky, what he or she has injected or ingested won't be harmful to the body. The individual will instead just be out the hard-earned cash. But many foodstuffs such as cooking oil or other items were not processed with intended use for intramuscular injection. Such a practice may lead to a severe infection that could even result in the need for amputation.

ABOVE: After the legislation, street dealers preyed on young aspiring body-builders who wanted to look like Arnold Schwarzenegger and Franco Columbu (shown here), and would take anything to achieve the physiques of their idols.

Photo by Art Zeller

• **ANABOLIC PRIMER** •

MAKING THE DECISION

"The vast majority of natural bodybuilders gain about 90 percent of their mass within the first five years of training. You'll never know what you're capable of until you've spent that time building your physique without going on the gear."

Despite the associated risks and potential side effects, some individuals simply won't be deterred from hitting the juice. This book isn't meant to be a tool to preach or impose judgment. Instead we'll summarize a few of the cardinal rules that should be closely followed if you want to ensure your steroid use is effective and, more importantly, safe. First, it's important to remember that many countries have reclassified steroids and numerous other performance-enhancing drugs as illegal substances. While quite a few prisons have excellent workout facilities, we're fairly certain you'd have much more fun training at the local gym rather than next to some guy named Bubba who thinks you have a nice behind. So, consider the pros and cons one last time before you decide to pop that pill or inject that needle.

RULE #1
Train naturally for five years before starting on steroids.
While five years may sound like a long time, trust us, this time frame is fairly short in the grand scheme of your life. The vast majority of natural bodybuilders gain about 90 percent of their mass within the first five years of training. You'll never know just what you're capable of achieving until you've spent that time building your physique without going on the gear. After that period, if you honestly feel you've reached your natural genetic peak, you can then consider whether using steroids might be your next step.

RULE #2
Refrain from use until you're at least 24.
No one, regardless of the situation, should contemplate using steroids until they're at least 24 years old. Your body is being naturally flooded with testosterone and growth hormone until you reach your mid 20s. During the teen years and into your early 20s, you don't need the boost from steroids to make great progress. If for some reason you can't achieve gains without drugs over those years, odds are that taking steroids won't even make much difference. Muscle stagnation or lack of growth is a clear sign you need to re-evaluate your entire training regimen and nutritional strategies. Something you're doing (or not doing) isn't working for your individual body. Another important factor to

take into account with regards to age is that steroids shut down the growth plates at the end of long bones. Using steroids at any point over the course of your teens or early 20s will only hinder your potential to reach your full height. Finally, steroids stunt your natural hormonal system, causing major fluctuations to your hormone levels. These effects are bad enough when you're older – you definitely don't want to be facing hormonal havoc while in your teens and early 20s.

BELOW: Building a strong, solid physique requires intense training, proper nutrition and time; steroids won't do the work for you.

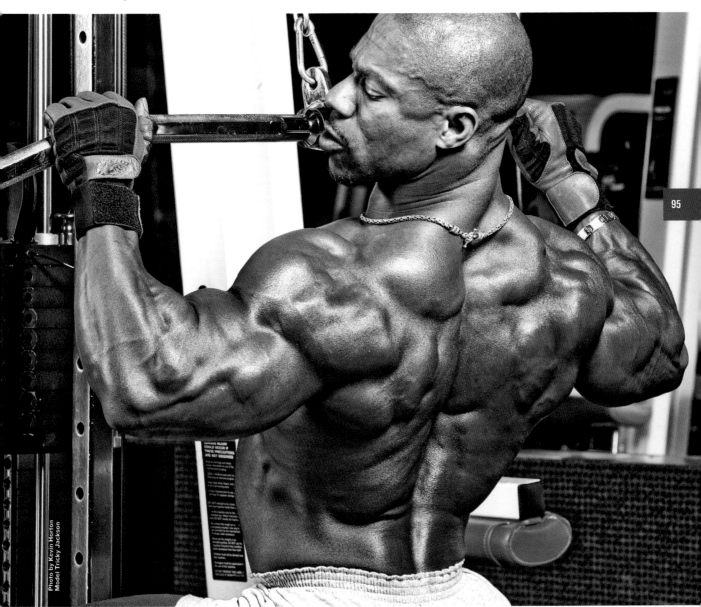

Photo by Kevin Horton
Model Tricky Jackson

95

RULE #3
Arrange to have ongoing medical supervision, if possible.

Despite the claims of some lawmakers and anti-steroid groups, moderate steroid use by healthy individuals is relatively safe. We use the term "relatively" because no one can predict how he or she will react to a given drug before actually taking it. Individual responses will vary, so if at all possible, try to plan ahead for a physician to monitor your use. Given the status of the medical system these days, you might have to exhaust quite a few resources and spend some time searching for a doctor, as most are hesitant about or outright avoid any involvement with steroids. The political climate is anti-steroid and doctors fear misinterpretation of prescribing steroids for non-medical use, as it could be devastating to their medical careers. There are some progressive doctors out there, however, so you're wise to put in the effort to find one. Getting periodic blood tests is another excellent way to see and track how your body is reacting to the drugs.

BELOW: The likelihood that side effects will occur is directly related to the amount ingested.

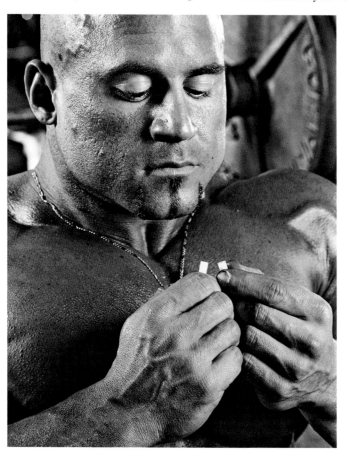

RULE #4
Limit your cycles to six to eight weeks at the maximum.

This rule may go against the norm, but shorter, more frequent cycles are more effective and certainly safer than going on the gear for years at a time. For one, the body's receptors tend to become desensitized with long-term use. Therefore, after a period of time you'll need to use higher dosages just to achieve the same effects. Longer cycles are also harder to come off of. Your body's endocrine system takes weeks if not months to normalize itself after an extended steroid cycle. You may even need drug therapy to kick-start the regulating process. After a short cycle though, your bodily systems will probably only need a few weeks to readjust to pre-steroid function and levels. The gains you make on short cycles also tend to be more permanent and easier to retain and maintain. Finally, as you might expect, the risk of side effects correlates with the length of duration. The vast majority of individuals who experience adverse side effects are those who stay on the drugs month after month, year after year.

Photo by Ralph DeHaan
Model Mike Morris

RULE #5
Take as small a dose as possible.

Given the amounts some of today's pros are using, you'd be shocked by the dosages most champions from the '60s and early '70s used. A typical cycle involved taking three or four Dianabol tablets per day (and this was mainly during the pre-contest season to hold muscle mass while preparing for a show). Consequently, these bodybuilders didn't experience the distended bellies, acne and bitch tits that we so often see displayed onstage at today's contests. The bodybuilders from earlier decades used the drugs to supplement their sound training and nutritional practices – they didn't rely on the drugs to do all the work. The potential for and severity of side effects is also closely related to dosages – more drugs equal greater risks.

RULE #6
Avoid 17-alpha-alkylated steroids.

Of the two primary forms of steroids – injectable and oral – those taken via injection tend to be safer. Most oral steroids have been chemically altered to ensure survival while passing through the digestive system. Unfortunately, it's this chemical modification that places additional stress on the liver, making this kind more detrimental to the health of your body. While certain oral steroids are harsher than others (e.g., Dianabol and Anadrol-50 are more potent than Winstrol and Anavar), all forms ingested orally will increase your LDL (bad) cholesterol and lower your HDL (good) cholesterol. If you decide to use orals, make sure your cycle is limited to no more than four to six weeks. Injectables are a better option whenever possible.

RULE #7
Quit using when your gains stop.

The human body is a complex system and will eventually build tolerance to steroids. The 250-milligram injection that initially worked will at some point need to be increased to 500 milligrams, just to maintain the same gains. Before long you'll again have to up your dosage to 1,000 milligrams or more. And even then your body may max out. When your gains come to a halt, it's time to cut your losses and come off the juice. Accept that you've gained more muscle than you could have naturally, and start cleaning up your system. Subjecting your body (and wallet!) to ever-increasing dosages in an effort to gain some additional pounds of muscle mass is simply not worth it: At the very least you'll be out the cash. Your luck may run out and you could get arrested. Or the outcome may impact your health: Your heart or liver may wear down to the point at which they

> "When your gains come to a halt, it's time to cut your losses and come off the juice. Subjecting your body to ever-increasing dosages is simply not worth it: At the very least you'll be out the cash. Your luck may run out and you could get arrested. Or the outcome may impact your health."

97

are no longer able to function properly. Continuing use may damage your health permanently and you may never again lead a normal lifestyle. Kidney dialysis at age 25 is not a pleasant experience.

RULE #8
Buy your products from a reliable source.
Admittedly, purchasing steroids from a reputable source is easier said than done. The reclassification of the drugs in the early '90s made obtaining real steroids a more complicated and difficult process. You definitely do not want to trust just any gym rat who offers to sell you some. The reality of the situation is that gym rats do sell real gear. Many also sell garbage that should under no circumstance be injected into your body. And the rule of Caveat Emptor applies here: There have been instances where "gym rats" were actually undercover FDA agents. We mentioned Bubba earlier – you likely still don't want to share a prison cell with him. If you have any doubt whatsoever as to the safety or legitimacy of a certain source, you're best advised to avoid it and move on.

RULE #9
Learn and get information
from reliable individuals.
Every gym has their "Danny Deltoids" and "Bobby Biceps." These are the guys whose lives revolve around the gym. They have few other interests in life, and their entire social networks are over at the squat rack. While the serious lifters are in and out of the gym in less than an hour, these guys hang around performing 20-plus sets of bench presses. Although these individuals spend quite a bit of time in the gym, most aren't very knowledgeable on the topic of steroids. As such, they're probably the last people you should be seeking advice from about using the drugs. Far better sources are available to consult. Veteran competitive bodybuilders are one suggestion. Obviously you'll need to be tactful in your approach, as you don't want to imply you think the guy is a juicehead. You also don't want to be too inquisitive and give the bodybuilder the impression you're an undercover FDA agent. Diplomatically introduce yourself and state your case (preferably out of earshot from other gym members). If you handle the situation with proper discretion, odds are he'll help you out. Other potential sources for information include doctors, nurses or other health practitioners, and print resources such as books and magazines. The Internet can also be a valuable tool for learning, but use caution when searching on Web sites. Anyone can set up a home page and there is a large amount of misinformation online. So if you're surfing the Web to find out about steroids, be aware that what sounds factual may not be backed by in-depth research or conclusive evidence.

"Pay attention to your body's signals. If your car was making an unusual noise, you wouldn't keep driving it until the noise got unbearable or a part fell off – you'd get your car checked. The same applies to steroids."

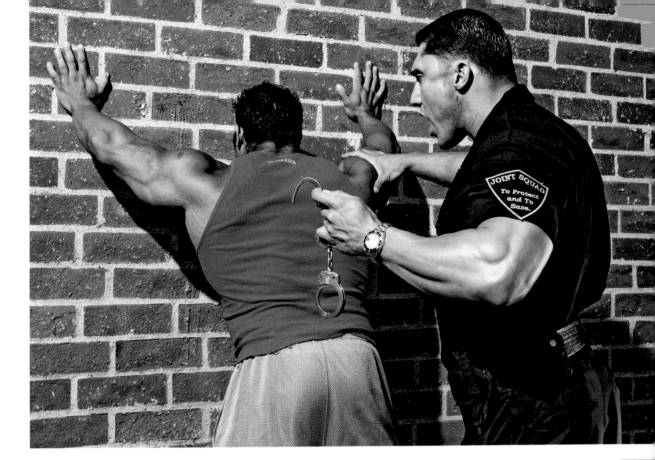

RULE #10
Do not share needles under any circumstances.

While this rule is a matter of using common sense, needle sharing does still happen. You may think you know your training partner or friend – but do you really? His blood carries a record of any disease he's ever had. It also contains traces of all his one-night stands and previous sexual partners. No matter how clean you think a needle is, the device is still capable of transmitting such lethal diseases as AIDS and hepatitis. Needles are very inexpensive to buy; if you don't feel comfortable getting them at the drugstore, simply go online and order them.

RULE #11
Stop your cycle at the first sign of trouble.

If your system isn't tolerating the steroids well, your body will almost definitely give you plenty of warning that something's awry. Pay attention to your body's signals. If your car was making an unusual noise, you wouldn't keep driving until the noise got unbearable or a part fell off – you'd get your car checked. The same applies to steroid use. If you start experiencing chest pain, or any other sign of discomfort, immediately go to your doctor or the emergency room depending on the severity of the pain. Likewise, any strange lumps need to be checked by a physician. Even a small, benign lump can grow to be a large, cancerous mass over a short amount of time. No trophy, whether from a local show or the Mr. O, is worth risking your life over.

ABOVE: When it comes to the market, it's imperative to buy from reputable sources. Trusting just anyone could get you into serious legal trouble.

Photo by Robert Reiff
Models David Hughes and Sam Sacker

● **ANABOLIC PRIMER** ●

COMING CLEAN

Given the more recent crackdown on steroids by the government and sports organizations, and the risk of potential side effects (often exaggerated but present nonetheless), many users may decide to come off the juice. Another important factor for users considering going clean is the amount of bogus steroids flooding the black market, as those products may be more dangerous than the steroids they're designed to imitate.

No matter what your personal reasons are for stopping, a few points need to be taken into account. As with most drugs, breaking a steroid habit can initiate the onset of certain health problems. One of your first priorities is to seek medical assistance. A physician ideally should have been monitoring your health over the entire course of your cycle, but it's an absolute must when you stop taking the drugs. Seeing a doctor may seem as simple as booking an appointment, but don't be surprised if many physicians turn you away because of the stigma attached to steroid use. Your best bet may be the direct approach – go to his or her office, disclose your situation and show a genuine desire to become steroid-free. Many professionals in the field will appreciate your honesty and honor their Hippocratic Oath.

On a more personal level, your close friends will play a big role when you stop your cycle. However, if this group of friends are themselves users and have no intentions of coming off, you may want to rely on another support system. Withdrawing from any drug is a highly emotional process where the individual requires constant care and consideration from others. Enduring side effects such as mood swings, depression and irritability becomes even more difficult if the closest people to you either show no support or try to talk you out of your decision.

Nutrition is another main area of concern when you cease taking steroids. Most users report that when coming off the gear

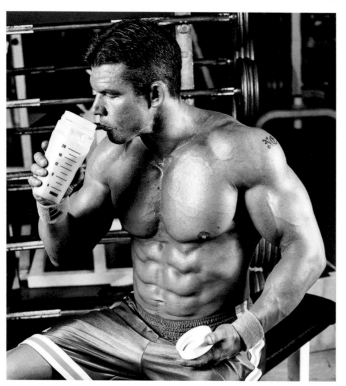

BELOW: Supplements in the form of protein shakes are an ideal solution to keep your calories up to meet nutrient needs when your appetite is lagging.

100

Photo by Ralph DeHaan
Model Dr. Nick Evans

they seem to catch one cold after another. Steroids seem to have a boosting effect on the immune system, but the body appears to become increasingly susceptible to illness after the drugs are stopped. The exact biological reason is unknown, but the immune system enters a state of depression, leaving the individual vulnerable to just about every minor cold, infection or virus that's going around. In addition to maintaining a balanced diet, stepping up your intake of antioxidants and nourishing your body with quality, nutrient-rich foods will help get your system back on track.

Proper nutrition is also critical as a means to help you retain much of the muscle mass and strength you gained while on the cycle. A certain amount of loss is inevitable, but you can hold onto a large percentage through smart training (see "Training – Getting Back In the Groove"), solid eating and additional supplementing. Nutritional supplements are a great way to get in the muscle-building calories without force-feeding yourself. While on the cycle your appetite was probably through the roof; once you come off, however, just trying to eat three square meals a day may be challenging. A helpful solution is to consume one or two daily protein drinks, as they're easy to get down and will ensure your calorie intake stays up. Don't forget the importance of vitamins and minerals either – they'll assist in normalizing your bodily systems and will provide a much needed boost to your steroid-abused endocrine system.

STEP BY STEP

The length of time required to fully recover from steroid use depends on a number of factors: the amount of drugs used, the duration of the cycle, how the drugs were stopped (cold turkey or with gradual tapering) and whether any post-therapy testosterone boosters were taken. While definite variation exists from individual to individual, there are three distinct phases associated with cessation of steroid use.

Phase I

Phase I is the easiest to endure but hardest to initiate. After months if not years of popping pills and injecting needles, the user decides to quit. For someone who has never engaged in the practice, this resolution may not seem like a big deal, but for the steroid user the choice is monumental. For some, the decision is nothing short of traumatic. And while there are good reasons for quitting the juice cold turkey (legal issues likely being the most pressing), a gradual tapering off will make for an easier recovery period.

Many individuals find the first couple of weeks off the juice to be the least difficult of the process. The reason is that most of the anabolic and anti-catabolic effects are still in the system, despite no new drug being added. This will be especially true if the individual was

"Steroids certainly increase muscle size, strength and even endurance. Anyone who denies this statement is not dealing with reality. The problem is that the user's innate resources cannot maintain the strength and size increases. The steroid user is thus faced with the constant need to go on the sauce in order to maintain the gains he made on steroids. The end result is a constant on/off series of cycles that systematically increase the risk of chronic-induced damage. Granted one does not lose all gains during off-the-sauce periods, but the loss is often so extreme that it becomes a psychological burden."

– Dr. George H. Elder, *MuscleMag International* contributor using long-lasting injectable steroids. It usually takes four to six weeks for the effects of the drugs to start wearing off – when they eventually do though, you'll be acutely aware of it. For starters, you won't be able to train like an animal for two or three hours at a time. Even if you could force your body through such a training marathon, you'll be extremely stiff and sore for a week, whereas steroids would have you ready for action in 24 to 48 hours. You'll also notice your appetite taking a nosedive. You're not building the same degree of muscle any longer (you'll in fact lose some) so the body doesn't need the same amount of calories to sustain itself.

Another obvious side effect will be a decreased sex drive. Most users report a high sex drive while on a cycle, but the exact opposite when they go off steroids. The absence of the drugs in your system, plus your depressed testosterone levels could leave you about as randy as a castrated 16th-century monk.

Finally, you'll have to expect a certain amount of weight loss to occur. There is no way to predict how much weight you'll drop after going off the drugs – some guys get lucky and retain just about all of their steroid-induced muscle mass while others lose virtually every ounce. Most individuals fall somewhere in between, losing an average of 10 to 15 pounds. Of course, the degree of weight loss is also relative to how big the individual was to begin with. A 250-pounder could lose 25 to 30 pounds while a 180-pounder might only lose 10 to 12. With regards to a time frame for this stage, you can generally expect to remain in Phase I for approximately 10 to 12 weeks.

No doubt many readers found the realities of Phase I depressing and disappointing. We hate to break it to you, but entering Phase II is no walk in the park – the challenges do get worse as your body re-adapts and recovers.

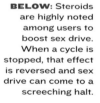

BELOW: Steroids are highly noted among users to boost sex drive. When a cycle is stopped, that effect is reversed and sex drive can come to a screeching halt.

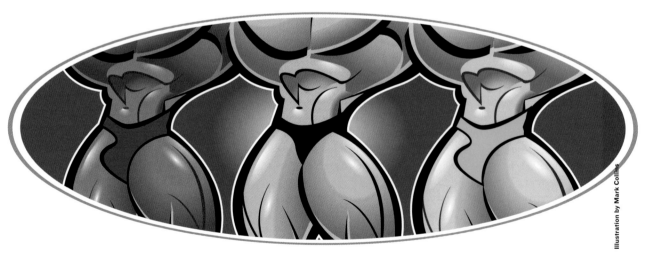

Illustration by Mark Collins

Phase II

About 12 weeks after taking their last dosage of steroids, most individuals can expect to enter Phase II of the recovery process. This stage involves hitting rock bottom, but after overcoming this lowest of lows, the battle is all uphill from here (though it's definitely a slow climb!).

If users found the weight decreases in Phase I difficult to endure, Phase II could very well be psychologically devastating. The specific amount varies, but further drops of 30 to 40 pounds can occur during Phase II as the steroids are virtually eliminated from the individual's system. All those months or years of heavy usage also will have likely depressed their natural testosterone levels to near zero.

Yet another challenging aspect of Phase II is strength loss. Much like weight loss, the degree of strength decrease is dependent upon a number of factors, but many individuals revert back to their pre-steroid levels.

Other noticeable changes that occur during this period are increased frequency of colds and infection, extreme sluggishness during and after working out, and an overall lack of desire to train.

This part of Phase II is probably the most crucial point of the entire recovery process: an individual can choose to take one of three roads. Many give up training altogether, as they can't come to terms with using lighter weight and can't shrug off the repeated comments from gym members about how "small" they're getting. Running into ex-bodybuilders years later who have given up training completely is not uncommon. After establishing themselves as one of the alpha males at the gym, they just can't handle being just another average gym member. The matter isn't helped by the fact that an entirely new generation of steroid users serve as a constant reminder of how far the previous user has "fallen." Discouraged and deflated, rather than focusing on building a great-looking and healthy body naturally, these guys avoid the gym scene entirely.

Photo by Irvin Gelb
Model Silvio Samuel

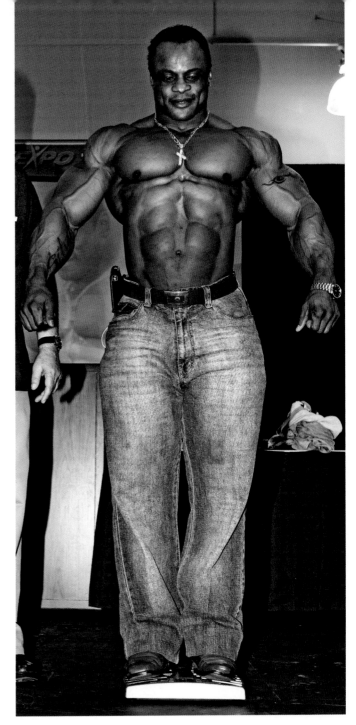

ABOVE: Once steroids clear the body, weight loss typically ensues. Initial drops of 10 to 15 pounds are average, and many guys see the scale plummet another 30 to 40 pounds during Phase II.

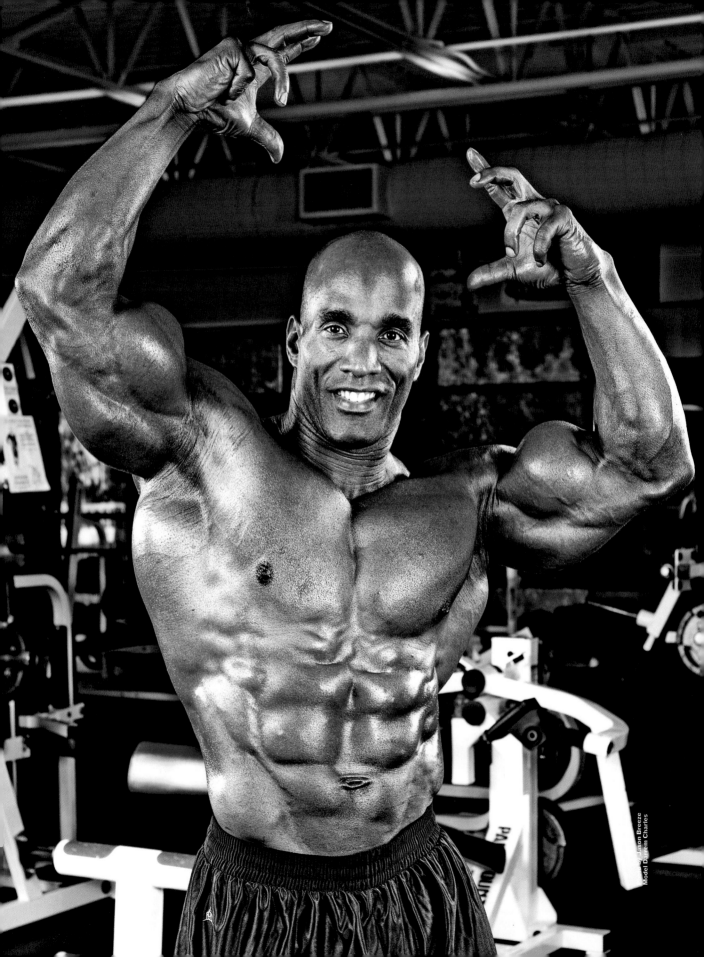

At the other extreme are those who just can't tolerate the physical and psychological changes, and react by going back on the juice. The unfortunate part of this decision is that if they had only waited another few weeks, they would have "bottomed out" and then again started to make some decent progress in terms of strength and size gains. By restarting steroids at this stage, however, these individuals are more likely to continue using over the long-term. Because their first attempt to get off the gear was unsuccessful, many users get deterred and see no point in making another effort to stop. As such, the addiction only gets stronger and the risks of serious side effects only increase as more time passes.

The third option, of course, is pressing onward toward becoming completely clean. Individuals who take this path will still have many challenges ahead, but working through the psychological and physical effects associated with Phase II is absolutely necessary to achieve full recovery.

Phase III

If you've managed to endure the adversities of both Phase I and II without throwing in the towel and going back on the juice, congratulations! You can now start pulling yourself out of the steroid-free rut. One positive aspect of Phase III is that this stage marks an upward turn on your road to recovery. Once your testosterone production kicks back in, you may find your levels will actually rise to a point higher than what they were pre-steroids. The process by which this occurs is called overcompensation. After years of making little or no testosterone, your body may start manufacturing as much as possible in a short time period. You can take advantage of this and gain back much of your lost muscle mass. Keep in mind though, at a certain point your testosterone levels will start to normalize and you'll have to adjust your workouts accordingly (see "Training – Getting Back In the Groove").

The specific time frames of these stages vary from person to person, but most individuals can expect to go through all three phases over the course of approximately six to eight months. Remember, the entire process is essentially a form of endocrine shock, so constant and close monitoring by a physician is highly recommended.

POST-STEROID DRUG THERAPY

Including a section on drug usage right after one on drug withdrawal may seem a bit unusual, but for many who've gone clean, some form of drug therapy is necessary once the body is without steroids. By now you should realize that tampering with your body's endocrine system is like risking it all in a high-stakes poker game. Many users can abuse the drugs to the max and suffer no ill effects. Others just dabble in

> "Phase II marks the most crucial point of the entire recovery process. Many give up training altogether, as they can't come to terms with using lighter weight and can't shrug off repeated comments from gym members about how 'small' they're getting. Running into ex-bodybuilders years later who have given up training completely is not uncommon. After establishing themselves as alpha males at the gym, they just can't handle being just another average gym member."

105

steroids and end up needing medical intervention. You can thank or curse your ancestors all you want, but there's no changing the cards you were dealt in the genetics department.

The primary drug used by bodybuilders after their steroid cycle is human chorionic gonadotropin (hCG). An entire chapter later in the book is devoted to hCG, so here we'll only give you the basics. This hormone is produced by the embryo in the placentas of pregnant women, and when injected into males, hCG acts like LH – leuteinizing hormone. Remember, LH is released by the anterior pituitary gland and stimulates the testes to increase testosterone production. Most bodybuilders can probably avoid the need for hCG if they gradually taper off their steroid usage rather than quit cold turkey. But for those who need to terminate their steroid usage quickly or are just genetically unlucky, short-term therapy with hCG may be required to kick-start the testes.

The other main post-steroid drug is Nolvadex. The name Nolvadex is the trade term for an anti-estrogen drug called tamoxifen citrate. Since estrogen production can sometimes accompany steroid use and post-use, many bodybuilders include an anti-estrogen drug to combat the effects of the female hormone. A lot of bodybuilders actually take the compound during their steroid cycle, but others only start using it in the last weeks of the cycle or just shortly thereafter. As with hCG, genetics often dictate whether the individual will need to add estrogen to their post-steroid treatment.

TRAINING – GETTING BACK IN THE GROOVE

After you work through the six to eight months of coming off steroids, you'll likely be ready to resume training. Take pride in the fact that the gains you'll make from here on will be natural and permanent. The first thing you need to realize, however, is that you won't be able train with the same intensity and duration as your "gear" days. Forget the two-hour sessions and six-day splits – that level is simply unattainable naturally. Ideally you should start off by performing a full-body workout two to three times per week. As basic as this may sound, this degree of training is all your body can handle at this point. And more importantly, this regimen is all you'll need. After being without regular workouts for so long, your body will be begging for any type of stimulation. You'll be surprised at just how little it needs to start growing again. After a few weeks using the full-body approach, you can consider switching to a split routine.

Your strength levels are another key factor to consider. Don't expect to pick up where you left off with three or four 45-pound plates on the bar. Not only are your post-steroid muscles incapable of lifting such heavy weight, but your recovery system will also be

"At the other extreme are those who just can't tolerate the physical and psychological changes, and react by going back on the juice. The unfortunate part of this decision is that if they had only waited another few weeks, they would have 'bottomed out' and then again started to make some decent progress in terms of strength and size."

106

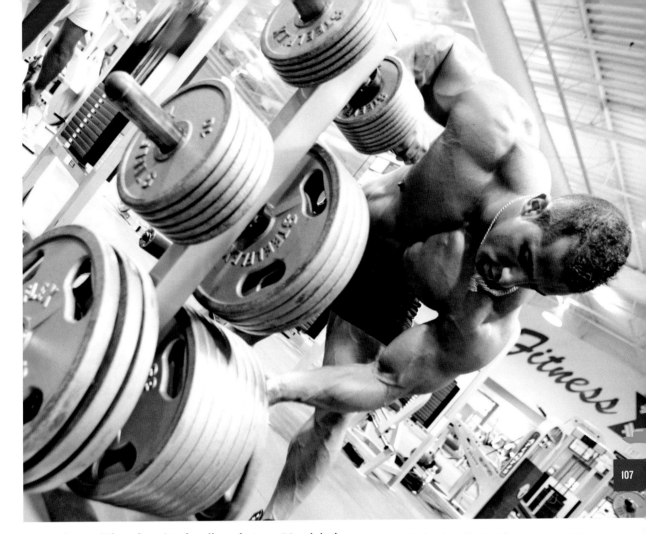

Photo by Paul Buceta
Model Fouad Abiad

extremely taxed if you force it to handle such stress. Most injuries after a layoff usually occur in the initial few days, and it's often because the individual attempted to hoist the same amount of iron as he would have mid-cycle.

Finally, don't expect the same degree of muscular weight gain as you did while on the juice – it just isn't going to happen. You were probably putting on a couple of pounds per week during your steroid days. Natural training on the other hand is a lesson in patience, and 10 to 12 years is about the norm for achieving your optimal physique. Of course you do have a big advantage over those new to training: You have what's called muscle memory working for you. Once a muscle reaches a certain size, your body somehow "files" the blueprints away for future reference. Regaining that lost muscle mass tends to be much easier than building it the first time around. Now, your odds for reaching the same size and strength as your steroid days are slim, but you'll likely be bigger and stronger than if you'd never taken steroids at all. And another benefit is that you'll be healthier – you'll have little reason to worry about elevated cholesterol, high blood pressure, acne and other problems associated with taking the drugs. (You won't run the risk of being the subject of a police sting either!) With time, patience and a commitment to consistency, you'll build a great-looking physique that will no doubt be the envy of others.

ABOVE: Coming off steroids means accepting that some of those weight plates will have to be unloaded – you simply won't be able to lift the same poundage as you did while on a cycle.

● ANABOLIC PRIMER ●

ESTROGENS, ANTI-ESTROGENS AND RELATED COMPOUNDS

Most individuals naturally tend to associate anabolic steroids with the male hormone testosterone. Despite the fact that estrogen is a female hormone, however, some evidence does suggest it may be a factor in promoting strength and size gains. Farmers have been aware of this for decades and routinely inject their livestock with estrogen as a means to significantly increase the muscular bodyweight of the animals.

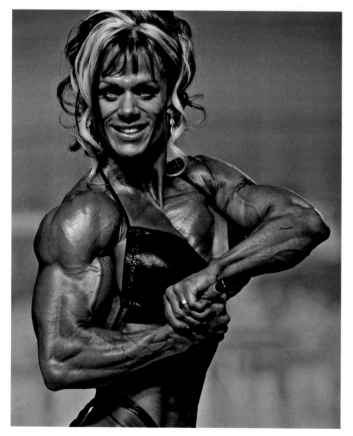

BELOW: Even though estrogen is labeled the "female" hormone, research indicates it may facilitate gains in strength and size.

With regards to anti-estrogens, bodybuilders frequently turn to these compounds both during and after their steroid cycles. The strategy behind taking anti-estrogens is to combat feminizing effects of excess estrogen produced from steroid metabolism.

ESTROGEN

The important roles hormones play within the human body cannot be underestimated. Estrogen is essentially considered the female equivalent of the male hormone testosterone. Keep in mind, however, that males and females each contain concentrations of both hormones – "male" and "female" are simply relative terms in this regard. The vast differences in actual hormone levels between the sexes are what have led testosterone and estrogen to become labeled as male and female, respectively.

The female ovaries secrete estrogen, which functions to regulate the female reproductive cycle and develop and maintain the secondary sex characteristics. The hormone also contributes to ensuring proper health and function of the liver, bones, arteries and skin.

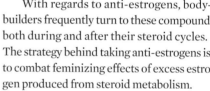

Photo by Gordon Smith
Model Cathy LeFrancois

ESTROGEN BLOCKING

The phrase "estrogen blocking" is fairly commonplace these days among bodybuilders and others in the athletic world. Generally speaking there are two ways to affect estrogen within the body: block the receptor site or interfere with the enzyme that converts testosterone into estrogen. When a molecule fits into the receptor but does not send out an estrogen signal, it's termed an antagonist. At the same time the molecule blocks naturally occurring estrogen and prevents it from binding and exerting its physiological effects. Such compounds are usually referred to as estrogen blockers. Conversely if a compound binds to a receptor and produces the same effect as the natural compound (i.e., acts like estrogen) the term agonist applies. At the most basic level, antagonists acts like an off switch while agonists function as an on switch.

ESTROGEN – BODYBUILDING APPLICATIONS

It was originally thought that muscle tissue was estrogen insensitive. But animal studies, particularly involving beef cattle, have proven otherwise. This research has demonstrated that estrogenic compounds can have anabolic effects, which are believed to be caused by the indirect action of estrogen on the pituitary. The presence of estrogen causes the gland to release bovine growth hormone and has a direct effect by stimulating skeletal muscle receptors. Evidence also indicates that estrogen can induce the growth of testosterone receptors. This would cause an increase in anabolic reactions without raising testosterone levels. Skeletal muscle in beef cattle is known to contain both androgen and estrogen receptors. Since only androgens appear to exert a direct growth effect on receptor sites, the combined injection of both estrogenic and androgenic drugs would explain the additive growth observed in these animals.

Despite the fact this research is limited to animal studies, a few bodybuilders consider it reason enough to try estrogen-containing compounds to increase muscle size and strength. While the anecdotal evidence is promising, keep in mind that no such investigations involving estrogen use to increase muscle mass have been conducted on human males, largely because of the ethics involved and the reluctance of most males to administer female hormones into their bodies. Those bodybuilders who have dabbled in estrogen use likely took either birth control pills or RU-486, which are two of the more popular estrogen-based compounds.

BIRTH CONTROL PILLS

While the presence of estrogen is usually viewed as problematic because of its gender-related actions (water retention, increased fat storage, gynecomastia), the right ratio of testosterone (or anabolic

"You'd be hard pressed to find a picture taken before 1975 in which anyone showed signs of gynecomastia, yet nowadays it's as common as fake boobs on a Hollywood starlet. What's even more intriguing is that back in the '60s and '70s, no one used anti-estrogens. That's because they weren't invented. Today anti-estrogens are considered a must as prevention against estrogenic side effects for anyone who uses anabolic steroids. Still, time and time again you'll see bad cases of gyno."

– Nelson Montana, *MuscleMag International* contributor

steroids) to estrogen may in fact promote greater muscle growth. While this medication's intended use is to prevent pregnancy, female bodybuilders often take birth control pills to time their menstrual periods. At a physiological level, there is some evidence that birth control pills may increase amino acid utilization. Although the exact biochemical mechanism is not known, it is believed that birth control pills may boost the ability of vitamin B-6 to moderate amino acid metabolism (vitamin B-6 functions as a coenzyme in the metabolism of most amino acids).

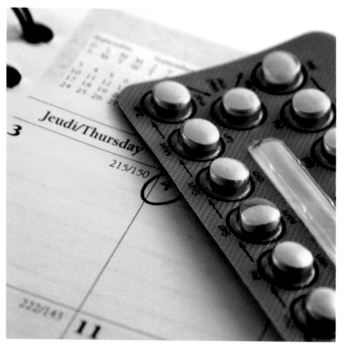

ABOVE: Birth control pills are primarily a contraceptive medication, but they may also boost amino acid utilization in the body.

RU-486

RU-486 is a European-designed compound that gained notoriety in the late 1980s as the "abortion" pill. It prevents (and can terminate) pregnancy by generating massive hormonal fluctuations in the female body that cause any developing embryo to abort. The moral implications of this have been the topic of much debate, and we'll leave that discussion for others to tackle. Our purposes are more focused on the physiological effects, as there have been reports of bodybuilders using RU-486 to promote muscle gains. Certain research has cited that the compound itself has anti-catabolic properties and protects muscle tissue from the negative effects of cortisol. On a basic level, this information sounds favorable, but other research has indicated the pill may decrease the sensitivity of testosterone receptors. So while the pill may be anti-catabolic, it's also potentially anti-anabolic. Reports from European bodybuilders (the drug is widely available in Europe) seem to confirm the findings, as most users noted little to no benefits from taking RU-486. Indeed the drug doesn't seem to have any detrimental health effects, but it doesn't seem to offer any performance-enhancing benefits either.

SIDE EFFECTS

Plain and simple, manipulating hormone levels has its consequences – if Mother Nature or the evolutionary process had meant for males to have high levels of estrogen, their bodies would have come equipped with ovaries! The simple fact that even small amounts can cause gynecomastia, or that transsexuals take estrogen as part of their sex-change therapy should be a clear indication of the potential outcomes associated with using estrogen compounds. Considering there is very limited conclusive proof of estrogen as an inducer of testosterone receptors, and despite the fact that estrogen-fed cattle do increase their muscular bodyweight, you're advised not to use estrogen for athletic purposes. The benefits are just not definite enough to justify the risks.

ANTI-ESTROGENS

While estrogen use is relatively rare in the sport, virtually all competitive bodybuilders have taken anti-estrogen drugs at some point during their cycles. If excessive estrogen is present in an individual's system (or the person just happens to be extremely sensitive to even small amounts of the hormone), numerous unpleasant side effects may develop. The most well-known and unsightly condition is gynecomastia – the swelling and feminizing of the breast region in males. Many bodybuilders add anti-estrogen drugs and supplements to their stacks as a means to proactively counter the condition either by decreasing the production of estrogen or blocking its effects. What follows is a brief description of some of the more common compounds used by bodybuilders to combat high estrogen levels.

NOLVADEX (TAMOXIFEN CITRATE)

Even though it's not classified as an anabolic steroid, few stacks these days are missing the drug Nolvadex. Many bodybuilders incorporate this compound in their pre- and post-steroid stacks believing its anti-estrogen properties will prevent the feminizing effects brought on by the aromatization of testosterone. This drug is also commonly used as a method to treat already existing conditions including gynecomastia. Nolvadex's primary mechanism of action is to compete with estrogen at the receptor sites, thus minimizing the hormone's gender-specific effects.

Unfortunately, Nolvadex isn't risk-free – it can produce adverse results opposite to what are desired. The drug's effects can be somewhat like a Catch 22: use may be counterproductive because the compound interferes with even small amounts of estrogen that may increase the effectiveness of testosterone. Other research, however, has suggested that estrogen may inhibit the enzymes necessary for testosterone production. Bodybuilders who use the compound during a cycle also need to account for the dreaded "rebound" effect. Like most hormone-based drugs, Nolvadex may cause an influx of estrogen when the user comes off the drug. Sky-high levels of the female hormone result, making the body susceptible to enormous water retention and the user at risk of looking like a water-soaked sponge on contest day.

A little-known aspect of Nolvadex is its interaction with growth hormone. The research findings on the relationship of the two are mixed. One particular study found that Nolvadex could block the

"Like most hormone-based drugs, Nolvadex may cause an influx of estrogen when the user comes off the drug. Sky-high levels of the female hormone result, making the body susceptible to enormous water retention and the user at risk of looking like a water-soaked sponge on contest day."

111

"What makes Teslac especially interesting is that it may also be anabolic in nature. Its anabolic potential is twofold: Teslac can boost testosterone production and increase mineral conservation."

GH increases produced by testosterone enanthate. Another study reported just the opposite: GH levels increased after enanthate and Nolvadex administration. These inconsistencies mean bodybuilders stacking Nolvadex to block estrogen effects and increase GH levels may actually be promoting just the opposite. And let's not forget that GH also has numerous interactions with insulin.

The primary sources for obtaining Nolvadex are by prescription and from the black market. While it was at one time a viable option to get this compound legitimately from a physician, the process is no longer so cut and dry. Use of Nolvadex is widely considered non-medical in nature, so most doctors will not hand out prescriptions for the drug very readily. Granted gynecomastia should be considered a valid reason, but many doctors counter that it didn't develop under "legitimate" or "normal" circumstances. Since professionals in the medical field relate the condition to steroid use, they are opposed to "abetting" an illegal drug user by writing a prescription. This state of affairs forces the hands of bodybuilders and others seeking the drug, and they are left no other option than to turn to the black market. Here again the anti-steroid movement has not improved the situation, but rather made it more dangerous.

TESLAC

Teslac is a byproduct that results from the metabolism of the female hormone progesterone. It functions by combining with cytochrome P450 to block the aromatase enzyme actions at receptor sites (aromatase is the primary enzyme responsible for converting testosterone into estrogen). What makes Teslac especially interesting is that it may also be anabolic in nature. Its anabolic potential is twofold: Teslac can boost testosterone production and increase mineral conservation. Teslac boosts testosterone by raising production of gonadotropin-releasing hormone (GnRH) in the hypothalamus gland. GnRH is secreted when hormone levels, particularly estrogen, fall. But since it also stimulates the testes to promote testosterone production, many bodybuilders consider Teslac a good option to try in their stacks.

The effects of Teslac on mineral conservation are more basic at the physiological level. By increasing retention of such minerals as potassium, nitrogen and phosphorous, the body remains in a more stable environment for protein synthesis. The outcome is thus a moderate anabolic effect. We draw the line at using the term "moderate" because Teslac is in no way comparable to steroids when it comes to promoting gains in muscle size and strength.

The FDA considers Teslac an anabolic steroid (even though chemically it's not), and as such the drug falls under the Draconian Schedule III status of illegal. Trafficking and/or possession could get you hard prison time.

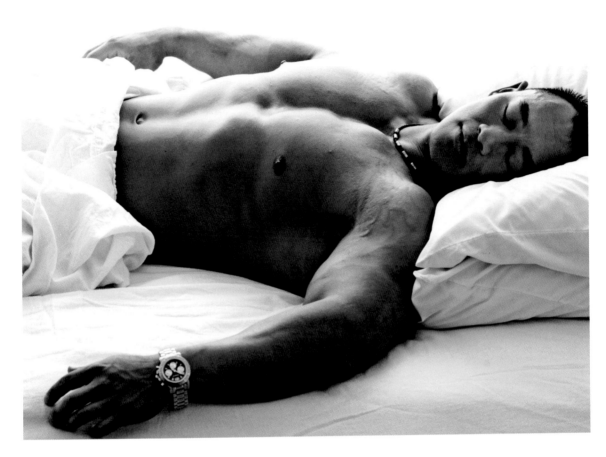

113

CYTADREN

Cytadren (the trade name used for aminoglutethimide) is a prescription drug primarily used to treat Cushing's syndrome, which is an endocrine disorder characterized by increased levels of cortisol in the bloodstream. Cytadren's main function is to block the various enzymes that convert cholesterol into pregnenolone, aldosterone, cortisol and estrogen hormones. The generally recommended dosages for treating Cushing's syndrome and related diseases is in the single-gram range, however, amounts as low as 250 milligrams have proven effective in controlling steroid-induced aromatization. If an individual is unable to get a prescription for whatever reason, Cytadren can be bought on the black market for relatively cheap (about $40 to $50 per bottle). The half-life of this drug is eight hours, so it is better taken in smaller dosages split throughout the day. The most common method is to take half a tablet upon waking, then a quarter tablet both six and 12 hours later. This dosing approach generally keeps levels fairly constant, but allows for a small drop in the few hours before you arise,

ABOVE: Those who take Cytadren often split the dosages, taking the largest amount upon waking, when levels have dipped overnight.

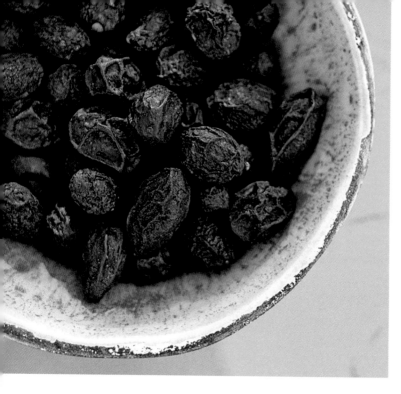

which is why the first dose in the morning is larger. Because this pattern spreads out the drug use, the inhibition of cortisol production is generally too low to be noticed, and the likelihood of a rebound effect on cessation is limited. When stopping, however, it is not a bad idea to taper off, first omitting the midday quarter-tab dose for a few days, then removing both quarter-tab doses, then reducing the morning dose to one quarter tablet, and finally stopping use completely. As for the length of time necessary for the tapering period, a week seems to be sufficient for most users.

ABOVE: Saw palmetto extract has become one of the most popular herbs among bodybuilders who want to stay natural. Though many of its proclaimed side effects aren't founded in solid research, many studies indicate this herb holds potential to fight inflammation.

SAW PALMETTO – IS IT A NATURAL ANTI-ESTROGEN?

Researchers (and many bodybuilders) are constantly looking for natural means to combat the side effects of performance-enhancing drugs. One of the most popular herbal options is saw palmetto. The extract of this plant species is commonly marketed to the general public as a "natural" means to counteract the problems men face as they age. It's been promoted as a cure for everything from hair loss and gynecomastia to prostate enlargement. But while certain studies make saw palmetto sound beneficial, the conclusive medical evidence is limited – especially as it applies to preventing hair loss and combating estrogen. The only area in which there is evidence of the herb's positive effects is prostate enlargement.

MECHANISMS OF ACTION

Saw palmetto is believed to exert its anti-baldness and prostate health benefits by preventing conversion of testosterone to the breakdown metabolite dihydrotestosterone – or DHT. Saw palmetto reportedly blocks the enzyme 5-alpha-reductase (5-ARD) from modifying testosterone into DHT. Unfortunately, the medical evidence isn't strong to back such claims. Most of the hype surrounding its efficacy is related to test-tube studies (called "in vitro") that did show saw palmetto to block 5-ARD in certain cells. However, animal and human studies have failed to prove the same results. These incongruent findings have led researchers to speculate whether it might work via another pathway.

SAW PALMETTO SEESAW

Further research also suggests that instead of blocking DHT conversion, saw palmetto may actually reduce its uptake by various tissues. One study reported that saw palmetto extracts blocked both testosterone and DHT uptake by upward of 40 percent in 11 different tested tissues. When the outcomes from this study began circulating, bodybuilders started tossing their saw palmetto supplements like yesterday's garbage. After all, what aspiring Schwarzenegger would want to inhibit his testosterone potential?

ANTI-INFLAMMATORY PROPERTIES

One of the most interesting areas of research on saw palmetto focuses on its potential to fight inflammation. Many researchers believe this is the only function where saw palmetto holds any merit. A number of studies have documented this herb's ability to block many enzymatic actions that cause the inflammation response, including those affecting the prostate. These findings are significant because many cases of prostate enlargement are not the result of DHT but rather enzyme-induced inflammation.

ANTI-ESTROGEN EFFECTS

Supplement manufacturers, in their quest to attract bodybuilders, try to promote saw palmetto as an anti-estrogen compound. However, buyers beware: while the herb may have some anti-estrogen effects on the prostate, the same effects don't necessarily carry over to other physiological occurrences such as preventing gynecomastia or bodyfat increases. The reason is that many compounds are "double agents" – they can act as agonists in some tissues and antagonists in others. Even anti-estrogen drugs can function in this manner, and a perfect example is the popular drug Tamoxifen. In women, the drug acts as an antagonist in breast tissue but an agonist in uterine tissue. This is why it's used to treat breast cancer, but unfortunately may at the same time increase the risk of uterine cancer. Saw palmetto could be another such example. As of this book's publication date, no credible research (large-sample, long-term, double-blind) has confirmed that saw palmetto can prevent or reduce the effects of increased estrogen in either the breast region or fat deposits.

FINAL THOUGHTS

The relatively cheap cost and lack of associated side effects are two pros that make saw palmetto appealing to bodybuilders. Based on the research, it probably wouldn't be harmful to use this extract if you have a history of prostate enlargement in your family. As for taking it to resist steroid-induced estrogen increases, we recommend you save your money. The evidence just isn't definite enough. The same holds true for the herb's role in preventing hair loss. If you're genetically challenged in the follicle department, saw palmetto probably won't do much to prevent your ensuing cueball look.

"The extract of this plant species is commonly marketed to the general public as a 'natural' means to counteract the problems men face as they age. It's been promoted as a cure for everything from hair loss and gynecomastia to prostate enlargement. But while certain studies make saw palmetto sound beneficial, the conclusive medical evidence is limited."

115

GROWTH HORMONE

For those readers too young to remember the early 1990s, a radical change took place that would forever alter the face of modern bodybuilding. From the late '60s to the early '90s, the biggest bodybuilders were tipping the scales at around 230 to 240 pounds. Sure, you had the occasional freak like Lou Ferrigno or Lee Haney, but for the most part, the largest bodybuilders maxed out at 240 pounds. It was in 1992 and 1993 when the average weight on the pro scene began to creep up. Guys who normally weighed in at 230 were now carrying 260-plus pounds of ultra-prime beef into battle. And it didn't take years for them to pack on the mass either. Many bodybuilders left the stage in late fall of '92 at the lighter weight and turned up for the next spring's shows 25 to 30 pounds heavier.

It wasn't so much the amount of muscular bodyweight that made people start to raise their eyebrows but the speed at which it was being gained. Most individuals achieve about 90 percent of the maximum amount of muscle mass they'll ever carry in the first five years of training. From that point onward it's more a case of shaping and refining. For the average pro bodybuilder who'd trained for 10 years or more, adding 25 or 30 pounds more muscle mass was unheard of – at least until the early 1990s. So what happened? What miraculous new training technique turned the previously "large" 230-pounders into the 270- to 280-pound freaks we see dominating bodybuilding stages these days? Well it wasn't so much a different approach or new piece of equipment that accounted for the unprecedented mass gains; the radical transformations rather, were a product of what was added to the needles.

During the 1950s bodybuilders began adding human growth hormone (HGH or GH) to their stacks when they heard about its powerful fat-burning and muscle-building properties. GH was touted as the almost-perfect anabolic compound – aside from its effects on fat and muscle size, it was also undetectable in a drug test. Even at the print date of this book, GH is still difficult to detect and as such remains a choice compound among athletes in drug-tested sports.

While the media may report otherwise, GH is not so much a drug as it is a naturally occurring hormone. GH was first isolated over 40 years ago and is a polypeptide-based (protein) compound manufactured and secreted by the pituitary gland. For those up to speed on molecular chemistry, GH contains 191 amino acids and

> "Many athletes using low-dose HGH report improved joint function. Of course not injecting into the joint, as most athletes do with HGH, means a greater whole-body effect and a lower concentration at the site of injury. Regardless it still appears to help with joint problems."
>
> – Will Brink, bodybuilding and nutrition writer

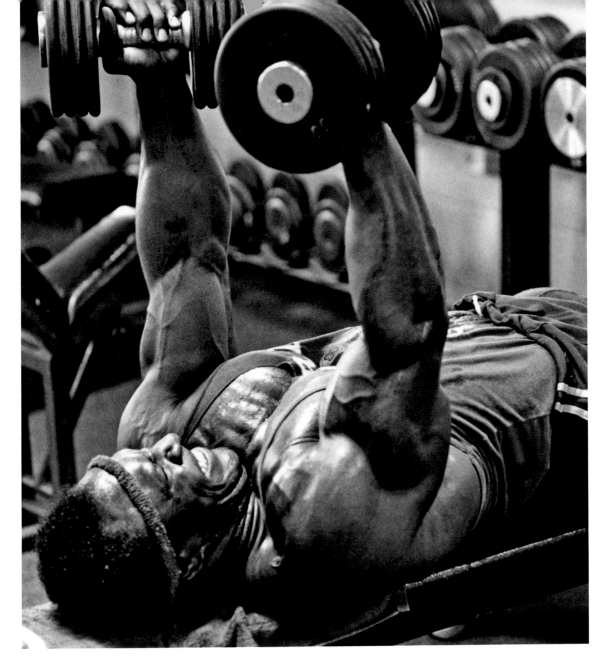

ABOVE: Lee Haney, pictured here, was one of the few mass monsters before his time. It wasn't until the early 1990s when competitors exploded in size.

comprises about 10 percent of the pituitary gland's weight. The average male secretes about 0.5 to 1 milligrams per day, and once in the bloodstream, the hormone has a plasma life of about 60 to 90 minutes. Although this time frame varies, most individuals release the maximum amount of GH during their first 60 to 90 minutes of sleep.

GH is fairly standard in that it's controlled by other hormones: growth hormone-releasing hormone (GHRH) and growth hormone-inhibiting hormone (GHIH), both of which are produced in the hypothalamus. Further to the influence from these two hormones, GH release is also determined by factors such as sleep, certain amino acids, low blood sugar, stress, and of course, exercise – but not just any form of exercise. Research seems to indicate that the greatest concentrations of GH are emitted following periods of short-duration, high-intensity exercise.

"Other variables such as a person's age and amount of bodyfat can also exert an effect on GH release. We know GH release begins to decline in healthy adults between 20 and 30 years of age. Researchers attribute this to aging alone. It is probably the result of a defect in the releasing mechanisms that control GH release from the pituitary gland, rather than a defect in the production or storage of the hormone in the pituitary. Our body still makes GH, but aging impairs our ability to release it into the bloodstream. This is also true for bodyfat as we associate higher levels of obesity with decreased GH release."

– Dr. Douglas M. Crist, expert on aging and growth hormone

MECHANISM OF ACTION

GH is probably the most important hormone for stimulating growth in children. But unlike anabolic steroids in which growth seems to be limited to the muscles, GH exerts its effects on most tissues. Receptors for this hormone have been found in the liver, kidneys, bones and muscles. Of particular interest is the impact of GH on the bones, especially when problems develop early in life. Excessive GH will cause abnormal elongation of the body's long bones, leading to a condition known as gigantism. Individuals affected by this health issue may reach heights of over eight feet; the tallest man ever in medical history was Robert Wadlow of the U.S. who stood at a towering 8'11". Of course, the opposite can occur if insufficient amounts of GH are released during the growth stages. The resulting condition is known as dwarfism and affected individuals may only stand two to three feet in height.

While GH's height-related effects are experienced in the early years, the hormone serves a role throughout life by continually moderating important metabolic processes like fat, protein and carbohydrate metabolism.

Although the exact mechanism of action is not fully understood, GH is believed to increase the transport of amino acids into tissues and also speed up their conversion into protein. Study findings also suggest that GH increases the cellular content of DNA and RNA. In these respects, GH is similar to anabolic steroids as a promoter of anabolic reactions.

GH is also an important contributing factor for fat metabolism. Just as insulin is the primary controller of carbohydrate metabolism, so too does GH have a major effect on fat storage. A number of theories have been put forward to explain the relationship between GH and fat cells, including: 1) GH reduces the rate of new fat storage and synthesis; 2) GH increases the rate of fat mobilization for energy; and, 3) GH increases the release of certain fat-burning hormones such as epinephrine and norepinephrine.

In existing fat tissue GH promotes the breakdown of stored triglycerides, thus increasing fatty acid plasma levels. Furthermore, because GH suppresses glucose uptake, the conversion of glucose into new fat is also inhibited.

The positive effects of GH are not limited to metabolic processes; this hormone also benefits the immune system in various ways. A number of studies have determined a correlation exists between high GH levels and circulating levels of various cancer- and virus-fighting cells. Other tests led researchers to discover that GH injections caused subjects' immune cells (called killer cells) to increase by up to 80 percent. Another notable outcome of these trials was that subjects gained three pounds of muscle tissue and

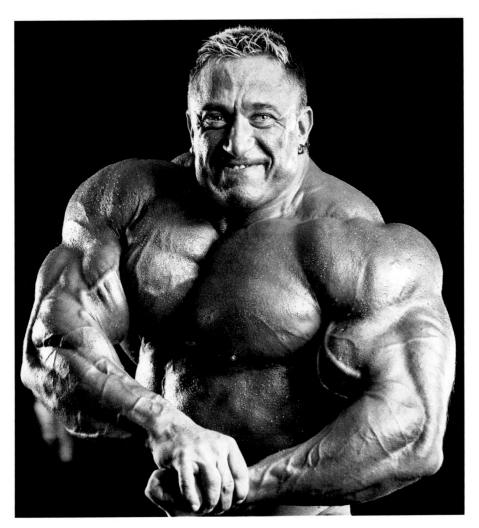

LEFT: The addition of growth hormone to stacks enabled many bodybuilders to pack on mass over very short time frames. More and more competitors were showing up onstage with physiques similar to giant Markus Ruhl.

Photo by Josef Aldt
Model Markus Ruhl

lost an average of five pounds of fat (all without even being on a specific health and training plan!).

The results of such research have led to a specific area of study in which doctors are exploring the effectiveness of GH as a means to combat the AIDS virus and other immunity-weakening diseases. Scientific and medical investigations are also being conducted to examine GH as a potential treatment for multiple sclerosis (MS). The theory is that GH increases production of another hormone called IGF-1 – a peptide growth factor capable of regenerating nerve tissue. MS is characterized by the degeneration of nerve tissue (specifically the outer insulating layer surrounding the nerves); any drug that can increase IGF-1 levels is worth further study to determine its potential value as an MS treatment option.

A TALE OF TWO SOURCES

Aside from physiological effects, GH has followed a similar evolution to anabolic steroids. Just as steroids were born from testosterone, GH was first isolated in natural forms before synthetic versions became available. The first sources were human cadavers (meaning dead people, for those not familiar with the term). The problem, however, was that extraction was very expensive, not to mention dangerous. Despite using the best-possible screening techniques, a number of viral Creutzfeldt-Jakob disease cases were transmitted from the cadavers. In the 1980s though, medical science came to the rescue with synthetic versions of GH based on the latest recombinant DNA techniques. Both Genentech and Eli Lilly manufacture synthetic forms of the drug available under the trade names Protropin and Humatrope. In terms of safety, Humatrope seems to get the nod – Protropin contains an extra amino acid in its molecular nucleus (192 versus 191), and a few individuals reported adverse reactions to the drug.

ABOVE: Cardio is the main approach used to burn bodyfat, but trainers often lose some mass at the same time – GH has been reported as an effective substance to spare muscle tissue while torching fat.

USE IN BODYBUILDING

Unlike the nearly 60-year history of anabolic steroids, GH use is a relatively new phenomenon. No doubt a few bodybuilders with the right contacts and cash dabbled in it during the early 1980s, but it wasn't until synthetic versions came on the scene in the late '80s and early '90s that GH use became widespread.

From interviewing numerous bodybuilders who have used GH, it seems the hormone plays a bigger role in fat loss than in promoting muscle gains. Anecdotal evidence indicates its greatest assets are helping the user hold onto existing muscle tissue and burn bodyfat in preparation for a contest. Despite their best efforts, most bodybuilders do lose some muscle mass during their pre-contest dieting and increased cardio phase. Many report that GH is a huge factor for sparing muscle tissue and burning bodyfat.

Numerous athletes outside the sport of bodybuilding also began using GH during the '90s. The increased sophistication of drug tests combined with steroids being reclassified as controlled drugs left many athletes looking for a legal, undetectable substitute. GH was what they found. Up until a few years ago, no test method could detect it. And currently the only possible way to identify its use is blood tests that can differentiate between natural and synthetic forms. Even these tests, however, are not foolproof. And further to validity, this form of test brings with it both legal and human rights implications – while getting an athlete to pee in a cup for a urine test is one thing, drawing blood opens up an entire Pandora's Box of controversies.

HOW EFFECTIVE?

The efficacy of GH is often questioned, largely because of the drug's short history in sports. While there is general acceptance that steroids produce major gains in muscle size and strength among users, the evidence on GH is still unclear. If we use theory as a model, any drug that speeds up fat metabolism and increases protein synthesis should be a perfect bodybuilding drug. But to date, few scientific studies have been carried out to examine the effectiveness of GH as an athletic drug. And unlike steroids, which boast over 50 years of user reports to back them up, GH use is still in its infancy. This hormone is also very expensive, with cycles costing thousands of dollars. As such, only top-rank athletes and a few "regular" folks can afford to use it. Existing reports are mixed – some users say it makes a huge difference; others claim strength and size gains are actually less than that of some of the better steroids.

One of the best insights regarding its effectiveness comes from bodybuilding expert, acclaimed writer and former *MuscleMag* columnist Dr. Mauro DiPasquale who called GH a "plateau buster." He suggests that GH alone has poor to moderate effects, but when it's used by experienced bodybuilders who have "maxed out" size-wise with steroids, this hormone enables them to easily add another 25 or 30 pounds of muscle mass. Dr. DiPasquale's perspective is seemingly on track – such results were witnessed in the early to mid 1990s when many 230-pounders started showing up onstage weighing 270-plus pounds. You only need to dig out some old back-issues of *MuscleMag International* to figure out who these guys were. Flip through enough copies and you can almost nail down the exact month when a certain pro started adding GH to his stack.

SYNERGISM WITH OTHER DRUGS

The reason behind GH's plateau-breaking effect is unclear, but many experts believe the drug is having some sort of synergistic effect with steroids. By itself GH is only moderately anabolic, but when stacked with steroids (and other drugs such as thyroid and insulin, as is the case nowadays), the results can be nothing short of spectacular.

> "As for the gut, it's generally accepted that high-dose GH over long periods of time causes some organs to grow, creating the beautiful distended 'GH gut' you often see displayed on-stage. However, I am not convinced that's the sole cause of this syndrome."
>
> – Will Brink, bodybuilding and nutrition writer

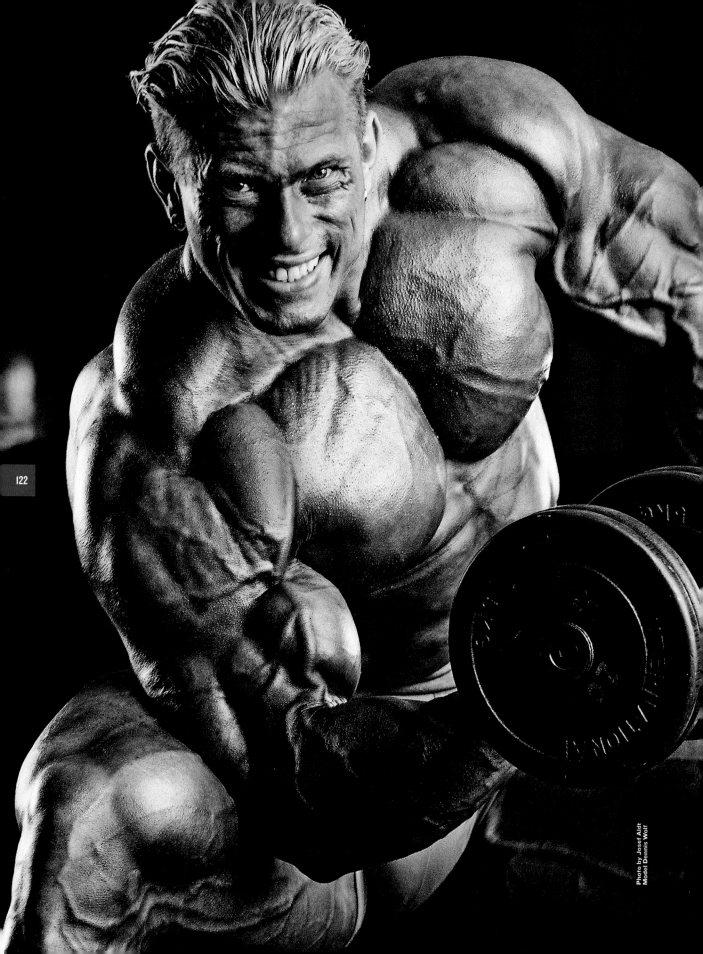

122

Photo by Josef Aldt
Model Dennis Wolf

Although testosterone doesn't seem to increase GH release, certain evidence suggests that GH may in fact increase the sensitivity of cell receptors to testosterone and anabolic steroids. The exact mechanism of action is not known, but one suggestion is that some of the excess testosterone is being converted to estrogen, and believe it or not, the excess estrogen is what increases receptor sensitivity. Another theory is that estrogen may increase GH production. For example, female bodybuilders with low bodyfat percentages tend to have GH levels comparable to their male counterparts. Some experts have posed that minimal bodyfat levels in females cause their bodies to compensate by increasing estrogen production. This in turn causes a ramped up production of GH. The reason that non-bodybuilding females are not as muscular as males is because estrogen also causes water retention and greater production of fat.

Drug interaction is further complicated by the fact that many bodybuilders stack GH with such drugs as insulin, thyroid and numerous other muscle- and fat-burning compounds. Some stacks are a virtual "pharmacopeia" of chemical agents. One reason modern bodybuilders are not only bigger but also much harder than their counterparts of 20 or 30 years ago is the use of fat-burning drugs like Cytomel and Synthroid. Because such practices began for the most part during the '90s, the long-term consequences of stacking all these drugs are still unknown. Some study findings support that excess use of thyroid drugs may blunt the body's ability to use GH. Other research seems to indicate just the opposite – elevated levels of thyroid hormones may increase the body's sensitivity to thyroid. Similar to anabolic steroid research, few controlled studies examining the effects of GH in bodybuilders and other athletes have been carried out. And you likely won't see much published on this hormone given current legislation and the political climate surrounding performance-enhancing drugs.

COSTS

Despite steroids being reclassified as controlled substances, it's still possible for individuals to do a six- to eight-week cycle for less than $500. Not so, however, with GH. Expectations were such that once synthetic versions of it came on the market, the price would drop. But this has not been the case. GH remains one of the most expensive athletic drugs sold on the black market. Although reliable estimates are difficult to confirm, it's guessed that the average pro spends anywhere from $5,000 to $10,000 for one cycle of GH. Even weekend warriors are reported to spend thousands of dollars for a short cycle.

> "Up until a few years ago, no test method could detect GH. And currently the only possible way to identify its use is blood tests. This form of test brings with it both legal and human rights implications – while getting an athlete to pee in a cup for a urine test is one thing, drawing blood opens up an entire Pandora's Box of controversies."

123

124

"In the late 1980s, a potentially dangerous form of GH made its rounds through the gyms of North America. It was advertised as 'Gorilla Juice,' and it is believed the concoction wasn't derived from synthetic sources or even humans, but rather South American rhesus monkeys. The very existence of Gorilla Juice is not in doubt, but exactly what the vials contained has never been proven."

THE GH BLACK MARKET

One of the reasons for the high cost of GH is its limited availability on the black market. There are dozens of legitimate and underground labs producing steroids, but only a couple of GH manufacturers. As with most high-demand items, there is a direct relationship between cost and availability. Another cost-contributing factor is the instability of the GH molecule. Most steroids can easily be stored at room temperature, whereas GH needs to be refrigerated. Extra care goes into the storing and transporting; time and effort is money, hence the higher price.

GH exists in many forms on the black market – this is a point you will likely want to keep in mind if you decide to buy the drug from some gym rat. If he offers to sell you GH for a few hundred dollars and has it stored in his locker or gym bag, odds are you're either getting a complete fake, a bottle labeled GH that actually contains steroids, or worse – improperly stored GH.

In the late 1980s, a potentially dangerous form of GH made its rounds through the gyms of North America. It was advertised as "Gorilla Juice," and it is believed the concoction wasn't derived from synthetic sources or even humans, but rather South American rhesus monkeys. The very existence of Gorilla Juice is not in doubt, but what exactly the vials contained has never been proven. Some have hypothesized that because extracting GH is so difficult – especially from rhesus or any other species of monkeys – odds are that bodybuilders were likely duped into buying one of the cheaper injectable anabolic steroids. As it turns out, bodybuilders may want to thank their lucky stars for being misled, as rhesus monkeys carry some of the most dangerous pathogens fatal to man. Viruses such as AIDS are believed to have originated in rhesus monkeys.

Other compounds, besides monkey GH, are also sold on the black market disguised as GH. Users have reported buying vials that held nothing more than saline (salt) solution and even plain old water. Some cases even exist of real GH being sold, but because of improper storage, the product was virtually useless.

Yet another synthetic version that continues to turn up is cadaver GH. During the 1990s a potent but potentially deadly form of the drug was being produced in the former Soviet Union. Lab tests later determined that much of those samples were contaminated with impurities, thus indicating that less than stellar hygienic precautions were being followed to eliminate viral contamination. So we ask: Do you really want to be injecting this stuff into your ass for the sake of a few more pounds of muscle mass?

There are other bogus forms of GH containing hCG. As noted, hCG is a hormone that stimulates the testes to increase testosterone output. It may give the user a slightly harder, fuller appearance, but hCG will only boost testosterone levels to whatever your body's upper

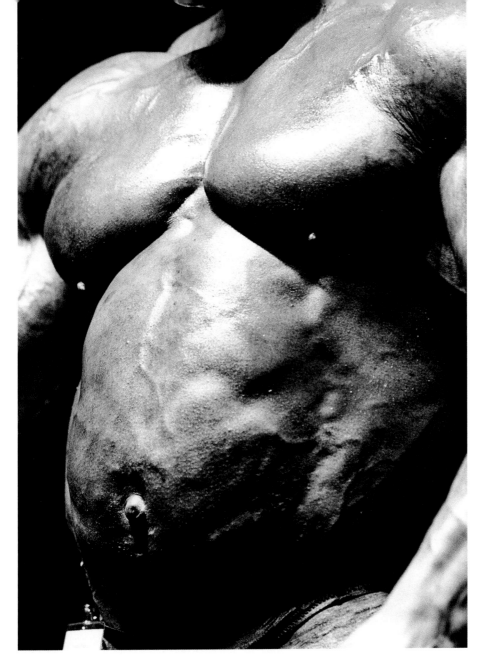

limit happens to be. Further, long-term use can wreak havoc with your body's endocrine system. This hormone should be used for only short periods of time after a steroid cycle, to kick-start the testes to produce testosterone. It should never be used on its own as an anabolic aid.

SIDE EFFECTS

GH use comes with its own set of risks and can produce unwanted side effects. In patients who are deficient to begin with, reports of side effects are rare. This outcome is logical because these patients are being closely monitored by physicians and receiving only replacement dosages of GH (i.e., what their body would normally produce). Bodybuilders and other athletes rarely have such safeguards in place. Many pump in over 20 times the recommended dosage and do so with no medical supervision.

Photo by Irvin Gelb

The most pronounced side effect of GH is a syndrome called acromegaly. The condition is characterized by an enlargement of the bones of the head, feet and hands. The long bones can also become affected sometimes and will take on a thick look. Children being treated with GH therapy rarely experience these problems since their growth plates are still soft and pliable. But once the plates fuse, the bones simply cannot lengthen and thus will thicken outward. Acromegaly sufferers may also exhibit the "Frankenstein" look where their foreheads become more pronounced. If you were to compare photos of the same bodybuilders spanning over a five- or 10-year period, you'll spot those whose experimentation with GH didn't turn out exactly as planned.

Another side effect of GH concerns its impact on many of the body's other hormones. Excessively high levels of GH have been shown to damage the pancreas, which is the body's primary insulin-producing gland. Short-term use may push the body into a coma; long-term consumption can lead to the onset of diabetes. Developing this condition may mean taking oral medication or injectable insulin for the rest of your life.

Furthermore, GH can affect the release of certain stress hormones such as epinephrine and norepinephrine (also known as adrenalin and noreadrenalin). While elevated levels are probably not dangerous for short periods of time, their long-term effects on heart rate and blood pressure could be life threatening.

Another hormone affected by GH is insulin-like growth factor 1 (IGF-1). Research indicates that GH increases production of IGF-1 in the kidneys, liver and other tissues. Here again, short-term elevation is likely tolerable, but the long-term consequences are unknown.

From a superficial and cosmetic perspective, GH can cause skin-related side effects. Acne – especially the large fluid-filled cyst types – is a common outcome of taking the drug. Although not fully understood, the condition is believed to be brought on by GH's increased fat-burning ability. And while this condition is not physically dangerous, it could be psychologically scarring especially for those already suffering from self-esteem issues. Our warning about steroids is herein worth repeating: under no circumstances should teens ever use GH.

One of the most dramatic cosmetic effects of GH is the enlargement of the midsection. The bloated look you see on some pro bodybuilders rivals that of females in their third trimester of pregnancy. While some experts blame the condition on insulin, others argue that GH, unlike steroids (which only increase muscle size) is causing many of the internal organs to swell. Narrowing the culprit, however, is difficult because of the complex drug cocktails used by some bodybuilders.

> "Acromegaly is characterized by an englargement of the bones of the head, feet and hands. Sufferers may also exhibit the 'Frankenstein' look where their foreheads become more pronounced. If you were to compare photos of the same bodybuilders spanning over a five- or 10-year period, you'll spot those whose experimentation with GH didn't turn out exactly as planned."

126

One of the most frightening forms on the black market is called research-grade GH. Unlike synthetic forms, which are an exact copy of natural human forms, research-grade has been modified and contains an extra amino acid. While this type is fine for research purposes, it's not intended for human use. If taken, up to 40 percent of users end up developing auto-immune diseases. For those not familiar with the term, this essentially means a person's immune system begins attacking its own body. Worse still is that cases have been reported in which individuals using research-grade GH developed an allergy to their own GH! At a basic level, one system of your body is treating another system as if it was an invading pathogen.

If you're still not dissuaded, consider this: Given its tissue-enlarging ability, some experts are suggesting that GH use could cause growth in existing tumors. Conclusive evidence to support this hypothesis is very limited. If the theory stands to reason, however, individuals with slow-growing tumors could have their lives shortened by using GH.

Some more "minor" afflictions and ailments round out the list of potential associated side effects: headaches, mood swings, excessive sweating, skin discoloration, and occasionally, visual impairment. Also worth noting is that some data indicates GH can negatively alter a person's ratio of HDL to LDL cholesterol. HDLs (high-density lipoproteins) help keep the body's arteries clear of fat buildup. Conversely, LDLs (low-density lipoproteins) build up on the insides of arterial walls, causing blockages that can lead to heart disease and stroke. Those with a family history of heart problems definitely need to think twice before using GH as an anabolic aid.

Photo by Paul Buceta
Model Paul Dillett

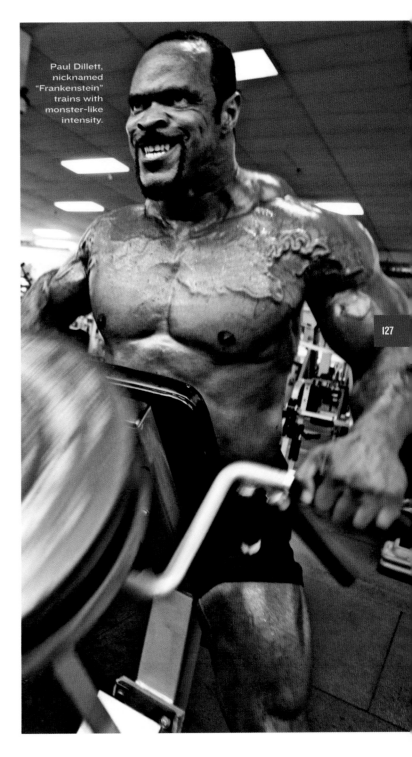

Paul Dillett, nicknamed "Frankenstein" trains with monster-like intensity.

127

INSULIN – NOT JUST FOR DIABETICS

128

> "Insulin saves lives. Insulin builds muscles. Insulin wrecks health. Insulin kills."
>
> – Richard Trent, *MuscleMag International* contributor

When Dr. Banting and Dr. Best first isolated the hormone insulin in the 1920s, they could never have envisioned that 70 years later, their life-saving discovery would be a hot topic in bodybuilding gyms. But the use of insulin by those within this sport is a perfect example of the win-at-all-costs mentality adopted by some bodybuilders. As an anabolic aid, insulin didn't really penetrate into the bodybuilding community until the early 1990s. Once word spread that the pros were adding it to their stacks, however, this hormone became the talk of gyms everywhere.

ORIGINS

Although this organ doesn't get the same attention as the lungs, heart, liver and kidneys, the pancreas is nevertheless vital to life. The pancreas is a small, five- to seven-inch organ located between the stomach and small intestine. Unlike most glands, the pancreas is both exocrine (secretes enzymes into special transport ducts) and endocrine (secretes enzymes into the bloodstream). This organ houses specialized tissues, called the islets of Langerhans, which contain four types of cells: alpha, beta, delta and F cells. This chapter will only cover the alpha and beta cells, as these two have the most relevance with regards to insulin and its impact on bodybuilders.

ALPHA CELLS

The primary hormone produced by alpha cells is glucagon. As blood-glucose levels fall within the body, glucagon is released to start the process of glycogenolysis – the conversion of glycogen into glucose (sugar). If glycogen levels are low, glucagon can convert other compounds into glucose including amino acids and lactic acid. Although both pathways are important, it's through glycogenolysis that most of the body's glucose is supplied.

INSULIN

Another hormone, insulin, works opposite to glucagon. Produced by the beta cells, insulin converts excess glucose back into glycogen. It

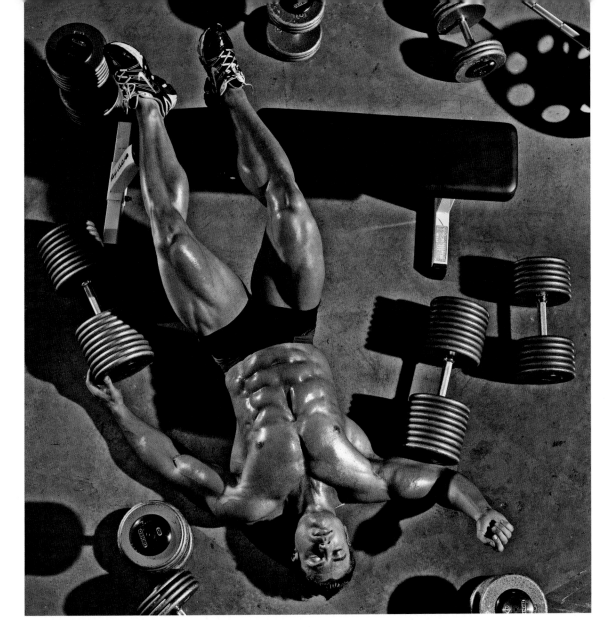

also speeds the rate of glucose transport across cell membranes. Once synthesized, glycogen is primarily stored in the liver and muscles as a future source of energy. It's insulin's third role, however, that has caught the attention of bodybuilders: transporting amino acids across cell membranes where they are then used to synthesize protein. Insulin also seems to suppress protein breakdown by catabolic hormones.[1] Further study findings suggest that insulin can increase the anabolic effects of individual amino acids such as glutamine.[2]

SUBSTRATE DEPENDENT

An interesting facet of insulin is that its performance of the actions noted above is dependent upon the nutrients available and the metabolic requirements of the individual. If overweight, sedentary individuals take insulin, they will gain fat; if bodybuilders who train intensely and consume large amounts of protein take insulin, they will instead gain lean muscle tissue.

ABOVE: For bodybuilders whose goals focus on muscle and strength gains, insulin is an attractive hormone. It carries amino acids across cell membranes to be used for protein synthesis and also helps inhibit protein breakdown.

Photo by Robert Reiff
Model Binais Begovic

TREATABLE, NOT CURABLE

All of the body's hormones are constantly changing – there are times when levels fluctuate, sometimes into dangerous ranges. If the beta cells produce too much insulin, blood sugar levels will fall rapidly, which can lead to the life-threatening condition of hypoglycemia. At the opposite end of the spectrum is diabetes – the condition where beta cells don't produce enough insulin. As a result, blood sugar levels become too high and this form is known as diabetes mellitus or Type I diabetes. When sufficient insulin is produced, but the body's receptors have trouble recognizing it, Type II diabetes is diagnosed. Type II, which is also categorized as adult-onset, tends to develop later in life, whereas Type I sufferers are born with the condition. Type I diabetics usually need insulin injections to regulate their blood sugar levels while Type II diabetics can often control it with dietary changes or medication.

The 15 to 20 million Type I diabetics living in North America can thank Dr. Banting and Dr. Best for their lives – prior to the discovery these doctors made in 1921, a diagnosis of diabetes was usually a death sentence. Most diabetics now, however, can lead relatively normal lives with modified diets and regular insulin shots. Routine exercise is also known to be largely beneficial for helping diabetics cope with the condition.

HEART ATTACKS

Insulin levels are related to diabetes, but insulin levels also affect heart health. If individuals continually ignore the importance of a proper diet and instead pig out on high-sugar foods like cakes, pies and doughnuts, their bodies literally become awash with insulin. This is because the body strives to keep blood glucose levels constant. While the increased insulin will reduce blood sugar, it also wreaks havoc with the arteries. The first to clog are the small arteries that supply blood to the heart. The heart, like all muscles, needs a constant flow of blood to receive oxygen and nutrients and at the same time remove the waste products of metabolism. If the transport of oxygen and nutrients is cut off, the person is at risk for suffering a potentially fatal heart attack. And even if the individual survives, the damage to the body is not 100 percent repairable. The problem is compounded by the fact that insulin raises the tendency for blood to clot. The combination of increased clotting and decreased arterial diameters leads to elevated blood pressure. Insulin also promotes the storage of excess iron in the tissues. High levels of iron in the body can also be damaging to the heart. A final area of concern is that insulin encourages fat storage, which in turn raises blood pressure and places even more stress on the heart.

"Besides such supplements as vitamin C, E, chromium and lipoic acid, just shifting away from simple sugars to complex carbohydrates has been shown to improve insulin sensitivity. High-fiber/low-GI lentils, oatmeal, brown rice, and beans should be your main source of carbs."

– Will Brink, bodybuilding and nutrition writer

Keeping insulin release to a minimum, therefore, is of great importance. The two best ways you can do this are restricting simple sugar intake and participating in regular exercise.

TYPES AND FORMS

There are two primary forms of insulin available for human usage. One type is made by converting animal insulin (usually from pork or beef) into human insulin. The second form is produced via recombinant DNA technology. Both versions are usually packaged in concentrations of 100 units per milliliter, and the two seem to be equally effective in regulating blood sugar. The only difference is that the synthetic forms seem to absorb slightly faster, resulting in a shorter duration of action in the body. Occasional incidence of allergic reactions to the animal form has also been reported.

Many bodybuilders who have tried both animal and recombinant DNA insulin find there is often a dramatic difference between the two with regards to muscle building. They also report that tolerance levels can build up, and they use cycling as a means to combat this effect.

Insulin can also be classified according to its rate of action. Fast-acting insulin (commonly called regular insulin) begins working within minutes and lasts for six to eight hours. This type is usually used in diabetic emergencies and for long-term treatment of diabetes. Slow-acting (or intermediate) insulin takes about two hours to function in the body, but the effects can last up to 24 hours.

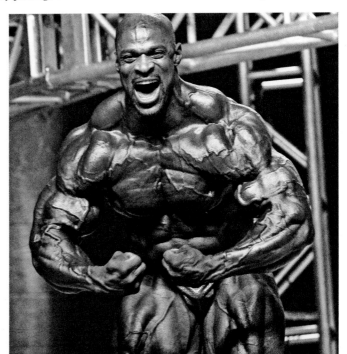

BELOW: Former Mr. Olympia Ronnie Coleman displays the physique of a champion-level bodybuilder.

131

TO THE OLYMPIA STAGE

By most definitions (and actions), insulin is a powerful anabolic hormone, and as such has made it into the stacks of many pro and amateur bodybuilders. Its widespread use in the sport is largely due to the fact that insulin is produced in huge quantities and is legally available without prescription.

Unfortunately, there have been very few, if any, studies of insulin use conducted on healthy (i.e., non-diabetic) subjects. The lack of published scientific and medical data means that the only "evidence" about use is the anecdotal reports from bodybuilders.

Photo by Irvin Gelb
Model Ronnie Coleman

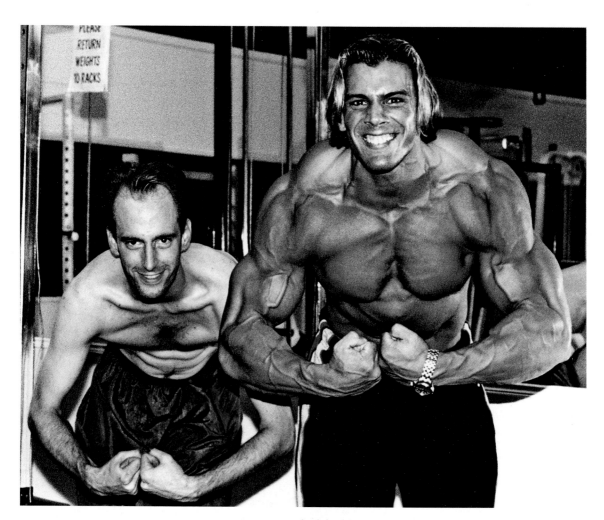

132

ABOVE: In general, the effects of insulin are as individual as the people that use the hormone. Some users report gains of 20 to 30 pounds while others claim it made no difference whatsoever.

Most bodybuilders who disclose information about insulin use report taking an average of 20 to 50 IUs (International Units) every day. Personal preference usually determines the type (fast- or slow-acting) consumed, but some over-ambitious individuals throw caution to the wind and take both types.

Another vital consideration when using this hormone is injection timing. Bodybuilders may be taking insulin primarily for its effects on amino acid transport and protein synthesis, but remember, the hormone also regulates blood sugar levels. If the injection is administered on an empty stomach, the insulin may drop already low blood sugar levels down to a dangerous point. And the result could be a state of hypoglycemia characterized by such symptoms as breathing difficulties, tremors and profuse sweating. In extreme cases the individual could become comatose or even die.

Model Frank Sepe with a fan

Smarter members of the sport ("smart" itself being a hotly debated word in this circumstance) take about 10 grams of sugar per IU of insulin about 30 minutes after the injection. Some bodybuilders take multiple shots throughout the day, and as such have to be ultra-strict with regards to diet and food choices – especially sugar intake.

Bodybuilders can be grouped into three categories based on their insulin usage. Some bodybuilders swear by its effects and claim the hormone helped them add 20 to 30 pounds onto their frames. They also find that it does wonders to facilitate the procedure of carb loading during the pre-contest phase of training. A second group have tried insulin and found it made no difference to their mass-gaining goals or pre-contest training. The third group, unfortunately, aren't alive to share their stories – these individuals rolled the dice with insulin and paid the price with their lives.

THE BIG THREE

Insulin is yet another "synergistic" drug – alone it only produces slow to moderate gains in muscle mass, but when stacked with other drugs, particularly GH and anabolic steroids, it contributes to huge increases in size and strength. Together, insulin, GH and steroids are know as "the big three" in bodybuilding circles and are believed to be the primary reason that today's pro bodybuilders can carry 50-plus pounds more than their counterparts of just 20 years ago. Given that such a practice is less than 20 years old, however, the long-term effects of this triple threat remain unknown.

SIDE EFFECTS

All drugs, even those developed for medical reasons, involve certain risks. Healthy individuals who inject insulin into their bodies are susceptible to negative reactions – the most serious of which can be life threatening.

The main side effects associated with insulin involve glucose regulation. Insulin, as was noted earlier, is non-selective in its effects. Bodybuilders may be taking it to speed up amino acid transport, but any glucose present will also get carried along. When individuals with normal insulin levels administer excess amounts of the hormone, they can easily throw off the delicate balance between blood sugar, insulin and glucagon. This triad is so sensitive that even minor changes to one element can have drastic consequences such as confusion, unconsciousness and even death.

Further to its impact on glucagon and glucose, insulin can interfere with the body's ability to regulate epinephrine (adrenalin). Its primary role is the fight or flight response, but epinephrine can also act to back up glucagon. Long-term use of insulin can interfere with this safeguard function, and thus potentiate the onset of hypoglycemia.

> "Together, insulin, GH and steroids are known as 'the big three' in bodybuilding circles and are believed to be the primary reason that today's pro bodybuilders can carry 50-plus pounds more than their counterparts of just 20 years ago."

133

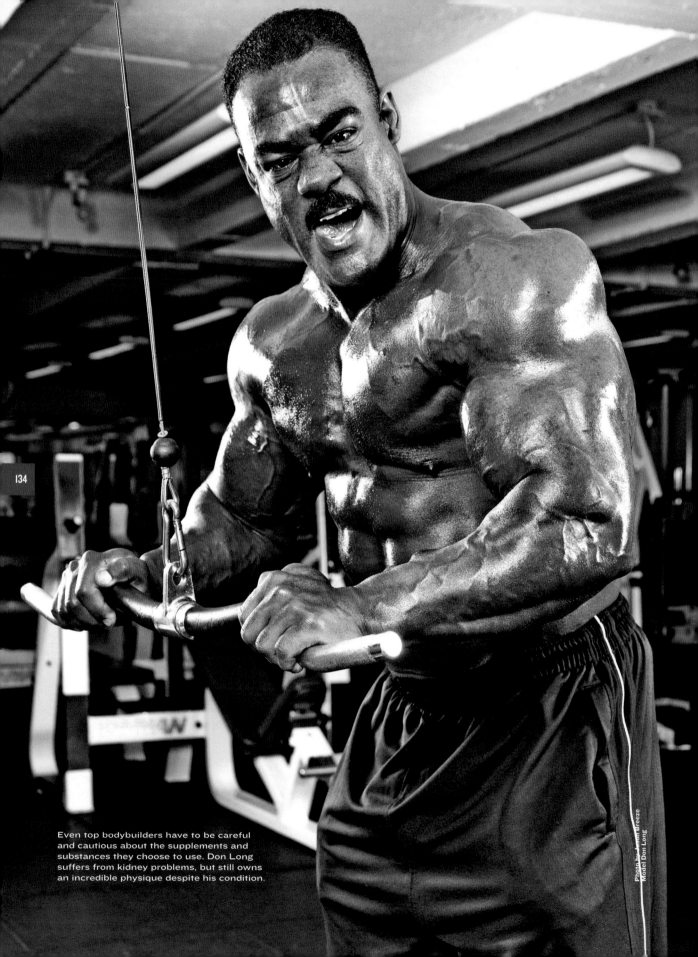

Even top bodybuilders have to be careful and cautious about the supplements and substances they choose to use. Don Long suffers from kidney problems, but still owns an incredible physique despite his condition.

134

One of the more rare side effects of insulin is its relationship to heart disease. Some research seems to indicate that elevated insulin levels can cause an increase in blood lipid levels. Of course, the reverse is possible: high fat levels may be causing insulin levels to increase. Until the cause-and-effect relationship is more fully studied and understood, bodybuilders with a family history of heart disease should be cautious about using insulin.

FINAL THOUGHTS – LITERALLY

Insulin use carries with it potentially deadly effects, so we strongly urge readers to avoid all types of this hormone. Unlike GH or steroids, one bad insulin experience could literally end your life in mere minutes. Just because some 250-pound gym rat swears by this substance doesn't mean it's safe for you. Unless your goal is to be remembered as the corpse with the great-looking physique, leave the insulin injections to diabetics.

References

1) DiPasquale, Dr. Mauro. "Are you insulin ignorant?" *Flex* magazine. 13:13 (Feb. 1996).
2) Yaraheski K., *et al*. "Short-term growth hormone treatment does not increase muscle protein synthesis in experienced weightlifters." *Journal of Applied Physiology*. 74:6 (June 1993).

BELOW: Insulin abuse is no joke – this hormone is highly dangerous and potentially deadly even in smaller dosages.

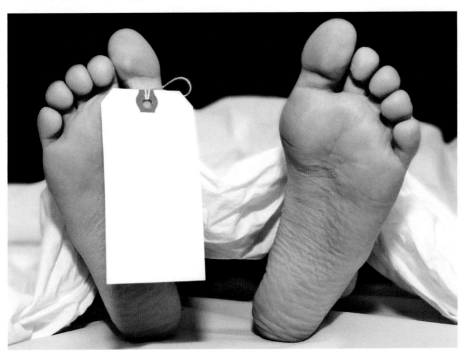

DIURETICS

"Competitive bodybuilders are known to use every trick in the book to make their muscles appear larger onstage. But even when bodyfat is reduced to incredibly low levels, the retention of excess water can blur a bodybuilder's ripped condition, so many competitors resort to the use of diuretics to obtain super-thin skin and eliminate water."

– John Gunstream and James D. Stockard, *MuscleMag International* contributors

There was a time when bodybuilders relied on diet and cardio exercise alone to get them ripped enough for a competition, but such an approach is no longer sufficient. The standards in this sport have become so high that only those bodybuilders bordering a near zero-percent bodyfat can hope to place in the top three of a major event. If each muscle is not crisscrossed with striations and veins, you might as well skip the competition altogether.

Bodybuilders generally use two strategies to achieve such an extreme degree of muscularity. The first is to drop their fat levels as low as possible using traditional diet and cardio exercise combined with thyroid drugs to boost their metabolisms. The second approach is to shed as much subcutaneous water as possible. Reducing salt intake and hitting the sauna was the old method, but today's bodybuilders more often opt for the drug route to really give their skin that paper-thin look.

Like all mammals, the human body is composed mainly of water. In fact, by weight the average person is 60 to 70 percent water. Even though our evolutionary ancestors left the oceans hundreds of millions of years ago, our bodies are still dependent on this simple life-giving liquid. Water is so vital to biological existence that it's one of the first compounds scientists look for when searching for signs of life on other planets. Humans can go a week or more without food, but can only survive a few days without water.

Further to giving the body support and structure, water serves as a medium for the transport of numerous substances including nutrients, waste products and oxygen. Water also carries electrically-charged ions that serve to regulate various systems in the body including the nervous, cardiovascular and muscular systems.

With so many crucial functions, water is essential to the body; for bodybuilders in the pre-contest phase, water is of central concern, but for a different reason. Instead of intake, their primary focus is to deplete water and minimize retention. Many bodybuilders seek the assistance of drugs to shed that extra ounce of water weight from their bodies. They use steroids and growth hormone to build muscle, thyroid medication to burn fat, so why not water-shedding drugs to get rid of H_2O? These pills are called diuretics and while highly effective for eliminating water, they may also drop the body's ion count to a dangerously low level.

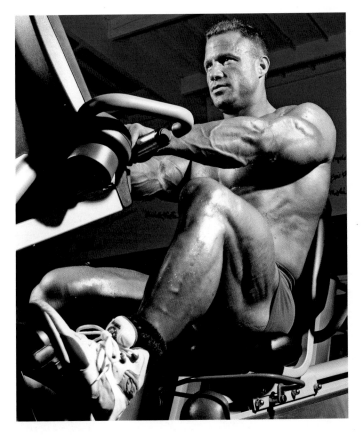

Photo by Irvin Gelb
Model Chad Ray Martin

LEFT: Bodybuilders rely on cardio as a means to get shredded and chiseled, but some use diuretics to amplify their ripped look.

WATER CONSERVATION

Water is essential to all living organisms, and the human body has evolved accordingly with various water-conserving systems to sustain life. As you might guess, the body's primary water-storing mechanisms are based on endocrinology.

The main hormone that functions to conserve water is ADH – antidiuretic hormone. ADH is a peptide-based hormone produced in the posterior pituitary gland that gets released into the blood where it then travels to the kidneys. Its primary mechanism of action is increasing the permeability of the kidney tubules. Through this process the kidneys can re-absorb water instead of letting it be excreted in urine. Such a control factor is absolutely vital for survival if the body ever begins to dehydrate. For example, if you start losing blood in large quantities, for whatever reason, the posterior pituitary releases more ADH in an effort to increase water conservation and help maintain blood pressure. Additional sources of ADH stimulation include exposure to heat, and physical or emotional stress may also elevate ADH levels.

138

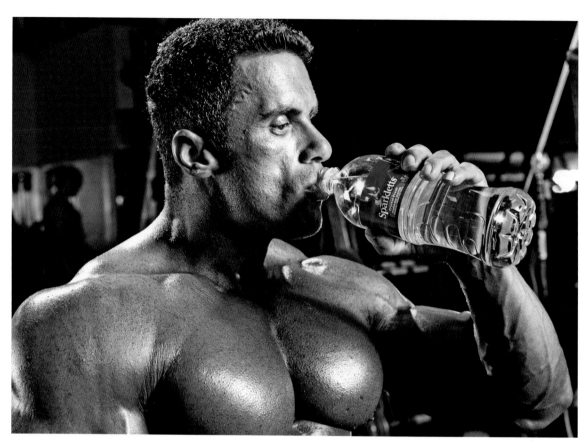

ABOVE: Staying hydrated is of utmost importance while training — water transports nutrients, oxygen and electrically charged ions to regulate various bodily systems.

Of course, the opposite response can also occur in situations of excess hydration. If you consume large amounts of water, your body shuts down ADH production to allow more water to be flushed out in the urine. Alcohol – especially beer – is famous for its diuretic effects, and its impact is twofold: The excess fluid contained in beer leads to water excretion, and alcohol itself is an ADH blocker.

MINERAL BALANCE

When discussing water conservation, mineral regulation in the body also needs to be closely considered. These two processes are tightly linked – taking diuretics to shed water invariably leads to mineral imbalances.

The body's primary hormone for controlling minerals is aldosterone, a mineralocorticoid that gets secreted by the adrenal glands located on top of the kidneys. The adrenal glands also produce other hormones, but this discussion will be limited specifically to aldosterone. Once released by the adrenal glands, aldosterone stimulates the tubules and collecting ducts of the kidneys to re-absorb sodium.

Photo by Robert Reiff
Model Oliver Adzievski

At the same time the hormone causes potassium ions from the kidney tubules to be lost into the urine. Aldosterone impacts the sweat glands in much the same way – they retain sodium and give up potassium to help maintain a normal acid-base balance.

HOW THEY WORK

Although diuretics are taken to promote water shedding, their primary mechanism of action is to decrease the kidneys' ability to conserve minerals (also called electrolytes). Sodium, potassium and zinc bind to water, so these minerals carry large amounts of water with them when excreted. So even though bodybuilders use diuretics to facilitate water depletion, H_2O is actually the secondary substance lost. Essentially then, the water loss is really a side effect.

The primary site where diuretics go to work is the nephron – the kidneys' main sub-unit of activity. There are over one million nephrons in each kidney and this high concentration greatly increases the surface area available for absorption. The nephron itself has two main parts: the renal capsule and renal tubule. Although both components serve as sites of absorption, most diuretics used by bodybuilders interfere with renal tubule function.

TYPES OF DIURETICS

Most diuretics fall into one of three categories: Loop, antidiuretic blockers or thiazides. Loop diuretics are aptly named because they interfere with electrolyte absorption in an area of the renal tubule called the loop of Henle. This type, of which Lasix is the most popular, are probably the most powerful diuretics and work by increasing excretion of sodium, magnesium and potassium. Loop drugs absorb very rapidly and begin functioning within 30 to 45 minutes; if taken orally they reach peak effect in one to two hours. In an emergency (such as pulmonary edema), however, they can be injected and as such start working in minutes.

The second group is antidiuretic blockers or potassium-sparing diuretics, the most common of which is Aldactone. This specific medication works by blocking ADH (the body's primary water-conserving hormone) receptors in the kidneys. Once blocked, ADH can't exert its mineral- and water-conserving effects on the kidneys. Of the three types, antidiuretic blockers are probably the safest since they help preserve potassium as water levels deplete.

The third form of diuretics is thiazides. When taken orally they begin to work within one hour and their effects can last up to 72 hours. Thiazides prevent sodium from being absorbed in the renal tubules. They also increase the excretion of both zinc and magnesium. One of the main advantages of thiazides is that they don't cause the same degree of calcium loss as the other two classes of diuretics.

"Diuretics are among the most dangerous compounds used by bodybuilders. Numerous bodybuilders including top pros have suffered short-term medical complications from diuretic use. Some have experienced uncontrollable cramps, while others had extremely flaccid and limp muscles. And still others have developed kidney disease."

– John Gunstream and James D. Stockard, *MuscleMag International* contributors

139

MEDICAL APPLICATIONS

Like insulin, steroids, growth hormone and thyroid drugs, diuretics were initially developed for legitimate medical purposes. Their primary use is in the treatment of high blood pressure, but diuretics are also prescribed to combat excessive fluid retention for those with heart and kidney disease. These drugs are also used to help with fluid buildup in the lungs of cancer patients.

ATHLETIC IMPLICATIONS

While shedding water prior to a contest is a main driving force, bodybuilders use diuretics for a number of different reasons. The high level of judging standards nowadays is but one factor competitors must consider – only the most muscular contestants have any chance of winning. Losing a few pounds of water to bring out that extra vein or striation could mean the difference between a first- and second-place finish.

Another purpose of dropping water is to lose a few pounds in order to enter a lower weight division. Instead of being at the bottom of one division, a bodybuilder could top the lower division. Rather than coming in as a fairly non-competitive small heavyweight, an

BELOW: While many competitors use diuretics as a tactic to bring out veins and striations, some athletes attempt to drop water to enter a lower weight division.

140

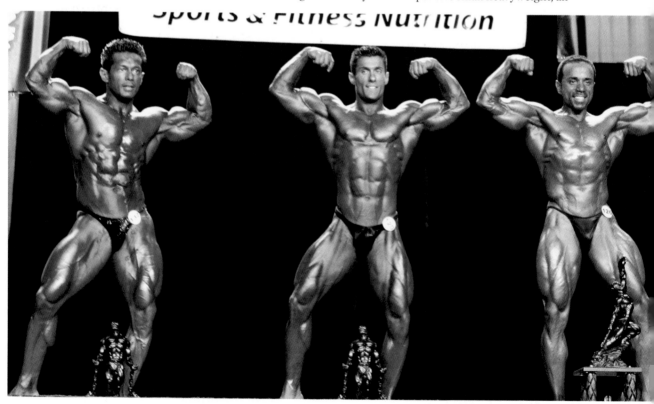

individual could shed a bit of water weight and make his mark as a large and highly muscular light-heavyweight.

A third reason athletes use diuretics is to dilute their urine before a drug test. Diluted urine contains lowers concentrations of drug metabolites, therefore lessening the chance an athlete would test positive for steroids or other banned performance-enhancing drugs. Various sports federations easily resolved this problem, however, by mandating that urine had to be of a certain concentration. As a secondary measure, many organizations also added diuretics to the list of banned substances.

FOR THOSE WHO DARE

There are many legitimate reasons for avoiding experimentation with diuretic drugs (which will be covered in the section that follows). Despite the risks though, there are no doubt a few readers who plan to use them regardless of the associated dangers. For those individuals, we offer a few points of consideration.

While starting diuretics a week or more out from the show may be tempting, don't. Try to limit use until a day or two before the contest because diuretics flush both water and electrolytes from the

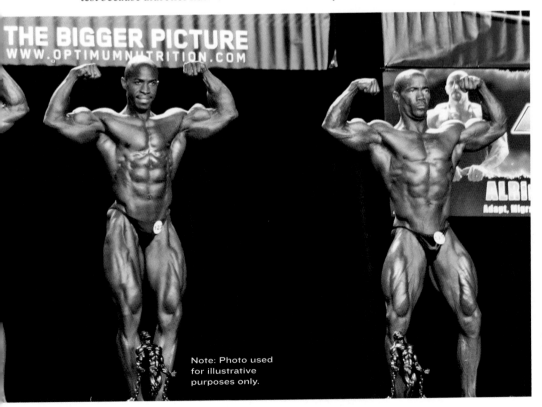

Note: Photo used for illustrative purposes only.

body. The longer you take them, the more depleted your system will become. Furthermore, because carbohydrate transport is facilitated by minerals – especially sodium – you risk interfering with the carb-loading process if your mineral levels drop too low. There is also evidence that diuretics reduce insulin's ability to transport glucose to muscles for storage as glycogen, again potentially throwing off the process of glycogen-loading. Our advice? Leave out diuretics until the last day or two. This time frame will still allow for flushing excess water from your body without interfering with the carb-loading process. Remember, this is assuming you take the drugs properly and that your body responds cooperatively. Diuretic use can be largely hit or miss when it comes to appearance, and more important, your health and well-being!

DANGERS OF DIURETICS AND ANTIDIURETIC BLOCKERS

Given their mechanisms of action, the primary side effect associated with both classes of drugs is dehydration. The human body is composed of over 60 percent water and even a minor decrease – such as on a hot summer's day – can lead to serious conditions like heat exhaustion and heat stroke.

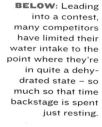

BELOW: Leading into a contest, many competitors have limited their water intake to the point where they're in quite a dehydrated state – so much so that time backstage is spent just resting.

142

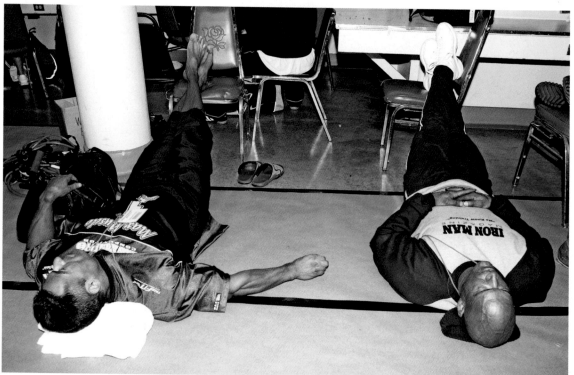

Photo by Irvin Gelb
Models Ahmad Haidar and Rusty Jeffers

Unfortunately, many bodybuilders tend to take diuretics in excessive dosages. Instead of shedding just enough water to highlight muscular detail, some guys end up in severely dehydrated states. You can't go to a bodybuilding contest these days without seeing at least one bodybuilder who cramps up onstage. This is because muscle contraction and relaxation is controlled by the nervous system and the relative concentrations of electrolytes such as sodium, potassium and calcium. Whenever these levels are imbalanced, muscle contraction is impeded. A cramp is really nothing more than a sustained, forceful contraction in a muscle that won't relax. The experience is very painful and may take minutes or even upward of one hour to subside. In severe cases, medical intervention may even be required to relieve the contraction.

Another major issue of diuretic use is its effect on the kidneys. When taken in high dosages over long periods of time, these drugs may lower your blood volume enough to impede kidney function. Further to interfering with the kidneys' various filtration systems, low blood volume can lead to actual tissue damage. And unlike the liver, which has some regenerative capabilities, kidney damage is permanent and irreversible. If these organs are harmed, you'll consequently have to take drugs, go on dialysis or need a kidney transplant (assuming you live long enough and can find a suitable donor).

Yet another factor to consider is the increased likelihood of developing gynecomastia. Many diuretics, especially ADH blockers such as Aldactone, are chemically similar to progesterone. For a few unlucky bodybuilders (teens are especially at risk), the progesterone receptors may kick in and produce a pair of the dreaded bitch tits.

If you're still not convinced about the negative aspects of using diuretics, consider the effects of these drugs on the cardiovascular system. Like the skeletal muscles, the heart is composed primarily of muscle tissue, with relaxation and contraction being heavily dependent on ion concentration. No doubt a muscle cramp in your calf is intensely painful, but you will survive; let your heart cramp, however, and you may be headed to the great weight-training pit in the sky.

Diuretic abuse may also throw the level of ions in your bloodstream out of sequence. For example, thiazides block the re-absorption of potassium. This can lead to a condition known as hypokalemia: low blood potassium. Such a state can cause muscular weakness, fatigue and actual muscle degeneration.

ADH blockers such as Aldactone can have the opposite effect and initiate hyperkalemia (high blood potassium). This is no trivial matter as high potassium levels can stop your heart. In fact, surgeons often use potassium (in medically controlled and monitored environments) to stop a patient's heart prior to open-heart surgery.

"Diuretics may in fact make your physique look softer instead of harder. Muscles after all are like most other body tissues in that they're primarily composed of water. If you go too heavy on the diuretics, you gamble with flattening out completely. Instead of appearing full and hard you'll look small and stringy."

143

Some bodybuilders choose to take both thiazides and Aldactone, rationalizing that if one increases potassium while the other drops it, then together the drugs will cancel out each other's effects. In theory this line of thought makes sense – at least as it applies to potassium levels. The problem, however, is that both drugs can increase the rate at which other electrolytes – especially sodium – are excreted. Pop enough pills and you'll be trading in your posing trunks for a hospital gown.

THE COCKTAIL EFFECT

Hopefully you now understand that, while not "hardcore" drugs, diuretics can have serious implications. Two of bodybuilding's young would-be future stars paid the ultimate price in their attempts to shed a few additional ounces of water. In 1982, Austrian bodybuilder Heinz Sallmeyer, winner of the lightweight class at the 1980 Mr. Universe contest, died of a heart attack believed to be brought on by diuretic use. In 1992, Algerian superstar Mohammad Benaziza died after complications following excessive diuretic use. While an official cause of death has never been conclusively determined, most in the bodybuilding world agreed that Benaziza depleted his electrolytes to dangerously low levels and consequently suffered a heart attack.

LASIX

As noted, Lasix is the most popular diuretic among bodybuilders, so its effects thus warrant a specific discussion. For starters, many people who are allergic to sulpha drugs are also allergic to Lasix. Use of this drug also carries a risk of salicylate toxicity if it's combined with aspirin. More specifically, this diuretic has been linked to a number of fetal abnormalities, so pregnant women or those intending to get pregnant should not use Lasix. Individuals considering the drug also need to understand exactly how Lasix works. Initially you'll find that you need to urinate every 15 to 20 minutes, but eventually the rate will slow down. Many bodybuilders assume the less frequent trips to the washroom mean the drug is wearing off, and they decide to take more. In reality though, the body is fighting against the water loss – it's trying to keep hydration levels within a healthy range (the importance of which has been ignored in competitive bodybuilding over the years). Unfortunately, adding more of the drug may be enough to push the individual into a state of extreme dehydration, resulting in minor to severe muscle cramps, or even to a life-threatening water-depleted state.

The effects of diuretics are not limited to your physiological systems; other implications of this drug's use shouldn't be ignored. For one, they may in fact make your physique look softer instead of harder. Muscles, after all, are like most other body tissues in that they're pri-

"As soon as the synthetic diuretics clear your system, the body's water-conserving mechanisms go into overdrive to restore water and electrolyte levels. Over the span of a few days you could go from looking shredded to appearing more like a large, waterlogged bag of sponges."

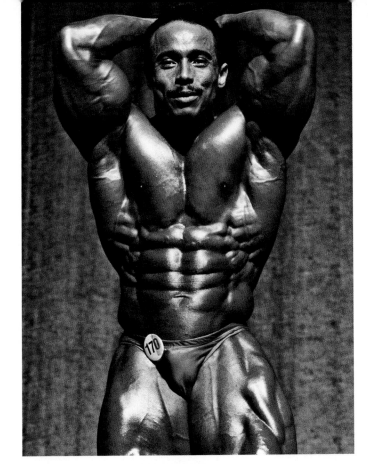

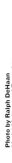
Photo by Ralph DeHaan
Model Mohammad Benaziza

marily composed of water. If you go heavy on the diuretics and shed too much water, you gamble with flattening out completely. Instead of appearing full and hard you'll look small and stringy.

The opposite can also occur after you come off the drugs. Just as testosterone amounts can rise above pre-steroid levels when you stop taking the juice, so too can your body overcompensate following diuretic use. As soon as the synthetic diuretics clear your system, the body's water-conserving mechanisms go into overdrive to restore water and electrolyte levels. Over the span of a few days you could go from looking shredded to appearing more like a large, water-logged bag of sponges. Now this post-use outcome wouldn't be a major issue if you were just competing in one contest. But if that first contest was a qualifier for a show the following weekend, you'd have a serious problem on your hands. You'd be left with somewhat of a Catch-22 choice: either try to shed the water naturally (which would probably be impossible given that your homeostatic systems are still recovering) or go back on the diuretics (which puts you right back at square one for risks and side effects).

Regardless of your competitive level in the sport of bodybuilding, we strongly urge you to avoid using diuretic drugs. Risking your health and well-being for the sake of a trophy is simply not worth it. If you're holding a few extra pounds of water a few days out from the show, you could instead try a mild herbal diuretic and perhaps a couple of extra minutes in a sauna. These methods should be relatively safe and effective for ridding water, while still leaving your muscles full and not interfering drastically with your electrolyte levels.

HCG AND CYCLOFENIL

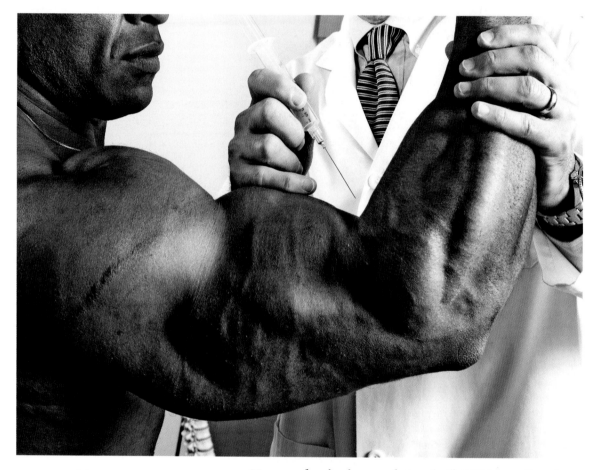

ABOVE: HCG is a naturally occurring hormone in females; males can't produce it and thus require injections to benefit from its positive muscle and strength effects.

Human chorionic gonadotropin (hCG) is another drug developed initially for legitimate medical reasons, not for increasing muscle size and strength. But yet again, the domino effect spread this drug across the bodybuilding community: once strength athletes and bodybuilders heard of its potential, hCG quickly appeared on the must-use lists in gyms around the world.

This hormone is a peptide hormone produced naturally in the placentas of pregnant women soon after conception. It is made by cells that form the placenta, later nourishing the egg after it has been fertilized and has attached to the uterine wall. HCG levels can first

Photo by Robert Reiff
Model Jerome Ferguson and Dr. Darrow

be detected by a blood test about 11 days after conception and by a urine test approximately 12 to 14 days after conception. In general, hCG levels will double every 72 hours. The level will peak in the first eight to 11 weeks of pregnancy and will then decline and become steady for the remainder of the pregnancy. For this reason, hCG is collected from the urine of pregnant women about two months after their last menstrual period, when the levels are at their highest.

As nature intended, hCG's function in women is to stimulate cell tissue, and the hormone also factors in egg development and ovulation. When a female gets pregnant, hCG effectively shuts down the menstrual cycle and increases the production of both estrogen and progesterone.

Males don't produce this hormone naturally, so it must be injected into their bodies. The reason bodybuilders and other athletes use hCG is because it's similar in structure and function to luteinizing hormone (LH). As you'll recall from Chapter 3, LH is the primary hormone in the male body for stimulating the testes to produce testosterone.

BODYBUILDING APPLICATIONS

The first generation of hCG users were probably introduced to the drug by physicians. Supervising doctors would give bodybuilders hCG shots during and after a cycle for two reasons: to block estrogen and to produce testosterone.

As we've discussed, during a steroid cycle many bodybuilders suffer feminizing effects due to high levels of estrogen (one of the breakdown products of steroids) in their bodies. Furthermore, elevated amounts of estrogen cause LH production to shut down, which in turn decreases testosterone production. By taking hCG during a cycle, testosterone is continually generated and the adverse effects of any excess estrogen are reduced.

The primary reason bodybuilders use hCG following a cycle is to increase their testosterone output. With regards to the hormone system, the body is fooled by the presence of steroids "thinking" they're the male hormone and responds by shutting down production. As long as the synthetic steroids are being injected into the body, all the desired effects of muscle strength, size and faster recovery times will remain. When the steroid cycle is terminated, however, the testes don't just switch on again overnight. If the individual was using high dosages of multiple steroids for an extended period of time it could take months, if not years, for normal testosterone production to resume. In cases such as these, medical intervention in the form of hCG therapy may be necessary.

Once steroids became illegal drugs though, most doctors refused to have any further dealings with steroid-using athletes – even to help them get off the juice. Consequently, many bodybuilders have been

"HCG is another drug developed initially for legitimate medical reasons, not for increasing muscle size and strength. But yet again, the domino effect spread this drug across the bodybuilding community: once strength athletes and bodybuilders heard of its potential, hCG quickly appeared on the 'must use' lists in gyms around the world."

147

driven to the black market to obtain hCG. While this has created all the same problems typical with the black market (legal issues, bogus drugs, no regulation), another issue surfaced when users began treating hCG as an anabolic aid rather than a hormone-normalizing drug. Instead of opting for small dosages to bring testosterone back within the normal range, bodybuilders began mega-dosing as a tool to increase muscle size and strength.

THE POWER OF hCG

When evaluating its effectiveness, hCG probably has more in common with growth hormone than with anabolic steroids. While virtually anyone who has had experience with anabolic steroids (the opinions of anti-steroid and law-enforcement groups aside) will readily admit the drugs produce significant gains in muscle size and strength, the same is not generally reported for hCG. Some users, however, say it seems to speed up fat loss close to a contest.

With regards to dosage, hCG seems to mirror growth hormone in that its results are not dependent on the amount: one dosage seems to elicit the same increases in testosterone production as multiple dosages. The prevailing theory to explain this occurrence is based on receptor sensitivity – many researchers suggest that hCG receptors are quickly desensitized, creating somewhat of an all-or-nothing effect. Essentially, one dose maximally stimulates the testes and further doses thus have no added impact.

SIDE EFFECTS

The common adverse effects of hCG use are the same as those experienced with any drug that increases testosterone output: acne, irritability, increased sex drive, and for some users, elevated aggression levels. These conditions can be reduced or eliminated with regular medical supervision, but again, most doctors are reluctant to treat individuals who use any type of performance-enhancing drug.

Elevated blood pressure resulting from increased water retention is potentially the most serious side effect associated with hCG. For healthy individuals this fluctuation is not likely to be a major issue, at least in the short term. But for those with a genetic history of stroke, raised blood pressure is not a situation to take lightly. There have been documented cases of young, otherwise healthy bodybuilders suffering strokes after a stint with hCG.

It's important to note that the risks of hCG use are heavily dependent on the dosages. Now, this may sound contradictory since we just finished explaining that results aren't linked to dosage amounts – bodybuilders don't need to take mega doses to obtain the desired effects. But when it comes to negative effects, however, the dosing becomes extremely critical. More hCG doesn't promote better results;

> "It's important to note that the risks of hGC use are heavily dependent on the dosages. Now, this may sound contradictory since we just finished explaining that results aren't linked to dosage amounts. But when it comes to negative effects, however, the dosing becomes extremely critical."

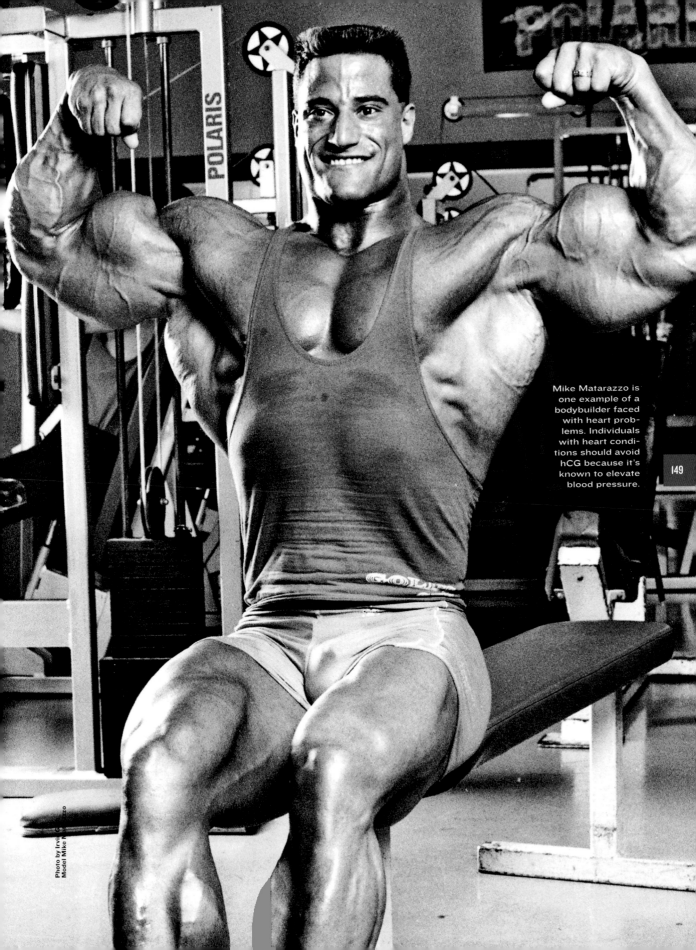

Mike Matarazzo is one example of a bodybuilder faced with heart problems. Individuals with heart conditions should avoid hCG because it's known to elevate blood pressure.

Photo by Irving G---zzo
Model Mike M---zzo

you're only risking your health with higher amounts. Knowing this, it kind of makes you wonder why any bodybuilder would take such large dosages in the first place.

While perhaps somewhat speculative, the answer probably lies within the realm of tradition. Many other performance-enhancing drugs do have a dosage-effect relationship: the higher the amount the greater the muscle size and strength results. (What many body-builders fail to recognize, however, is that they'd likely achieve the

RIGHT: Mr. Olympia title holder Dexter Jackson exudes all the features of a contest-winning physique that many guys would do anything to achieve: proportion, shape, symmetry and relative size.

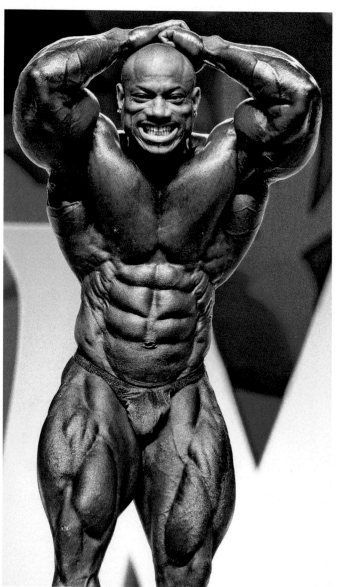

Photo by Rich Baker
Model Dexter Jackson

same gains by taking half or even one quarter of the drugs they're using.) But the "more is better" frame of thinking does indeed hold some merit with certain anabolic compounds and many bodybuilders automatically assume the same applies to hCG – even if they don't need to. And as long as this mindset exists, and medical practitioners are reluctant to get involved, bodybuilders will continue to use high dosages of hCG, consequently increasing their risk of experiencing side effects.

CYCLOFENIL

Cyclofenil is another drug bodybuilders use to modify their hormonal systems. Unlike hCG, which acts like LH increasing the output of testosterone from the testes, Cyclofenil acts by shutting down the feedback loop that decreases LH production. The theory is that by never allowing the body to reduce the rate at which LH is generated, testosterone levels will elevate.

Cyclofenil also functions as an anti-estrogen compound. The drug itself is a very weak estrogen, but it has a higher affinity for estrogen receptors. As such, Cyclofenil prevents stronger estrogens from bonding to the receptors and causing estrogenic effects. This action is so potent in the body that some bodybuilders use Cyclofenil during a steroid cycle to maintain low estrogen levels. Such use also results in less water retention and a decreased chance of developing gynecomastia. Many bodybuilders who use it attest to having a harder appearance and thus consider Cyclofenil an ideal pre-contest drug. The drug is also popular with so-called "natural" bodybuilders because technically it's not an anabolic steroid. With regards to performance enhancement, however, the increased testosterone levels attributed to Cyclofenil don't seem to produce substantial improvements. The majority of individuals who take it report slight gains in strength, a small increase in bodyweight, noticeable additional energy and faster recovery times between workouts. These results also seem to be more typical in advanced athletes who have little or no previous experience with steroids.

Most users report that the most effective dosage ranges from 400 to 600 milligrams per day. Lower dosages usually do not elicit the desired results and higher dosages only increase the potential for side effects to occur. Specifically in terms of side effects, some users experience mild acne, increased sexual desire and a flushed feeling on the skin. The first two symptoms are actually welcomed by most users as these signs indicate the efficacy of the compound. It's important to note that after cessation of use, some individuals experience a depressed mood and a slight decrease in physical size and strength. Those who take Cyclofenil as an anti-estrogen may also experience a rebound effect when use of the compound is discontinued.

"More hCG doesn't promote better results; you're only risking your health with higher amounts. Knowing this, it kind of makes you wonder why any bodybuilder would take such large dosages in the first place."

FAT
BURNING

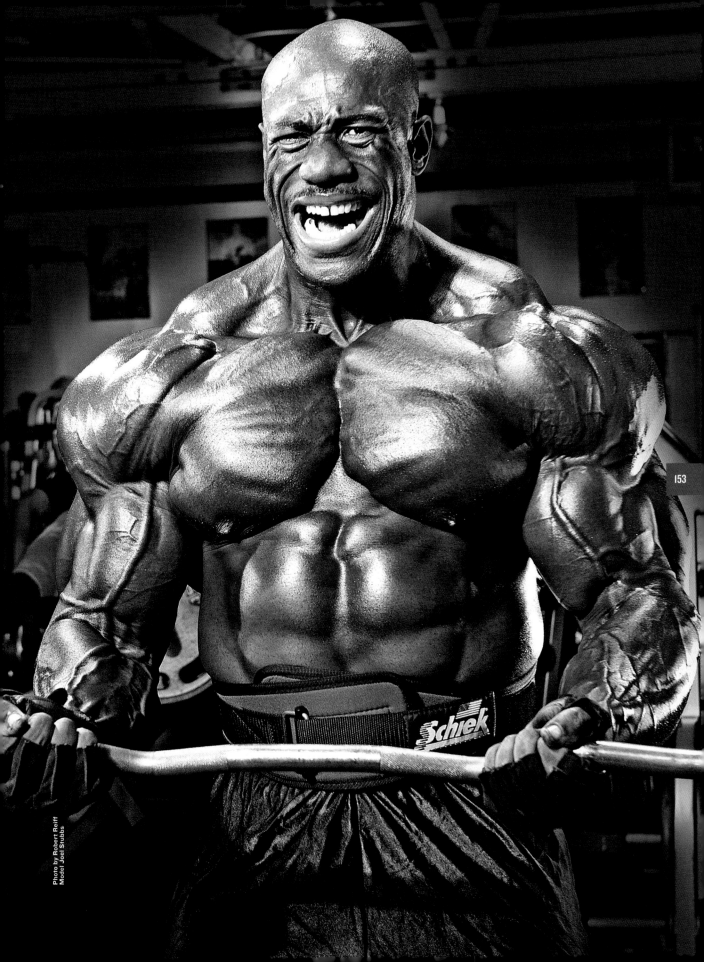

Photo by Robert Reiff
Model Joel Stubbs

INTRODUCTION

In many respects, aspiring competitive bodybuilders almost need a Master's or Doctorate degree in pharma-cology to successfully compete. While they may lack the formal educational credentials, however, most current bodybuilders know more about performance-enhancing drugs than the average pharmacologist or endocrinologist.

Once bodybuilders began to master the art of increasing muscle size, their next course of action was to investigate ways to drop bodyfat percentages. Starting in the 1970s, judges made it evident that they were looking for more than just muscle size. Only competitors who sported the hardest physiques were making it to the winner's circle. What the first generation of ripped bodybuilders such as Frank Zane, Chris Dickerson and Mohammed Makaway gave away in size to larger bodybuilders, they made up for and won with their lower bodyfat levels and superior conditioning. It wasn't long, however, before the 240- and 250-pounders got in on this trend. Guys like Lee Haney, Mike Christian and Berry DeMey were a few of the top competitors who led the way carrying 240-plus pounds of chiseled mass into battle.

From the end of the 1980s into the early 1990s, the average weight of pro bodybuilders went from 230 to 240 pounds to over 260. And while bodyweights increased, bodyfat percentages simultaneously dropped considerably. This trend has continued and has reached a point where a 280-pounder who competes today has decreased his bodyfat level down in the range of two to three percent. For readers who assume extra cardio and some sort of miracle diet have accounted for the drops, think again. The freaky states of hardness and vascularity that you see on a lot of guys are instead the result of certain drugs. Most of these specific substances function based on thermogenesis, but a few work by manipulating the body's energy-producing systems.

THERMOGENESIS

You can't easily flip through the pages of a bodybuilding magazine or surf a supplement Web site these days without coming across the word thermogenesis. It's one of the industry's fat-loss buzz words and despite the sci-fi ring to it, the actual process is not all that complicated. Thermogenesis is the term applied to the physiological state in which the body converts excess calories to heat rather than fat. It has also come to mean the process whereby existing fat stores are converted to heat energy.

Thermogenic drugs work in a number of different manners. When taken an hour or so before exercise, they increase the rate at which stored fat is burned as an energy source. These drugs also speed up the release of stored fat into the bloodstream, again causing more to be used for energy. Yet another characteristic of thermogenic drugs is their ability to boost the levels of other fat-burning compounds, particularly hormones.

The following chapters will cover some of the more popular fat-burning compounds and drugs used by bodybuilders these days in their efforts to get ripped. Most of the substances are legal, many are indeed effective, but a few could end your life.

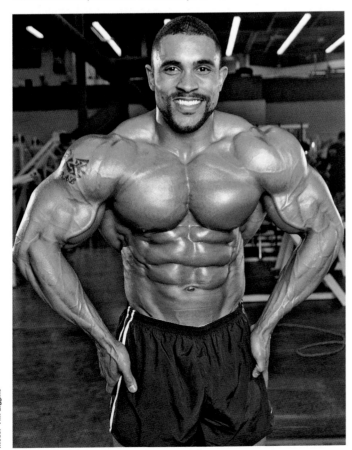

Photo by Jason Breeze
Model Tim Liggins

LEFT: Building an exceptional physique requires a delicate balance between increasing muscle size and dropping bodyfat; that's why bodybuilders are so up to speed on the many fat-burning products.

THYROID DRUGS

The next time you're at a bodybuilding contest – whether pro or amateur – take a close look at how the competitors place. All things being equal, bodybuilders sporting the lowest levels of bodyfat usually finish the highest. And unlike years ago when you only saw extreme degrees of muscularity in the bantam and lightweight divisions, now you'll see 280-pounders with two to three percent bodyfat. Innovative approaches to diet and training (especially cardio) have indeed contributed to the much-sought-after ripped look, but like many other aspects of modern bodybuilding, the primary tool to achieve that ultra-shredded appearance is drugs. And for most bodybuilders the top choice for stripping fat from their physiques is thyroid medications.

The thyroid hormones are produced in ... you guessed it, the thyroid gland – a small butterfly-shaped structure with two lobes, one located on each side of the windpipe (trachea). The thyroid gland has a well-developed circulatory system that enables substances such as amino acids, ions and hormones to be transported both toward and away from it. The bulk of the gland is made up of hundreds of thousands of spherical sacs called follicles. These sacs are filled with colloids, a gelatinous substance used for storing the thyroid hormones.

Two primary types of cells make up the thyroid gland. The most numerous are the follicular cells that secrete the thyroid hormones thyroxine and triiodothyronine. The thyroxine molecule contains four atoms of iodine and as such is often referred to as T4. Similarly, triiodothyronine is abbreviated as T3 because of the three iodine atoms in its base molecule.

Although not pertinent to our discussion, the other cells contained in the thyroid gland are called parafollicular cells (C cells) that secrete the hormone calcitonin. This additional hormone is one of the primary regulators of calcium in the blood.

T3 AND T4

Despite the fact that T4 makes up 90 percent of the thyroid's secretions, T3 is just as effective due to its higher bioactivity. Both hormones mainly consist of the amino acid tyrosine bound to iodine. The importance of adequate iodine in the diet has been known for decades – individuals whose dietary intake is deficient in iodine often develop a goiter. The condition is easily recognized by the pronounced swelling in the neck region when the thyroid gland becomes enlarged as it attempts to increase hormone output. However, goiter is extremely rare in Western societies because iodine has been added to water and salt supplies.

Although there are subtle differences between T3 and T4, both hormones essentially carry out the same functions. Arguably, their most important is to increase the rate at which cells use oxygen and organic molecules to produce heat and energy. In simple terms, they control the body's overall metabolism and the rate at which calories get burned. Of course, there is considerable variation among individuals with regards to metabolic rates. Two people eating the same number of calories and performing the exact same amount of cardio exercise may have drastic differences in their levels of stored bodyfat. Some individuals may be able to lose weight while consuming 3,000 calories per day while others will gain fat despite eating only 1,500.

Further to their metabolic role, the thyroid hormones also make the body more sensitive to the actions of epinephrine and norepinephrine – the end result of which is increased cardiac output. Additional functions of T3 and T4 include controlling homeostasis, modulating the nervous and skeletal systems, stimulating protein synthesis and helping control the body's water balance.

In terms of potency T3 is about five times more active than T4, and the body has the ability to convert T4 into T3 when needed. This is a function that bodybuilders need to be aware of if they take huge dosages of T4. Many guys opt heavily for T4 – anecdotal reports from users suggest that T4 doesn't have the same catabolic effects on muscle tissue as high amounts of T3. This could, however, be related to abuse of the drug and not the hormone itself.

CONTROL

Thyroid production is controlled by way of a feedback loop and the involvement of two hormones – thyroid-stimulating hormone (TSH) released by the anterior pituitary and thyrotropin-releasing hormone (TRH) released by the hypothalamus. When thyroxine levels drop in the blood, TSH is released. When these levels rise, TSH production is reduced. The response is reversed with regards to TRH: when thyroxine levels fall, TRH levels elevate which in turn stimulates the anterior pituitary to release TSH. As such, the outcome is greater thyroid gland activity and more production of thyroid hormones. Again here, the hormonal system monitors and controls its own levels. As long as there's no external interference, the system generally runs smoothly.

"The thyroid's central role in controlling the body's metabolism – especially with respect to fat burning – is a main reason that thyroid drugs have made it into the pre-contest stacks of many competitive bodybuilders."

157

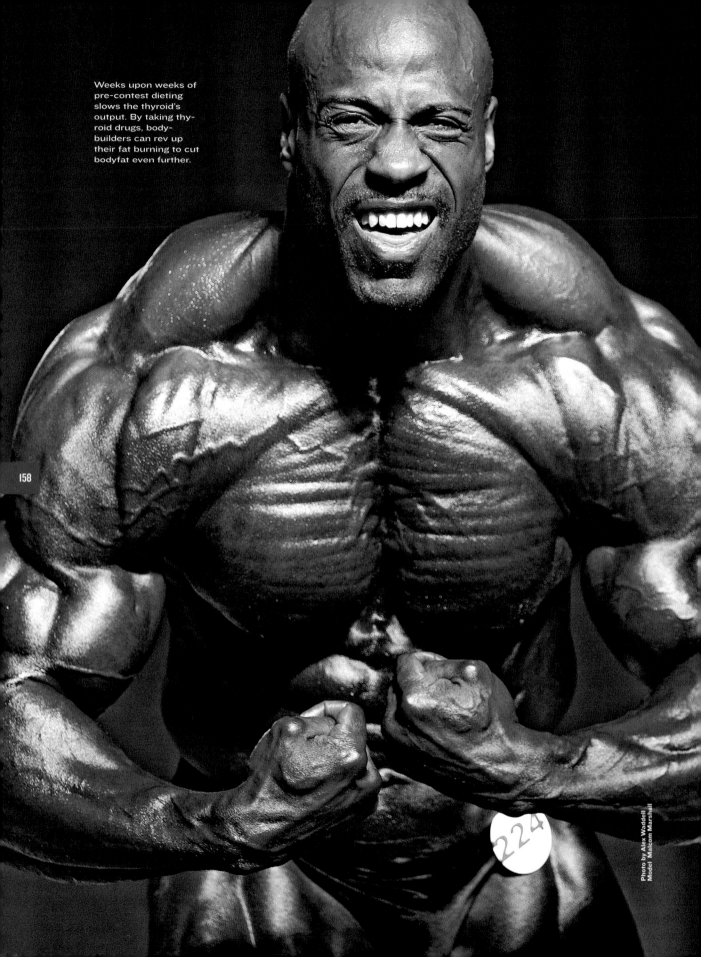

Weeks upon weeks of pre-contest dieting slows the thyroid's output. By taking thyroid drugs, bodybuilders can rev up their fat burning to cut bodyfat even further.

158

224

As soon as an individual starts introducing extra thyroid drugs into the equation, however, problems are bound to occur.

BODYBUILDING APPLICATIONS

The thyroid's central role in controlling the body's metabolism – especially with respect to fat burning – is a main reason thyroid drugs have made it into the pre-contest stacks of many competitive bodybuilders. Regardless of whether or not a person has the best genetic makeup, diet plans and training routines, there is a lower limit to where individuals can drop their bodyfat percentages. The body will fight tooth and nail to hang on to that last five or so pounds. But thyroid drugs allow bodybuilders to push past the cutoff point and turn their bodies into fat-burning furnaces, creating the near-zero percent bodyfat physiques we see on pro bodybuilding stages these days.

There are numerous contributing factors to why thyroid drugs are appealing to competitive bodybuilders. One of the "side effects" of long-term pre-contest dieting is the decline of the thyroid's output. This decrease in turn slows the person's overall basal metabolic rate (BMR), making further fat loss even more difficult. Although other factors are involved, the sluggish thyroid function is mainly due to less T3 production. Symptoms of reduced T3 production include lethargy, increased sensitivity to temperature fluctuations and a constant feeling of tiredness.

Another problem that arises with strict dieting is the inhibited functioning of the body's thermogenic systems. Thermogenesis facilitates the conversion of excess calories into heat, consequently preventing fat storage. As soon as there are fewer calories in the diet, however, the body senses the change and thinks it's entering a state of starvation. In response, the body automatically cuts back thyroid functioning, which then debilitates metabolism and leads to more calories being stored as fat. Humans developed this survival mechanism because it was necessary throughout our evolution when our ancestors went days without food. And while such reactionary systems aren't required these days, this biological feature is still part of our bodies and will activate if internal conditions call for it. There's a touch of irony in the fact that a behavior intended to reduce bodyfat levels may actually have the opposite impact.

Increased training is another strategy bodybuilders use to reduce their bodyfat percentages. Most competitors drastically increase their cardio frequency and duration in the months leading up to a contest. If cardio training becomes extreme though, the body may respond by decreasing the rate of calorie burning and fat loss. Here again, a practice aimed at dropping bodyfat may not only be ineffective, but counterproductive as well.

159

"Another problem that arises with strict dieting is the inhibited functioning of the body's thermogenic systems. Thermogenesis facilitates the conversion of excess calories into heat, consequently preventing fat storage. As soon as there are fewer calories in the diet, however, the body senses the change and thinks it's entering a state of starvation."

Because bodybuilding is a relatively small and close fraternity, most guys know who's doing what and are eager to get whatever competitive edge they can. Given the current trend in this sport toward the ripped look, many individuals turn to thyroid drugs such as Cytomel and Synthroid to obtain that extra degree of hardness. Use of these drugs might be justified if it was just as a means to boost thyroid output back to normal levels, but yet again, the "if some is good, more is better" mentality applies with thyroid drugs – some bodybuilders throw all caution to the wind in their attempt to achieve the best physique, taking as much as they can get their hands on.

SIDE EFFECTS

The degree and severity of side effects associated with thyroid medication is usually related to both the size of dosages and the duration of use. And while they are dosage-dependent compounds, both T3 and T4 may cause fat loss, muscle wasting or a combination of the two. This is because there is an optimum level in the body by which proper metabolic functioning takes place. Excessive thyroid hormones in the blood interfere with protein synthesis and thus may cause a loss of skeletal muscle tissue. Even more serious is the fact that high levels of these hormones can damage heart tissue (because this organ is primarily composed of muscle tissue).

The impact of thyroid medication on the liver is also of significant consideration. As we discussed in Chapter 8, the liver is the body's primary detoxifying organ. Any time excessive amounts of drugs – whether natural or synthetic – are introduced into the body, the liver has to work overtime to metabolize them. Similar to alcoholics who drown their livers with booze, athletes and other individuals who use thyroid and other performance-enhancing drugs may also develop liver problems.

HORMONE INTERACTION

Regulation of the thyroid system takes place via a process of biofeedback. As soon as outside sources of T3 and T4 are introduced into the body, the pituitary and hypothalamus will start decreasing the production of their natural thyroid-related hormones. And because the thyroid hormones interact with both insulin and growth hormone, the effects aren't isolated and invariably lead to problems with other hormonal systems. The internal bodily processes all function in delicate alignment – a balance that can very easily be thrown off.

ADRENAL HORMONES

In addition to the response from the pituitary and hypothalamus, excessive thyroid hormones can spark the adrenal gland's production of androstenedione – a hormone that's easily aromatized into

"T3 is a drug that must be taken with caution. If you don't know how or when to use it, T3 can permanently shut down your thyroid and you can end up on thyroid medication for the rest of your life. It can also be life threatening in rare cases because of its effects on the heart."

–Daniel De Grande, *Musclemag International* contributor

estrogen. Elevated thyroid hormones can also increase the production of a blood protein called sex-binding globulin. This circulating protein has a very high affinity for testosterone, essentially latching on and making it less available for use. The net effect of this is an imbalanced testosterone-estrogen ratio in the body, and gynecomastia can often be a resulting condition.

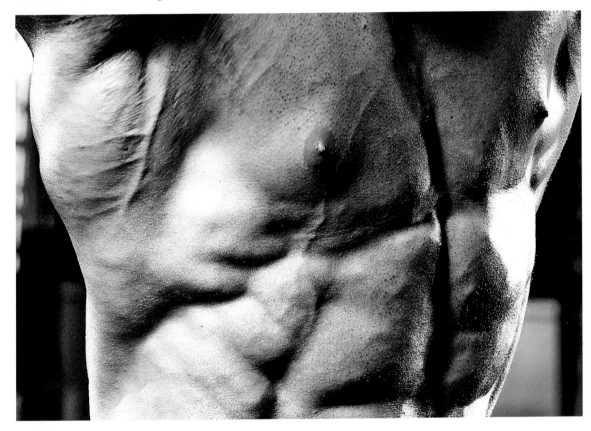

161

IGF-1

Also worth noting is that excessive use of thyroid medications may decrease the amount of IGF-1 levels in the blood. This process happens in a similar manner as the decrease of testosterone: high thyroid levels increase the amount of special proteins that bind to and neutralize IGF-1, which is a protein hormone that has been linked to promoting muscle-tissue synthesis. This growth factor is very similar in molecular structure to insulin; it carries the same number of amino acids as insulin (79) and is responsible for much of the anabolic properties of HGH. Proper production of IGF-1 in the body is important as this hormone is a key factor for growth during childhood and is highly anabolic in adults.

ABOVE: Taking too much thyroid medication can lead to an imbalanced testosterone-estrogen ratio, leaving the user more likely to develop gynecomastia.

Photo by Robert Reiff

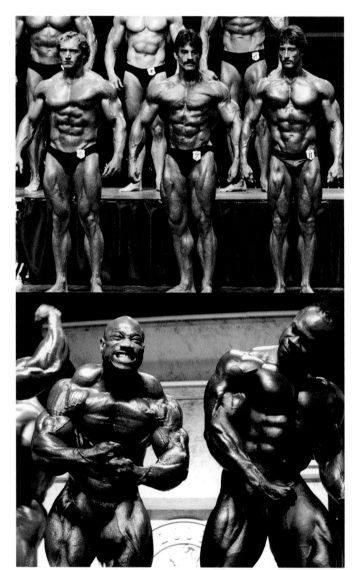

ABOVE: The bodies of bodybuilders from 30 years ago and today's pros are like night and day in many respects – GH use accounts for much bigger and harder physiques.

HGH/GH

Most readers are aware that human growth hormone is as much a part of modern bodybuilding vocabulary as steroids, creatine and whey protein. HGH, or GH, is one of the primary reasons that modern bodybuilders are so much bigger and harder than their counterparts of 20 or 30 years ago. Our discussion here will be limited to the relationship between GH and the thyroid hormones, particularly T3; for a more detailed description, please refer back to Chapter 14.

Research has shown that thyroid hormones increase the number of GH receptors in the liver. When an adequate number of calories are consumed in the diet, GH seems to increase T3 levels – a finding that's been put forward to explain how GH mobilizes fat stores and speeds up metabolism. You'd expect then that adding GH to a stack during a diet phase would also elevate T3 levels, but such doesn't seem to be the case. One study showed that food deprivation raised GH levels but decreased T3 and IGF-1 production.[1] And because GH is heavily influenced by IGF-1, it can actually be catabolic in a restricted diet.

INSULIN

Another primary hormone that influences the thyroid is insulin – in its presence, thyroid-stimulating hormone (TSH) encourages the thyroid to secrete more T3 and T4. A number of studies have confirmed that TSH, insulin and IGF-1 are connected in that they all interact to keep the thyroid gland functioning properly. During periods of food reduction, both IGF-1 and insulin levels decrease, thyroid activity becomes sluggish and metabolic rate slowly lowers – hence why strict diets rarely lead to meaningful fat loss. Extreme diets also elevate levels of the catabolic hormones cortisol and glucagon, which promotes muscle loss.

CLENBUTEROL

Clenbuterol is a member of the family of drugs called specific beta-2 agonists. Unlike ephedrine which is a nonspecific beta-2 agonist, clen-

Photo by Irvin Gelb

buterol binds to beta-2 receptor sites almost perfectly. Consequently the body burns fat at a much accelerated rate – but this effect only lasts for approximately two to three weeks as beta-2 receptors become desensitized to clenbuterol very quickly. Even increasing the dosage (and risking the associated side effects of taking more) doesn't seem to elicit added results. Furthermore, chronic use of clenbuterol seems to debilitate the body's own beta agonists like adrenalin and noradrenalin. When the beta-2 system is impacted in such a way by clenbuterol, normalization may take weeks if not months – a time frame that often involves a rapid gain of bodyfat.

So where does T3 fit into this picture? Experiments have shown that in order for clenbuterol to have a positive effect on body composition, thyroid levels must be optimal. Because T3 increases the number of beta receptors on fat and muscle cells, and clenbuterol is a beta-receptor agonist, it stands to reason that T3 gives clenbuterol more sites to work on. Unfortunately though, the process isn't so straightforward – clenbuterol also has a nasty habit of decreasing the level of free T3. So the body is left in somewhat of a win-lose situation: high levels of T3 increase clenbuterol receptor sites, but clenbuterol counteracts this effect by reducing T3 production.

PRECAUTIONARY MEASURES

For those readers who have decided to use T3 despite the risks and potential outcomes, we offer a few words of caution. Before you start anything, get your levels checked. If your T3 levels are naturally low (which is more common among the general population than people realize) there's a good chance you'll be able to get a prescription. As such you'll be spared from having to face the various pitfalls and dangers of buying the drug on the black market. But if your levels are normal, unfortunately you're on your own.

With regards to dosage, start out by taking just one 25-microgram T3 tablet daily. And as long as you continue to lose bodyfat, resist the urge to increase that amount. Consuming more, as we've discussed, doesn't necessarily mean you'll lose even more fat – you're instead more likely to inflict damage upon your thyroid gland. If after a few weeks you're still not losing fat, however, double the dosage to 50 micrograms per day. Regardless of the dose, make sure you limit use of T3 to no longer than six to eight weeks. Gradually tapering down the dosage is also a good idea over the last couple of weeks, as doing so gives your body a chance to start normalizing its own T3 production. Much like with steroids, exogenous levels of T3 will suppress TSH secretion, so quitting cold turkey should definitely be avoided – your body would be left without any form of available T3. You'd go from ripped and diced to the Pillsbury Doughboy within weeks!

"Experiments have shown that in order for clenbuterol to have a positive effect on body composition, thyroid levels must be optimal ... but clenbuterol also has a nasty habit of decreasing the level of free T3."

164

ABOVE: Individuals who take thyroid drugs are not immune to becoming addicted. And when use is stopped, the associated weight can send some guys into a depressed and discouraged state.

OVERCOMING THE VICIOUS CYCLE

While we discussed addiction in detail in Chapter 9, the topic warrants further attention. Most drugs have the potential to become addictive, and thyroid medications are no exception. As soon as an individual starts reaping the benefits of a certain drug and becomes accustomed to their new "look," getting clean becomes quite challenging. It will take a concerted effort on the part of the user and his support system of family and friends. Even under the best circumstances, it could still be months or years before the person's natural hormonal systems are completely back to normal. Matters are only complicated popular as it clears the system much faster than most anabolic steroids. Before drug-test methods improved, bodybuilders used to report being able to pass the test while using clenbuterol up to 48 hours beforehand.

Anecdotal evidence seemingly supports that most bodybuilders prefer the tablets of clenbuterol over the bronchial spray. In reference to amount, surprisingly the gym dosage is only approximately double the therapeutic dosage – about 50 to 100 micrograms per day (normal prescriptions are usually 20 to 60 micrograms a day). Given that its efficacy seems to diminish after about three weeks, most bodybuilders follow a three-weeks-on/three-weeks-off type of cycle. During the on weeks, most users take the drug for two days and then go off for two days. This approach, bodybuilders have discovered, seems to be the most effective for getting three full weeks of fat loss and muscle enhancement.

The iron warriors made another key finding about clenbuterol: unlike steroids, in which some gains are maintained after the cycle is stopped, virtually all progress made while taking clenbuterol is lost after the drug is discontinued. This is the primary reason that clenbuterol is most often used only as a pre-contest fat-burning drug and not relied on for meaningful growth of muscle tissue.

EVALUATIVE DIFFICULTY

Assessing the effectiveness of clenbuterol presents the same challenges as human growth hormone: Users are reluctant to talk about it. This "vow of silence" is even more pronounced if the athletes in question are involved in sports where the drug is officially banned. Any attempt to determine how well this compound works is further complicated by the issue of drug interactions. Most bodybuilders who use clenbuterol also use numerous other performance-enhancing drugs. Determining exactly whether the physical changes are caused by clenbuterol, the other drugs or a combination of all of them thus becomes quite difficult. The role of synergism must be accounted for – many drugs taken separately produce little to no effects, but when stacked together, they produce outstanding results on fat loss and muscle gains.

The relatively short history of clenbuterol use is yet another factor that inhibits assessing its effectiveness. Unlike steroids, which have been documented and studied for over 50 years, clenbuterol use really only started in the 1990s. There just simply aren't any "old-timers" to talk about their user days – little to no hand-me-down information exists. Granted in 20 or 30 years firsthand data from former clenbuterol users will become available, but until then, much is left to speculation. This shortage of knowledge is especially true in relation to side effects – many conditions and outcomes often take 20-plus

"During times of strict dieting, the drug seems to be highly effective for decreasing body-fat and sparing muscle tissue. And for bodybuilders who compete in drug-tested events, clenbuterol is even more popular as it clears the system much faster than most anabolic steroids."

169

> "There are volumes of research on clenbuterol use in animals. The question has to be asked, though: how relevant are the observations collected from a rat running in a cage to a 250-pound bodybuilder?"

years to manifest and present themselves in drug users – a frustrating reality for physicians and coaches trying to counsel athletes about clenbuterol use.

Perhaps the biggest obstacle faced by researchers and athletes alike concerns the lack of scientific data from studies done with human subjects. There are volumes of research on clenbuterol use in animals. Considerable data is also published specifically on the use of this compound as an asthma medication in Europe. But those all-important studies that examine the effects – both performance and health related – in athletes are virtually nonexistent.

It is possible to extrapolate data from animal studies – such practice is done all the time in medical research. The question has to be asked, though: how relevant are the observations collected from a rat running in a cage to a 250-pound bodybuilder? Comparing the anti-constriction effects of clenbuterol in monkeys and humans may be applicable, but is there merit in drawing a straight animal-human link when it comes to the drug's effects on protein synthesis and lipolysis?

Animal studies are also less credible in that the dosages tend to be dozens (and in some cases hundreds) of times greater than what humans can tolerate. Even if researchers were to somehow get permission to conduct the experiments on humans, there's no way they could morally use the same drug amounts on human subjects.

We must also remember that clenbuterol is not approved by the FDA for human consumption. Legally speaking, researchers can't just go into a gym and recruit 20 or 30 bodybuilders to start experimenting on. Labs may get funding to conduct studies on animals, but even then the odds are against it because research dollars tend to be allocated proportionately to the drug's potential use in humans. Therefore, because the drug isn't approved for medical use in the U.S., researchers are strictly prohibited from studying it in a human capacity.

SIDE EFFECTS

The lack of available scientific data on use by bodybuilders and other athletes means that we have to rely on the results of animal studies and asthma patients being treated with clenbuterol.

There are two general groups of people who are exposed to clenbuterol (not counting athletes): those directly treated with the drug and those indirectly exposed to it from eating clenbuterol-infused meat. In regards to the latter, liver meat is the most common culprit – as the body's primary detoxifying organ it tends to contain the highest concentration of any drugs that have entered the system.

The most common side effects associated with clenbuterol use are headaches, nausea and insomnia. In fact, the three are most often exhibited together – a lone symptom is rarely seen without the other two. Serious side effects have also been reported, the most severe of

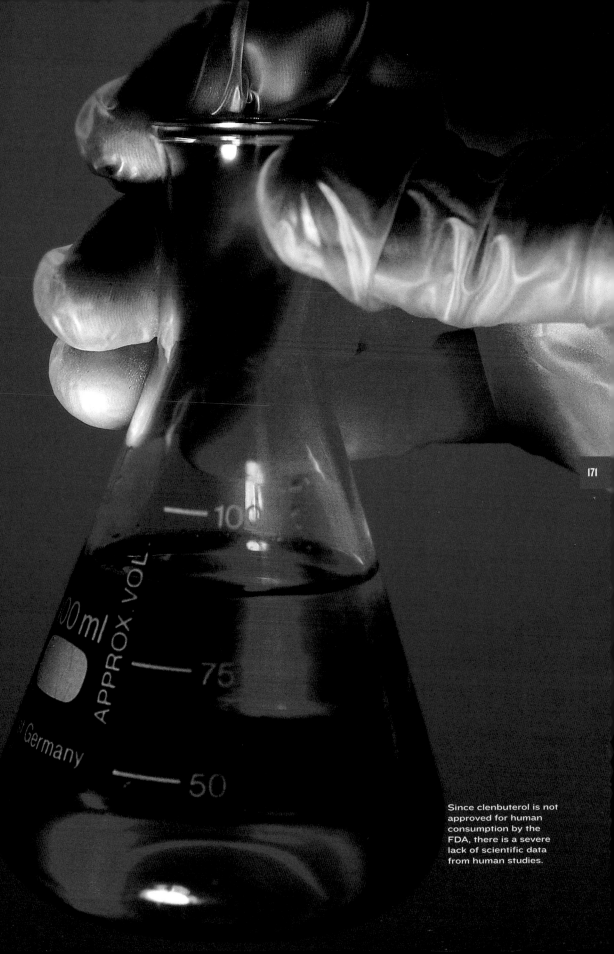

Since clenbuterol is not
approved for human
consumption by the
FDA, there is a severe
lack of scientific data
from human studies.

ABOVE: Drug cocktails can be as individual as each bodybuilder, but users need to be particularly cautious of which combinations put them at increased risk for serious side effects.

which is tachycardia: the medical term for a rapidly beating heart. And although rare, there have been cases of deaths attributed to clenbuterol use. (Keep in mind, however, that determining whether the cause was clenbuterol or another drug is difficult.)

Because drug cocktails are so popular among bodybuilders, they're at an increased risk for developing tachycardia. Competitors often take diuretics and other fat-burning and water-shedding drugs in the weeks leading up to a contest to shred their physiques. Besides the water loss, valuable electrolytes may be depleted, which is problematic because many of these charged ions are vital for regulating the cardiovascular and nervous systems. Clenbuterol also increases the excretion of many of these same electrolytes, thus making an already potentially dangerous situation that much more severe.

Studies with animals show that further to speeding up heart rate, clenbuterol may also enlarge the actual organ (creating a condition call myocardial hypertrophy). This situation can be deadly in

Photo by Irvin Gelb

humans as an enlarged heart can potentially lead to vascular obstruction. Clenbuterol's effects are exerted on the heart primarily because this organ contains a large number of beta receptors. When such a condition is present, the common heart medication propranolol, which is a beta-receptor antagonist (blocker), is prescribed to stabilize and slow the heart.

The list of side effects associated with clenbuterol use in animals doesn't end there. A few other potential outcomes from taking this drug are tremors, seizures, cardiac arrest, hemorrhaging and extreme feelings of nervousness.

LEGAL STATUS

Although not classified as an illegal drug (i.e., it isn't categorized under the Anabolic Control Act), virtually all sports organizations have it on their banned substance lists.[1] In addition, while possession for personal use probably won't get you jail time (in most U.S. states the charges would be classified as a misdemeanor for the possession of a prescription drug without a valid prescription), importing it from another country would be considered smuggling. This act will definitely do more than raise the eyebrows of the feds and you'd be facing serious federal drug-smuggling charges.

A few words also need to be mentioned about clenbuterol and the black market. With the combined crackdown on steroids and increased popularity of clenbuterol, genuine copies of the drug are becoming harder to find on the black market. Many bodybuilders report having bought fake versions for $100 to $200 per bottle. Others claim they've received oral anabolic steroids thinking it was clenbuterol. This mix-up became obvious when guys started experiencing the side effects normally associated with steroids (e.g., acne, increased aggression levels, water retention). We don't want to belabor the point, but the take-home message with regards to the black market is worth reiterating: the risk of buying fake or dangerous copies of the drug increases as you move further and further away from legitimate sources. In simple terms, that shadowy guy you meet in the gym parking lot may be profiting at your expense.

Even after this discussion, we admit that the jury is still out with respect to clenbuterol's impact on healthy human subjects. It may still be another 10 years or so before side effects in humans can be definitively linked to the drug. Until then, bodybuilders and other athletes using or considering clenbuterol should pay close attention to any warning signals from their bodies. If you ever have any doubts about potential problems with use, play it safe and pass on the drug.

Reference
1) http://www.deadiversion.usdoj.gov/drugs_concern/clenbuterol.htm.

"Legally speaking, researchers can't just go into a gym and recruit 20 or 30 bodybuilders to start experimenting on. Because the drug[clenbuterol] isn't approved for medical use in the U.S., researchers are strictly prohibited from studying it in human capacity."

EPINEPHRINE

174

Although most medical literature uses the term epinephrine, its more familiar name is adrenaline.
Epinephrine is secreted by the adrenal medulla of the adrenal glands (two small glands, one located on top of each kidney). What makes epinephrine unique is its dual action as both a hormone and a nervous system neurotransmitter – a characteristic that allows the two to function together in times of stress or danger.

Epinephrine is a known primarily as a "fight or flight" hormone and plays a crucial role in the short-term stress response (the autonomic reaction that occurs when a person is faced with a potentially dangerous situation). The human body will respond to the trigger in one of two ways: stay and confront the danger (fight) or flee (flight). In either case the nervous system kicks into overdrive and stimulates the adrenal glands to pump out huge amounts of epinephrine. The result is the "adrenaline rush" we experience when faced with a sudden shock or a threatening or exciting situation. The jolt of adrenaline is characterized by symptoms like elevated heart rate, sweating and increased mental alertness. This surge also produces a "side effect" – it frees up more fat stores for use as an energy source. In fact, research has indicated that with regular exercise, one of the primary causes of fat loss is the higher amount of epinephrine in the body. When you break it down, exercise is after all a form of stress and it does trigger the autonomic nervous system to fire up (albeit in a much reduced capacity than if you were ever confronted by a wild animal or armed intruder).

It is believed that epinephrine mobilizes fat stores via two primary mechanisms. The process can be slow and controlled involving the gradual release of epinephrine by the adrenal glands. Alternately, fat cells can be directly stimulated by the sympathetic nervous system.

At the cellular level, epinephrine binds to receptors on fat cells producing an intracellular messenger called cyclic AMP (cAMP). A cascade of further reactions then occurs and activates a hormone that breaks down triglycerides into free fatty acids and glycerol (hormone-sensitive lipase). The fatty acids are then transported to the muscles for use as an energy source.

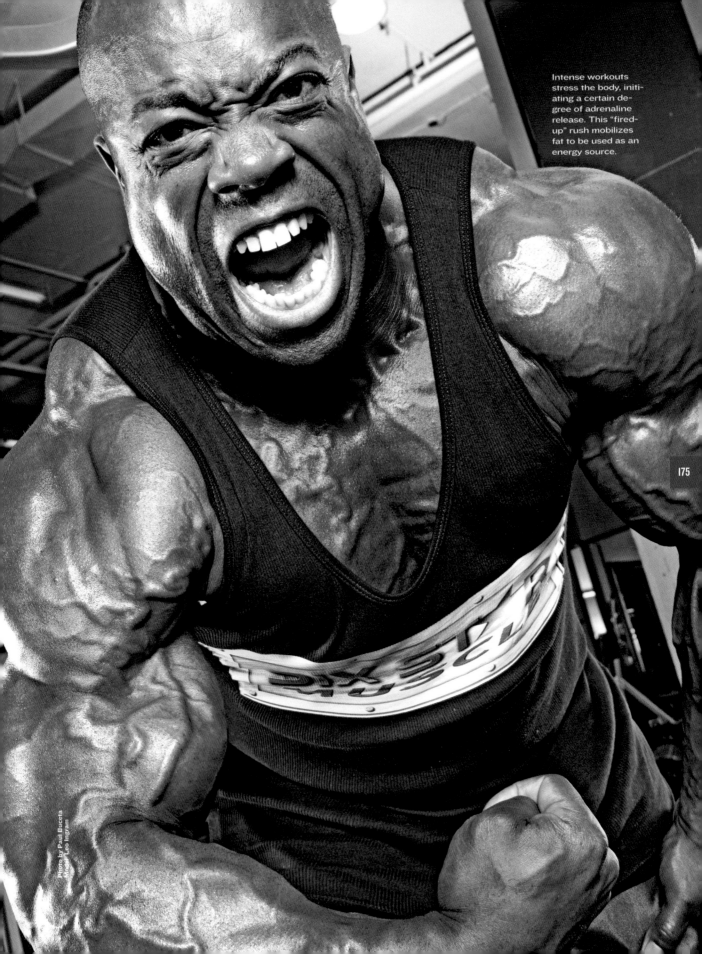

Intense workouts stress the body, initiating a certain degree of adrenaline release. This "fired-up" rush mobilizes fat to be used as an energy source.

175

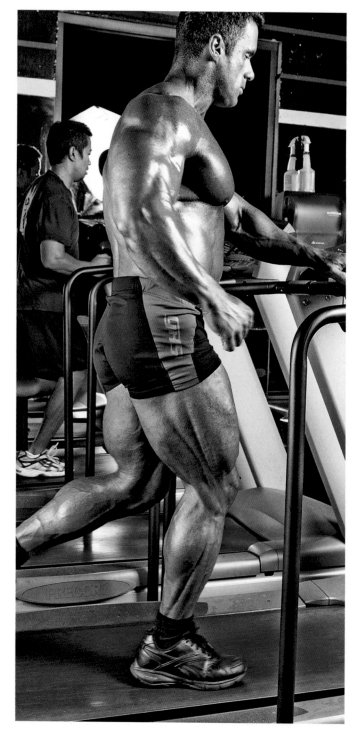

BODYBUILDING IMPLICATIONS

These fat-burning properties of epinephrine have not escaped the undivided attention of competitive bodybuilders. While not generally as popular as thyroid drugs or even certain steroids, some bodybuilders use epinephrine in the months before a contest to obtain that extra degree of hardness the judges seem to reward these days. Diet and cardio alone will enable most guys to shed away excess fat – a few months on epinephrine, however, could mean the difference between first and second place.

Many competitors also find the months preceding a contest to be very physically and mentally demanding. Increased cardio combined with a strict diet leaves many individuals energy-depleted and feeling just plain dragged out. While a lot of guys opt for caffeine to give their systems a kick, some bodybuilders go the extra step and take a shot of epinephrine before their workouts. Similar to caffeine though, the high is usually followed by an exhaustion crash as the body tries to normalize its own chemistry. In the span of a few hours you'll be trading in sets and reps for a blanket and pillow.

SIDE EFFECTS

Because epinephrine acts as a stimulant, its side effects can potentially be quite serious. The human body did not evolve to sustain a continual state of stress in the central nervous system. The "fight or flight" response is a mechanism for emergency situations only. Those who use epinephrine on a regular basis force their heart rate, blood pressure and a whole host of other systems into a constant state of stimulation. Even individuals of excellent physical health put themselves at risk for dangerous side effects.

The feedback mechanism must also be considered – like most hormones epinephrine release is controlled by a feedback loop. When outside sources are detected, the body responds by shutting down its natural manufacturing of the hormone. When the external source is no longer present, it takes the body weeks and sometimes months to resume normal production and regulate natural levels – if you're lucky. Here again, long-term use may necessitate medical intervention to kick-start the body's hormonal system.

It's important to note that while many bodybuilders use epinephrine, finding a licensed medical practitioner who'll prescribe it (or even monitor your use) for non-medical reasons is near impossible. We're going to replay the black market broken record – you've read about the risks in previous chapters and the same applies to epinephrine: buyers beware.

LEGAL ASPECTS

Epinephrine is classified under the same category as clenbuterol: it's a prescription drug, and as such applicable laws relate to possession of the drug without a valid prescription. To reiterate from Chapter 19, you probably won't be charged for possessing small amounts, but if the law enforcement agent is a stickler, he may try to nail you for possession with intent to traffic. If you have prior trafficking convictions, you'll likely get charged. Specifically with respect to drug testing, virtually all sports organizations include epinephrine on their lists of banned substances. While testing for a natural hormone is still tricky, the test methods are becoming more advanced every year. Translation: odds are you'll test positive.

"Some bodybuilders use epinephrine in the months before a contest to obtain that extra degree of hardness the judges seem to reward these days. A few months on epinephrine could mean the difference between first and second place."

177

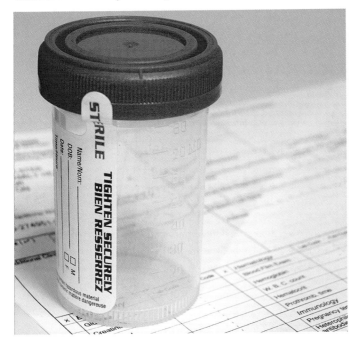

LEFT: Drug-testing methods have become so effective that even natural hormones can be measured – epinephrine is one such banned substance that will likely be detected.

EPHEDRINE

Though used in Chinese medicine for many centuries, ephedrine (EPH) is another athletic aid that didn't get mainstream attention until the late 1990s – and even then it was for controversial reasons. Bodybuilders use ephedrine for its stimulant and fat-burning properties. Research has determined that it also has the potential to increase strength levels. Until the substance was banned in 2004, ephedrine taken in conjunction with caffeine and acetylsalicylic acid (ASA) was the most popular fat-loss compound in OTC diet products. And despite its restricted status, ephedrine still remains a top choice among pre-contest bodybuilders.

Ephedrine is a naturally occurring compound (classified as a sympathomimetic amine) found in plants belonging to the genus Ephedra. The Chinese herb má huáng is probably the most well-known product containing EPH. At the molecular level, ephedrine is structured similarly to epinephrine and amphetamines and produces the same benefits and side effects.

MECHANISMS OF ACTION

In much the same way as clenbuterol and epinephrine, EPH functions by stimulating beta adrenoreceptors. However, unlike many other beta agonists, which are selective (they stimulate only one type of beta receptor), ephedrine interacts with a multitude of different beta receptors. In low doses ephedrine produces a greater sense of well-being and a seemingly unlimited energy level. In high doses, however, it can cause tachycardia, high blood pressure, and in very extreme cases, stroke or heart attack.

Its stimulant effects are only half of the equation though – ephedrine is also a powerful thermogenic compound. This characteristic is the primary reason that ephedrine became such a popular pre-contest aid for bodybuilders and fat-loss drug among the general public. And because ephedrine has a strong scientific pedigree, it has the upper hand on many bodybuilding supplements, which only offer empty promises and marketing gimmicks. Study after study appears to confirm that when ephedrine is combined with caffeine and ASA, the results are nothing short of outstanding for an OTC fat-loss product.

The exact mechanism of action is not fully understood, but scientists believe that when the three compounds are taken together they synergistically cause the body to increase production of norepinephrine (noradrenaline) – a hormone that's very similar in structure and function to adrenaline and causes similar thermogenic effects. Further research findings also indicate that ephedrine increases the output of T3 and T4 by the thyroid gland.

Another appealing feature of ephedrine is its ability to preserve muscle tissue when individuals are following a strict diet. One peril that bodybuilders often face when cutting calories and increasing cardio exercise during pre-contest training is losing some of their muscle tissue. As muscle mass decreases, the person's metabolism begins to function less optimally, which makes trimming additional bodyfat near impossible. Anecdotal reports from competitive bodybuilders seem to support that ephedrine is quite effective in counteracting this muscle loss. The result is somewhat of a double bonus for the user: he can carry more muscle mass onstage and can lose even more bodyfat. In the eyes of many bodybuilders, EPH is a supplement that facilitates entering a contest with a bigger and harder physique.

Ephedrine's popularity among athletes is further boosted because of its effects on strength. Again we must remain somewhat critical of the so-called "proof," because anecdotal reports are the main source, but most users note strength increases of 10 to 20 percent during a typical workout. Though not conclusive, the prevailing theory is that ephedrine, being a stimulant, increases action in the sympathetic nervous system.

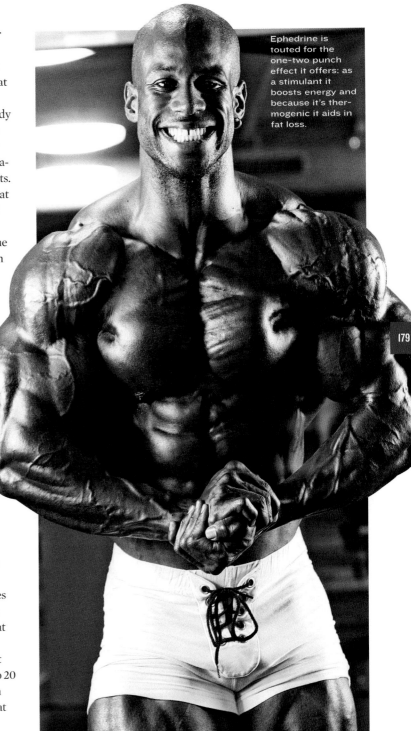

Ephedrine is touted for the one-two punch effect it offers: as a stimulant it boosts energy and because it's thermogenic it aids in fat loss.

179

Photo by Ralph DeHaan
Model Stephen Frazier

> "Because ephedrine has a strong scientific pedigree, it has the upper hand on many bodybuilding supplements. Study after study appears to confirm that when ephedrine is combined with caffeine and ASA, the results are nothing short of outstanding for an OTC fat-loss product."

As we discussed in the previous chapter, the SNS is responsible for the "fight or flight" response. Under conditions of stress or danger, additional nutrients and oxygen are being delivered to the muscles, and the body is also being flooded with stimulant hormones like adrenaline. Take, for example, news stories you've likely heard at one time or another about an individual of average weight who has lifted an enormous object to save a person trapped underneath. The feat itself sounds as though it would be impossible under normal circumstances, but there may in fact be a scientific explanation to this. Now you probably won't ever be hoisting 2,000 pounds in the gym, but evidence does give credit to the claims that one or two ephedrine tablets will definitely give your workouts a kick.

SIDE EFFECTS AND THE MEDIA

Few other bodybuilding supplements have received as much media attention as ephedrine. When MLB Baltimore Orioles pitcher Steve Bechler died during spring training in 2003, a media frenzy rivaling that of the 1988 Ben Johnson drug scandal was set into motion. Bechler died less than 24 hours after taking three tablets of a fat-loss product containing ephedra. The exact cause of death was never established, but it was believed a combination of heat exhaustion, the stimulant effects of the ephedra and Bechler's weight (he tipped the scales at a hefty 240 pounds at 6′2″) all played a role. The press had a field day, jumping all over the ephedra link, and making it sound like Bechler was in top-notch shape. The intense heat in Florida at the time, dehydration and Belcher's lacking physique were all but omitted.

Bechler's fate is a tragic example of what can happen when use of this drug goes terribly wrong. Taking ephedrine involves certain risks, though most of the side effects are dose related. A few individuals may be allergic to the drug at any dosage. Others who have heart conditions are susceptible to the stimulant effects. For the most part, however, healthy individuals who don't abuse the drug in high doses have little to worry about. Consuming one of the old 25-milligram tablets (or three of the new 8-milligram tablets) two to three times per day poses limited risk to the majority of individuals. It's when guys pop pills like candy or take EPH while doing physical activity in extreme weather conditions (as in the Bechler case) that severe side effects are more likely to be experienced. By no means are we attempting to promote use of ephedra, but we want to clear the air of the smokescreen created by the legal community and media: both outlets have focused excessive attention on a few hundred cases, blowing the risks associated with ephedrine use out of proportion. The fact remains, however, that millions of individuals use the compound as a drug or diet aid without any serious side effects.

The most prevalent symptoms of ephedrine use are those related to stimulant effects. As a beta agonist, EPH is capable of elevating a person's heart rate and blood pressure. For healthy individuals a slight increase in either is not a large concern. The elevated state only lasts a few hours after taking the drug and tends to diminish after use has been continued for a few weeks. Those with a history of stroke in their families, however, are especially at risk and should refrain from using any ephedra products.

Ephedrine's thermogenic properties are rarely the cause of health problems. Users just need to be cautious about their training environment because the substance causes a slight increase in body temperature – individuals who plan to exercise outdoors on a hot day may want to pass on the product or, at the very least, drink plenty of water and pay close attention for any symptoms of dehydration.

BELOW: Ephedrine users who train outdoors in hot and humid climates need to pay close attention to signs of dehydration, as this drug is thermogenic and raises body temperature.

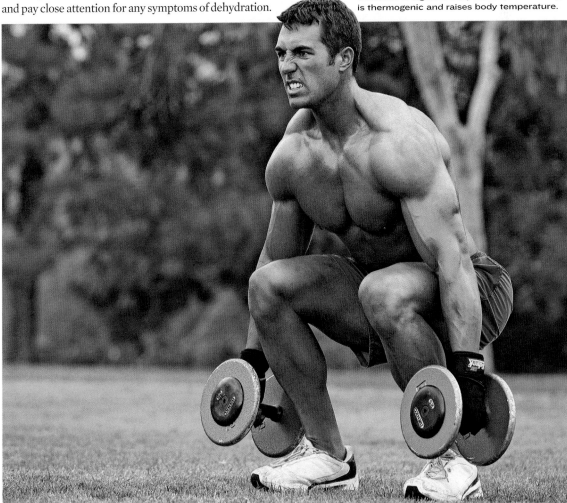

Photo by Alex Ardenti
Model Sean Glassman

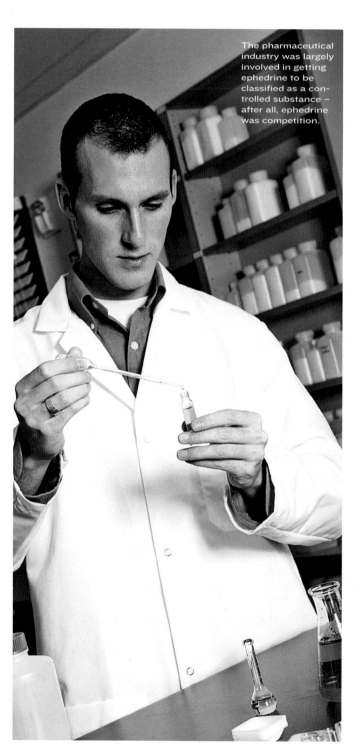

The pharmaceutical industry was largely involved in getting ephedrine to be classified as a controlled substance – after all, ephedrine was competition.

Finally, there have been a few cases in which individuals experienced slight hand tremors when using ephedra products. For bodybuilders and most other athletes, a shaky hand isn't a serious issue. Those in sports such as darts and archery, however, or those who work with their hands for a living (watchmakers, electronics) need to consider how use of EPH would impact their performance and/or livelihood.

LEGISLATION

When *Anabolic Primer* was first published in 1998, we warned that it would only be a matter of time before products containing ephedra would be reclassified as controlled substances. The situation hasn't quite reached the Draconian levels of steroid legislation, but ephedrine isn't the over-the-counter product it used to be. As of the print date of this book, ephedrine is not banned outright by the FDA; the substance is highly regulated though, because it's a precursor for several scheduled drugs (methamphetamine and methcathinone). Possession of ephedrine is legal, but sales of large quantities are closely monitored and many U.S. states govern how it's sold.

In early 2004 the FDA prohibited the sale of all OTC dietary supplements containing ephedrine. Although the ban temporarily came into question when a federal judge ruled it invalid, the U.S. Court of Appeals for the Tenth Circuit sided in favor of the FDA. In August 2006, a restriction was put on marketing any product containing ephedrine or ephedra-related compounds. Since then, retailers in the United States are required to collect the signatures and view a photo ID of every person who purchases products containing pseudoephedrine. This procedure must take place on every purchase of any product for which the entire box contains more than 60 milligrams of pseudoephedrine. What many people don't realize is that pseudoephedrine is one of the primary ingredients in many cold medications – so catching a cold and requiring medication now means you may be under the ever-watchful eyes of big brother.

CORPORATE PRESSURE

A major driving force behind the new legislation against ephedrine was large pharmaceutical corporations. Consider this chain of events: Bodybuilders and millions of others discovered that when combined with ASA and caffeine, ephedrine was one of the safest and most effective fat-loss compounds. It was also very cheap to buy. The pharmaceutical industry viewed this as a direct threat to their profits from similar fat-loss products. Why would individuals spend hundreds of dollars on a prescription diet-drug such as dexfenfluramine (which was later banned after it was linked to heart valve damage) when they could buy a month's supply of aspirin, caffeine and ephedrine for $25? The answer: consumers simply wouldn't. Faced with such competition, numerous pharmaceutical giants began lobbying the FDA to make ephedrine a controlled substance. And as noted, their pressure paid off in 2004.

FINAL COMMENTS

The U.S. government continues its plight in the "War on Drugs," so odds are slim that laws opposing ephedrine use will be relaxed any time soon. Consider the prohibition laws from the 1920s, for example; it took 13 years and billions of dollars in damages – both human and property costs – before the ban on alcohol was reversed in 1933. Now, the Canadian legal system isn't quite as strict as its U.S. counterpart – in Canada you can still buy ephedrine in 8-milligram tablets. For bodybuilders, this simply means you just take three tablets instead of one of the old 25-milligram tablets. American bodybuilders also have the option of buying the herb form of ephedrine, as doing so is still legal. Keep in mind though that the herbal medicine industry is poorly regulated so you can never be exactly sure what you're receiving and in what dosage. Considering all the loopholes, the logic behind ephedrine regulations seems cloudy. The inconsistency is especially apparent in comparison to alcohol or tobacco laws: you can still buy as much of these substances as you want – both drugs are legal to anyone over the age of 19 to 21 (depending on the state), despite having decades of research behind them outlining the dangers. Tobacco alone kills millions of individuals every year. So how do those drugs escape the government's attention while ephedrine gets the legal spotlight?

183

"Bodybuilders and millions of others discovered that when combined with ASA and caffeine, ephedrine was one of the safest and most effective fat-loss compounds. The pharmaceutical industry viewed this as a direct threat to their profits from similar fat-loss products."

MISCELLANEOUS FAT BURNERS

In Chapters 18 to 21 we covered the more popular drugs bodybuilders take to develop eye-popping stria-tions and veins. While most of the substances we've discussed are highly effective at burning fat, they're also controlled or regulated by the government. Obtaining these compounds thus becomes difficult and the black market maximizes on such situations – users end up risking their health and freedom all in the name of achieving a ripped physique.

As soon as ephedrine, the most popular fat burner, became controlled, supplement manufacturers began searching for legal alternatives. Some of the replacement compounds they found had actually been around for decades but underwent a revival thanks to strategic marketing techniques. Others were products of the latest scientific research. Still others had no solid basis in science, but bodybuilders swore by them.

Before looking in depth at these various compounds we need to clarify one important point: If you're currently carrying too much weight, simply adding a fat-burning product to your diet will have little to no effect; you also need to modify your eating habits and incorporate more cardio exercise into your workouts. Proper nutrition and training are the cornerstones for losing fat. The greatest fat-burning compound in the world will be useless if it's coupled with a bad diet. And fat burners cannot substitute for a well-rounded exercise program. Focusing your gym time at the bench press doing singles will offer limited benefits to your waistline. Aerobic activity – particularly cardio exercise – is the primary stimulus for fat loss.

CHARACTERISTICS OF A QUALITY FAT-BURNING SUPPLEMENT

While personal preference is an influencing factor in the selection of a fat-burning product, there are a few general recommendations to consider. For starters, in the supplement should contain ingredients that stimulate both the thyroid and adrenal glands. It should also contain components that speed up the rate at which fat deposits are made available for burning as an energy source. And it's an added bonus if the product also regulates sugar and insulin.

HYDROXYCITRIC ACID

Hydroxcitric acid (HCA) was a creation of the mainstream fat-loss industry and became one of the substitutes in bodybuilding fat-burning products when ephedrine was restricted. HCA is derived from citric acid in the Garcinia, a fruit that's native to Indonesia. While perhaps not as effective as ephedrine, it doesn't have the beta agonist's stimulant effects either.

Mechanisms of Action

Before examining how HCA may speed fat loss, a brief introduction about how the body metabolizes and stores fats and carbohydrates is needed.

When carbohydrates and sugars are consumed in the diet, both are reduced to the simple sugar glucose. Insulin then transports the sugar from the bloodstream to the body's various cells, and a certain amount gets stored in the liver and muscles as glycogen. During times of increased energy demands, the glycogen is quickly converted back to sugar. Other glucose supplies are broken down by way of the citric acid cycle into even smaller sub-units. (See Appendix pg. 522.)

For example, if you were to eat multiple chocolate bars in one sitting, the excess sugar would be converted into fat by a process called lypogenesis (literally "fat creation"). Although humans don't generate a great deal of fat from carbohydrates, any amount that gets produced is significant – it takes very little excess to impede the fat-burning process.

The real centers of glucose breakdown are the mitochondria – small energy producing organelles located in the body's cells. Mitochondria are often referred to as the cell's furnace or power-house because their primary function is to generate energy, especially ATP. As glucose is broken down inside the mitochondria, a product called citrate is created. Citrate is then released to be broken down into other sub-units that ultimately form fat. And it's here that HCA becomes relevant.

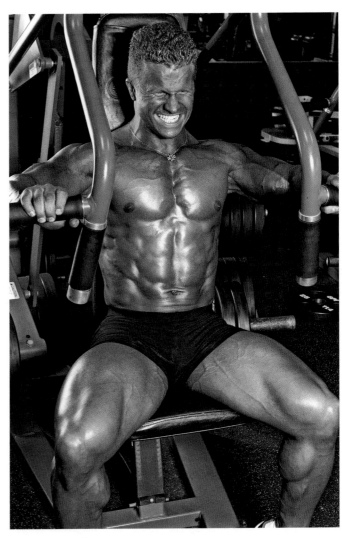

ABOVE: To effectively burn fat, you need to utilize three key principles: proper nutrition, focused training and quality supplementation.

185

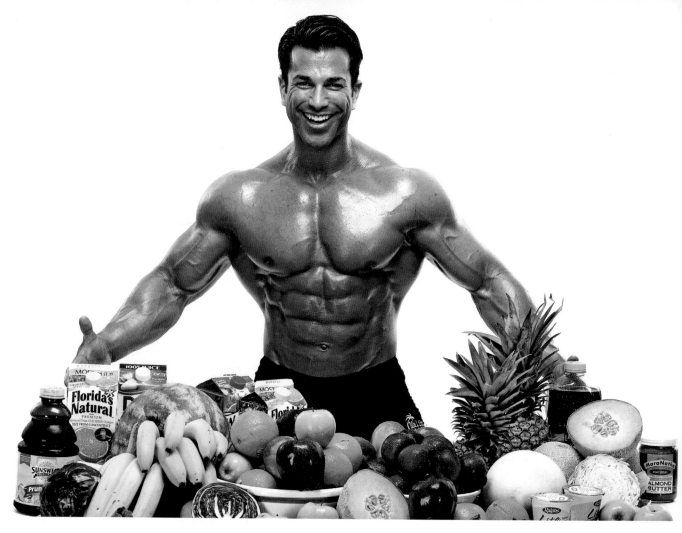

In order for citrate to be broken down, the enzyme ATP citrate lyase must be present. HCA appears to have the ability to block the actions of this enzyme and alter the body's fat and glucose metabolism in three main ways. First, the pathway for glycogen production becomes easier than conversion of glucose into fat. Second, with fat production slowed, the body begins to burn more stored fat as a fuel source. Finally, pyruvate – the enzyme that enters the mitochondria to be converted to citrate – ends up either completely burned in the citric acid cycle or gets recycled to form lactate and phosphoenolpyruvate. These two substances can also fuel the production of glucose and glycogen, and the increased glycogen supplies then get stored in the liver and muscles.

Besides the direct impact on fat burning and storage, HCA has the added benefit of suppressing appetite. After all, in the presence of HCA, the body thinks it has sufficient available energy resources so the brain decreases feelings of hunger.

The Research

Current investigations on HCA as a fat-loss product show definite promise. One three-month study conducted at Purdue University involving 89 overweight females showed that the group who used HCA lost more weight (8 pounds versus 5 pounds) than subjects given

Photo by Alex Ardenti
Model Sagi Kalev

an inert placebo.[1] Another study presented at the Experimental Biology 2002 meeting also confirmed the potential of HCA for fat loss. In that particular study, 48 subjects received either HCA or a placebo. Both groups maintained 2,000-calorie daily diets and exercised regularly. The subjects taking HCA lost almost five percent of their total weight after eight weeks. Those in the placebo group lost just less than two percent.[2]

An eight-week clinical trial published in *Nutrition Research*, a peer-review journal, revealed similar results. The study consisted of 30 participants divided into two groups. The first group received HCA, while the second group was given a placebo. The supplements were taken daily in three divided doses 30 to 60 minutes before meals. Both groups followed a diet of 2,000 calories per day and engaged in a 30-minute supervised walking program, five days a week. After the eight-week period, those taking HCA had lost over 12 pounds. By contrast, the individuals using the placebo had only lost 3 pounds.[3]

It's important to note, however, that most of the cited research on this topic involved overweight test subjects living sedentary lifestyles. There are few published studies specifically on bodybuilders who used HCA for pre-contest fat loss. In addition, most of the studies tend to be funded by companies that market HCA products. Because of this funding source, an enormous amount of pressure is put on the experimenters to "conclude" that HCA does in fact contribute to fat loss. Even the best of studies can be manipulated to create a biased outcome.

Side Effects

The lack of known side effects of HCA use is largely due to its relative newness as a fat-loss agent (the compound is less than 20 years old). While no one can unequivocally conclude whether individuals will experience issues down the road, the odds are remote that problems will arise after long-term use – HCA comes from a fruit, and compounds derived from natural foods rarely cause health problems in healthy individuals.

In general the only consistent side effect reported by users is slight stomach upset, which is fairly typical seeing as some individuals find most acid-derived compounds hard to digest. (This is why many people can't eat citrus fruit such as oranges or grapefruit on an empty stomach.) If you really want to use HCA but find it to be harsh on your stomach, you can either take the supplement with extra liquid or cut the recommended dosage of 1,000 milligrams in half. After a few weeks as your body adapts, you may be able to gradually increase the amount you take.

Using HCA

HCA is one of few products currently on the market that in theory prevents new fat formation. Most fat-loss supplements are based on

"If you're currently carrying too much weight, simply adding a fat-burning product will have little to no effect. The greatest fat-burning compound in the world will be useless if it's coupled with a bad diet."

> "Theoretically speaking, inosine should provide bodybuilders with more energy. More oxygen creates better muscle contractions which thus facilitates more productive workouts. The end result: increased muscle mass and decreased bodyfat."

188

the process of thermogenesis – when the body generates heat or energy thereby burning existing fat deposits. While this all sounds promising, keep in mind that scientific evidence to support HCA's effectiveness is quite limited.

Most HCA supplements are available as calcium salts and usually average 1,000 milligrams per serving. Anecdotal reports suggest that it produces the best results when taken about 30 to 60 minutes before meals; those with sensitive stomachs may want to take it with a small snack or copious amounts of liquid to avoid upset.

References

1) Mattes R.D., Bormann L. (2000). Effects of (-)-hydroxycitric acid on appetitive variables. *Physiology and Behavior*. 71, 87–94.
2) Preuss H.G., Bagchi, D. Sanyasi Rao, C.V., Echard B.W., Satyanaryana S. & Bagchi D. (2002). Effect of hydroxycitric acid on weight loss, body mass index and plasma leptin levels in human subjects. F*ASEB Journal*. 16, A1020.
3) Preuss H.G., Bagchi D., Bagchi M., Sanyasi Rao C.V., Satyanarayana S., & Dey, D.K. (2004). Efficacy of a novel, natural extract of (-)-hydroxycitric acid (HCA-SX) and a combination of HCA-SX, niacin-bound chromium and Gymnema sylvestre extract in weight management in human volunteers: a pilot study. *Nutrition Research*. 24, 45–58.

INOSINE

Those who read the pages of *MuscleMag International* and *Muscle and Fitness* back in the 1980s may recall articles on inosine. During those years, inosine was touted as another "natural" anabolic steroid replacer. While the claims about its muscle-building properties were grossly exaggerated, inosine does hold some merit as a fat-burning supplement.

Inosine is a nucleoside that comes from the family of molecules known as purines. Together with pyrimidines, the two make up the bases for the building blocks of DNA. First discovered in the 1840s, inosine was one of the first organic substances to be chemically isolated. Researchers initially assumed it was just another waste product of metabolism, but further investigations narrowed down its true function.

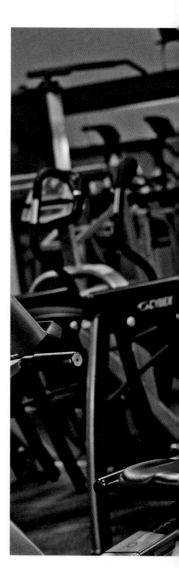

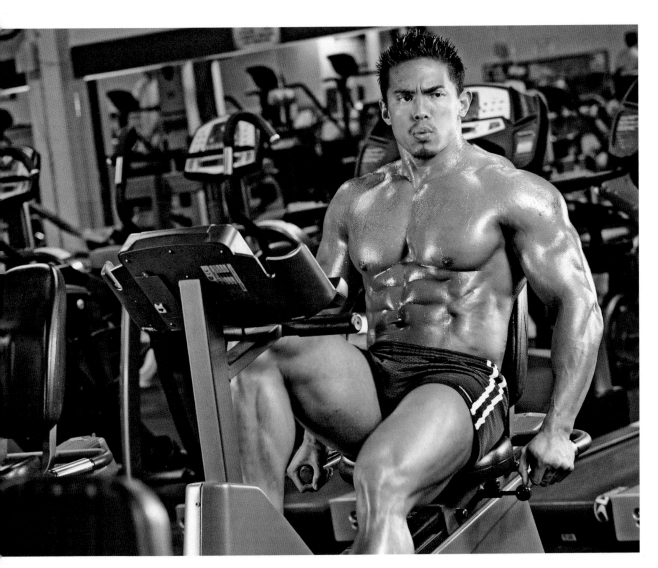

Photo by Alex Ardenti
Model Stan McQuay

ABOVE: Cardiovascular training offers many heart-healthy benefits – interestingly, inosine has been shown to generate stronger heart contractions.

Mechanism of Action

When scientists started examining the role inosine played in metabolism they uncovered a whole host of other effects. The molecule seems to have an impact on liver function, especially as it relates to enzyme regulation. They also found that inosine helps maintain ATP levels in bone marrow and enhances cardiovascular functioning. One of the most important effects on the cardiovascular system is the promotion of stronger muscle contractions in the heart. Unlike many substances, which don't seem to have much of an impact on heart function, supplementing with inosine appears to increase cardiac contractions. Numerous theories have been put

189

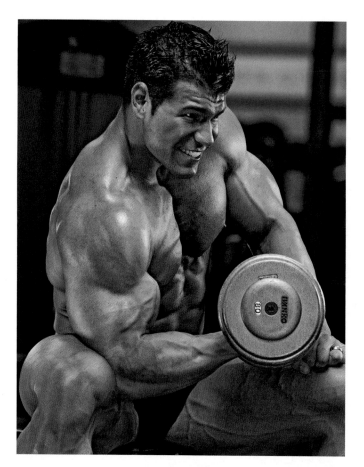

ABOVE: Bodybuilders who take inosine generally report that best results are achieved when the capsules are taken 30 minutes pre-workout.

190

forward in an effort to explain this, but the most accepted belief is that inosine can easily cross cell membranes and trigger the release of chemicals that free up more oxygen from red blood cells.

In addition to its actions on the cardiovascular system, inosine also assists carbohydrate metabolism. Again here, the process is not completely understood, but scientists believe that when ATP and oxygen levels are low, inosine can activate certain enzymes to speed up the rate at which carbohydrates are used as an energy source. And since intense exercise is a common cause of a drop in ATP and oxygen levels, it's easy to understand why the compound has received much interest in bodybuilding and other sports.

Bodybuilding Applications

Inosine received its first wave of attention in the former Soviet Union. After the Iron Curtain years, however, it was revealed that the Soviets had done quite a bit of research on natural substances to boost performance levels, as former Eastern Bloc athletes were using much more than inosine.

Most bodybuilders who use inosine report getting a "kick" during their workouts. Anecdotal evidence seems to demonstrate that the best effects are achieved when the product is taken about 30 minutes before the workout. Because there's limited available research on this supplement, it's difficult to conclude whether the boost is a result of the placebo effect or a legitimate biochemical action. Theoretically speaking, inosine should provide bodybuilders with more energy given its impact on the cardiovascular system (especially in relation to heart contractions and oxygen delivery to muscle cells). More oxygen creates better muscle contractions which thus facilitates more productive workouts. The end result: increased muscle mass and decreased bodyfat.

Administration and Dosages

When used medically, inosine is most often administered as an intramuscular injection (the standard dosage is 250 milligrams) one or two times per day. Admittedly, bodybuilders usually take more than the recommended amount, with 800 to 1,000 milligrams being their

Photo by Alex Ardenti
Model Steven Kuclo

typical dosage range. Investigations from the former Soviet Union found that Soviet athletes often took 2,000 to 4,000 milligrams of inosine per day.

When inosine became popular in North America, manufacturers released an oral version, which was made available in 500-milligram capsules. Most bodybuilders take two capsules, twice daily. Inosine is relatively inexpensive, as compared to other products, with a month's supply costing about $20.

Usage

The shortage of published research on athletes and insosine use complicates any attempt to draw firm conclusions on the supplement – instead we must again rely on anecdotal reports from users. Most bodybuilders report getting the best results when they take inosine about 30 minutes prior to working out, with the effects seemingly lasting about two to four hours. These claims are comparable to those of users who take ephedrine and caffeine supplements.

Side Effects

Since its mainstream introduction in the 1980s, inosine has received little attention for any side effects – even users who take five to 10 times the recommended dosage have reported few adverse symptoms.

Having said this, however, there is one group of individuals who should not use inosine: gout sufferers. Gout is a form of arthritis in which affected individuals either produce too much uric acid or their kidneys don't remove it fast enough. In either case the uric acid combines with sodium to form sharp, needle-like crystals that settle in the body's soft tissues causing intense pain and inflammation. The most common sites of pain for those with this condition are the big toe and along the rim of the ear.

High uric acid levels in the body can also increase a person's risk of developing kidney stones. With that in mind, those with a history of gout or kidney stones in their families should avoid using inosine.

CHOLINE

Choline is another supplement that underwent heavy promotion in bodybuilding magazines starting in the 1980s. Together with inositol, it was touted as an alternative to steroids and fat-burning drugs. Even without much scientific research to back it up, many bodybuilders swear by choline as a pre-contest fat-burning supplement.

The human body possesses the capacity to make choline, so for years nutritionists debated whether people actually needed to supplement their diets with this nutrient. In 1998, however, an expert panel was convened by the Institute of Medicine (IOM) in Washington, D.C., and they concluded that diets low in choline might be a precur-

> "The human body possesses the capacity to make choline, so for years nutritionists debated whether people actually needed to supplement their diets with it. It appears, however, that most Americans aren't getting a healthy amount."

sor to serious health problems. The IOM recommends 550 milligrams of choline per day for men and 425 milligrams per day for women to ensure adequate intake. It appears as though most Americans aren't getting a healthy amount though, as a study published in April 2005 in the *American Journal of Clinical Nutrition* discovered that average consumption in the U.S. is just 314 milligrams per day.

Natural dietary sources of phosphatidyl choline (PC) include eggs, beef liver, marine fish, soy lecithin and nuts. Free choline is found in vegetables such as cauliflower and green leafy vegetables. Small amounts are also used in processed foods, most commonly as lecithin and as an emulsifier.

Mechanism of Action

Choline is a member of the class of compounds called phosphoglycerides and is also a member of the B-complex vitamins. This nutrient is vital for many bodily functions including building cell membranes, mobilizing fat stores, decreasing cholesterol levels and increasing the liver's ability to metabolize fats. Choline also combines with fatty acids and phosphoric acid to form lecithin – one of the body's primary fat-burning compounds. Specifically with regards to the nervous system, choline boosts the integrity of myelin sheaths that cover and insulate the body's nerves. Like the plastic covering on electrical wires, myelin sheaths keep the nerves from short-circuiting (the best example being multiple sclerosis). Together with vitamin B5, choline also produces the brain transmitter acetylcholine, which facilitates muscle contractions and improves mental alertness and memory. This last function is especially noteworthy as there was a period of time in which choline was touted as a brain food and a whole cottage industry of books were published on the topic. However, the scientific community never did establish whether choline actually increased memory or just increased alertness, enabling individuals to better memorize information and thus achieve higher test scores.

Bodybuilding Applications

The body does have a certain level of ability to manufacture choline, but most needs to be consumed in the diet. Because some of its health-promoting effects specifically target the liver and kidneys – the two primary organs that can be damaged by heavy steroid use – bodybuilders on the juice may want to take choline in supplement form. The typical dosage is about 3 grams of choline and 1 gram of vitamin B5 (to help the body manufacture acetylcholine). This amount of vitamin B5 is relatively high, but reported side effects in healthy individuals are minimal even at that dosage.

"The Institute of Medicine recommends 550 milligrams of choline per day for men and 425 for women – the average consumption in the U.S. is just 314 milligrams per day."

192

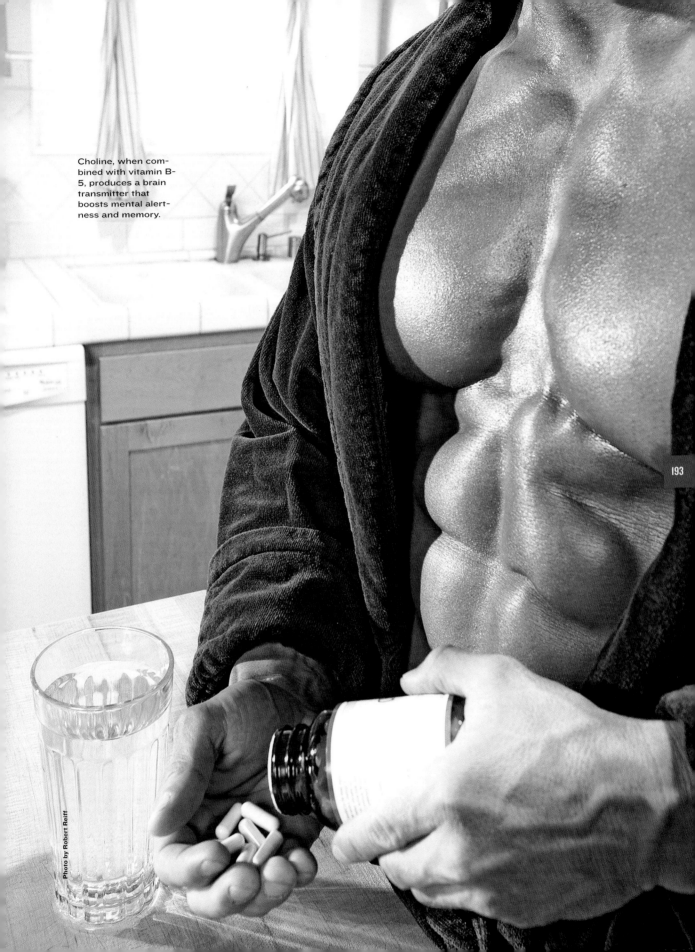

Choline, when combined with vitamin B-5, produces a brain transmitter that boosts mental alertness and memory.

193

Photo by Robert Reiff

194

INOSITOL

This compound was one of the first discovered that seemed to play a role in fat metabolism. When the human body is deficient in inositol, fat can accumulate in the liver. And while some people consider it a vitamin, inositol is not essential in the human diet and the body can manufacture it, which means it can't be considered a true vitamin.

Inositol is necessary for the formation of lecithin, and as such, functions closely with choline. Inositol is also a fundamental component of cell membranes and is necessary for proper functioning of the nerves, brain and muscles. To prevent the buildup of fat in the liver, inositol works in conjunction with folacin, vitamins B-6 and B-12, choline, betaine and methionine. This compound also exists as the fiber component phytic acid, which has been investigated for its cancer-preventing properties.

Specifically with respect to medical conditions, inositol is primarily used to treat liver problems, depression, panic disorder and diabetes. It also aids in the breakdown of fats and helps reduce blood cholesterol. From a psychological standpoint, inositol is an important compound, as brain neurotransmitters such as seratonin depend on it to function properly. Low levels of this nutrient may result in depression and some research has demonstrated that increased levels of inositol appear to be a promising treatment for depression. A final area of study on inositol concerns its anti-cancer properties in relation to diet. Certain research has demonstrated that because fiber is abundant with inositol, this may in part explain why populations with high-fiber diets often have a lower incidence of certain cancers.

As far as health benefits go, inositol seems to be a vital nutrient that positively contributes to numerous body systems. But for all the promise it holds as a treatment for depression and high blood cholesterol, and as a potential anti-cancer compound, inositol loses all scientific credibility when it comes to fat loss. It got a lot promotion as a fat-loss product, but that was just because supplement manufacturers capitalized on the fact that it plays a role in fat metabolism. When you get down to the actual science though, no proof exists to confirm that taking extra amounts will increase the body's fat-burning abilities. If you're deficient to begin with, then taking inositol would be an obvious choice to raise levels, but for those following healthy eating practices, there are more proven fat-burning compounds to use.

CARNITINE

Carnitine was discovered by Russian scientists in the early 1900s – now you'd think a compound with a history spanning over 100 years would be classified long ago, but such is not the case. Some biochemists consider it a member of the B-complex vitamins. Others categorize it strictly as a nutrient. Still others in the science field

"Many experts have suggested that carnitine does not in fact increase the rate at which fat is shed, but rather could improve the fat-to-muscle-loss ratio by preserving muscle mass during periods of increased cardio and strict dieting."

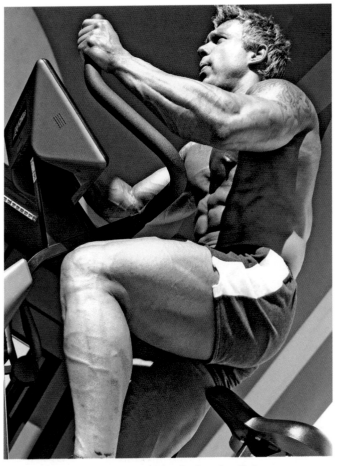

LEFT: Even when following a demanding cardio regimen, many bodybuilders seek a fat-burning supplement to aid their training efforts.

195

place carnitine in the amino acid family (but classify it as a nonessential amino acid because our bodies can naturally produce it).

Carnitine has been labeled a fat burner because it's required to transfer fatty acids across cell membranes into mitochondria. It accomplishes this by activating an enzyme called carnitine acyltransferase (CAT1), which then transfers the fatty acyl group of the fat molecule to the hydroxyl group of the carnitine molecule. This new complex crosses the membrane only to get broken apart by another enzyme called acyltransferase (CAT2). The end result of this complex process is ATP.

Carnitine has received a great deal of attention in the weight-loss industry and among competitive bodybuilders because of its impact on fatty acids and role in creating ATP. Many experts, however, have suggested that carnitine does not in fact increase the rate at which fat is shed, but rather could improve the fat-to-muscle-loss ratio by preserving muscle mass during periods of increased cardio exercise and strict dieting. Research also suggests that if carnitine levels are not optimal in our bodies, the amount of fats in the bloodstream may be higher, which could then actually interfere with the burning of existing bodyfat.

Despite what supplement companies would have you believe, there just isn't the research to support carnitine as a potent fat burner. Some studies have demonstrated that a carnitine deficiency may result in lower ATP levels – because carnitine turnover is increased during exercise, such a shortage could impede the energy available to muscles. Under these conditions, a rapid onset of fatigue and subsequent compromised recovery would result. With these findings in mind, recent research on fat burners has revealed that individuals who supplement with carnitine while engaging in intense exercise programs are less likely to experience muscle soreness and fatigue than those who do not.

Most anecdotal reports indicate that for the purposes of fat loss and increased energy during exercise, about 2,000 to 4,000 milligrams (usually divided into two dosages per day) is optimal.

BELOW: Despite what supplement companies advertise, no product can replace a proper training program.

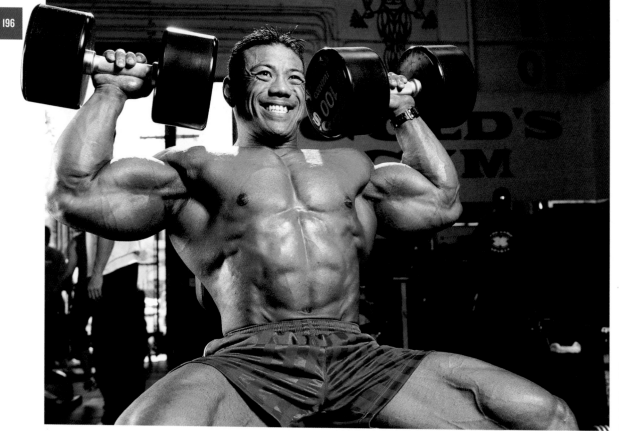

196

CHITOSAN

You have to give the supplement companies credit for their strategic marketing of chitosan. The ads for this supplement make it appear to be some sort of miracle cure for fat loss, and chitosan has quickly become extremely popular as a fat burner among those seeking a quick fix for weight loss. Most of the marketing caters toward those who want to eat like crap and still lose bodyfat. Advertisers claim you can chow down on foods like pizza, deep-fried chicken and doughnuts, and then take chitosan to counteract any storage of fat. Some of the claims got so outrageous that the FTC had to step in and set guidelines to deter companies from using such marketing.

Chitosan is a fibrous compound derived from the shells of marine animals such as crab and shrimp. Upon entering the stomach chitosan turns into a gelatinous substance, which then acts as a fat burner and attracts fat like a strong magnet. Chitosan functions in this manner because it's positively charged while most fats are negatively charged – the laws of physics apply, as the two naturally have a strong attraction to each other.

In theory this tight bond of fat and chitosan means they'll travel as a unit through the digestive system and be eliminated from the body. Chitosan is said to attract three to six times its weight in fats as it passes through the digestive tract, thereby causing less ingested fat to be stored. So while it's not a true fat burner, this supplement facilitates weight loss by preventing new fat cells from attaching to existing deposits.

Is this magic supplement too good to be true? In a word – probably. While chitosan has been shown in studies to bond to fat and lower levels of blood fats (i.e., triglycerides), it doesn't appear to have a notable impact when it comes to actual fat loss – at least according to findings from human research. Of even greater importance is that this fat burner has been proven to leach vital nutrients including fat-soluble vitamins and essential fatty acids from the body. It seems chitosan can't distinguish between fat molecules – whether they're unwanted saturated fats or essential fatty acids and fat-based vitamins. Finally, as unpleasant as the thought of this may be, you have to consider what happens to all the unabsorbed fat when it binds to chitosan and moves through the body. Many users have reported cases of diarrhea that rival the worst stomach and intestinal flu bugs. Those considering the supplement have to decide whether it's worth going through all that bodily torment with no guarantee that chitosan is really helping you lose bodyfat.

PYRUVATE

Pyruvate (also known as pyruvic acid) is a chemical compound formed by the breakdown of glucose during glycolysis – one of the

> "Most of the marketing [for chitosan] caters toward those who want to eat like crap and still lose bodyfat. Is this magic supplement too good to be true? In a word – probably."

197

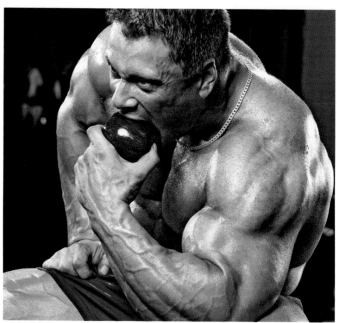

RIGHT: An apple a day keeps the doctor away, and the red varieties may help your fat-loss efforts.

198

Photo by Robert Reiff
Model Mark Erpelding

pathways the body uses to generate energy and make ATP. Essentially, the process starts with a glucose molecule. A sequence of reactions then occurs, and the output of this series of metabolic steps is pyruvate. ATP (energy) is formed during the process.

Though it can be generated by the body, pyruvate also occurs naturally in certain foods – fruits and vegetables contain the greatest amounts. Red apples, for example, are one of the best sources as each has a concentration of approximately 500 milligrams of pyruvate. Whole-food sources, however, contain much less pyruvate than you'd find in supplements.

Despite the fact that pyruvate's "15 minutes of fame" seems to have come and gone, it has the potential to again become popular as a fat-loss aid. More recent research on fat loss indicates that supplementation may be beneficial for individuals who wish to lose weight. There is evidence that pyruvate may help boost resting metabolic rate and improve the body's use of fuel – both ATP and blood sugar. The one area of contention, however, is exactly how much is needed to optimize these fat-loss effects. Study dosages range from as little as 6 grams to a very high 30 grams per day.

Pyruvate's fat-burning effects seem closely linked with its potential to increase resting metabolic rate. In simple terms, more fat is used as an energy source, thus speeding up metabolic rate. This in turn means more calories are burned throughout the day – even if you're fairly sedentary (that's why it's so appealing to couch potatoes). But keep in mind that most of the noted studies demonstrating fat loss used dosages that are too high to be considered safe for daily consumption.

Unfortunately for consumers, there is no solid evidence to back up the marketing claims of pyruvate. Although early animal studies using rats did show that pyruvate increased resting metabolism, the same results have never been confirmed with human subjects. In fact, in a recently published study on the compound, the group of people who did not receive pyruvate actually had a higher resting metabolism at the end of the study than those who did receive the pyruvate!

Until more conclusive research is available, all we can say is that pyruvate is another questionable fat-loss product that *may* hold promise. It's relatively cheap to purchase and is generally safe, so experimenting with it isn't overly risky – don't be surprised though if the results fall short of your expectations.

5-HTP (5-HYDROXYTRYPTOPHAN)

5-HTP is naturally derived from seeds of the West African Griffonia simplicifolia plant. It is also made in the body from the amino acid tryptophan. 5-HTP is a precursor to serotonin – a neurotransmitter that signals our brains to feel "happy and content." Among 5-HTP's main functions are to induce sleep and fight depression. Although not usually considered a fat-loss supplement, in recent years it's been marketed to help decrease cravings for sweets and other carbohydrates. This type of promotion helped 5-HTP make a quick jump onto the labels of numerous fat-loss products. With regards to weight gain, it's been suggested that many individuals add fat because their bodies have a decreased conversion rate of tryptophan to 5-HTP, and therefore have lower levels of serotonin. By providing the body with 5-HTP, serotonin levels increase and essentially turn off those feelings of hunger.

In a similar fashion, 5-HTP is also believed to cause a feeling of fullness earlier when you eat. Simply put, you'll feel like you ate a big meal before you actually do. This premature sense of satiety will result in less eating. This effect makes 5-HTP beneficial for people who have a difficult time controlling how much they eat, specifically high-sugar and carbohydrate foods.

While there is no debate that low serotonin levels can increase cravings for high-sugar foods, the jury is still out as to whether 5-HTP can or should be used by bodybuilders to drop bodyfat. To date, most studies have been conducted on obese women who tended to have poor eating habits to begin with. This data is incongruent with the lifestyle of bodybuilders – most guys in the sport have no problem following a healthy eating plan. They also probably don't need a compound that could decrease their appetites. Individuals need to remember that the key to real fat loss is not so much decreasing calo-

> "There is evidence that pyruvate may help boost resting metabolic rate and improve the body's use of ATP and blood sugar. The area of concentration is exactly how much is needed to optimize fat loss. Study dosages range from as little as 6 grams to a very high 30 grams per day."

199

> "The large-scale gravitation toward green tea isn't simply because it has a nice flavor when prepared – scientific data defends some astounding benefits when it's used as a supplement for immune system enhancement and fat-burning."

rie intake as it is consuming the right type of calories and increasing cardio exercise. For a 350-pound obese person trying to curb his or her appetite in an effort to shed a couple of hundred pounds, 5-HTP may hold promise. Conversely, given the current research, this supplement probably won't offer much benefit to competitive bodybuilders trying to get cut for a contest. For those who do decide to try 5-HTP though, reports confer that optimal dosages range from 50 to 300 milligrams per day, one to three times daily before meals. Of note is that the amounts used in the weight-loss studies were 700 to 900 milligrams.

GUGGULIPID (GUGGULSTERONES)

Guggulipid is a resin (yellowish sap) that comes from the bark of the Commiphora mukul. This plant sterol (containing guggulsterones) is currently being marketed as the latest, greatest fat-loss compound. The broken record about lack of evidence, however, must play again here. There just simply isn't the founded research to back the grand claims made by supplement manufacturers. This doesn't necessarily mean guggulipid is an entirely useless supplement – solid medical data demonstrates that it can in fact lower circulating levels of LDL (bad) cholesterol.

Animal studies conducted using guggulsterones suggest that the plant sterol works by enhancing thyroid functioning. As you'll recall, the thyroid gland produces hormones required to regulate metabolism. The presence of gugglsterones in the system may change thyroid hormone metabolism by elevating levels of circulating T3 (triiodothyroxine). In theory this should help the body burn significantly more fat, but the results have yet to be observed in any human studies.

While there is limited evidence that guggulsterones may lower bodyfat accumulation, the data is much more promising with respect to the compound's effects on the cardiovascular system. Numerous studies have found that supplementing with guggulsterone products can lower LDL and triglyceride levels in the bloodstream.[1]

You may want to consider adding guggulipid to your supplement regimen, given its beneficial cholesterol-lowering properties (and low cost and relative safety). Again, just don't expect any profound loss of bodyfat with this supplement.

GREEN TEA

For those history buffs out there, the earliest reference to green tea dates back some 4,000 years ago. The tea has come quite a long way since the ancient days when it was reserved only for emperors and the Chinese elite. This popular beverage has become one of the most sought after products for millions of individuals seeking greater health and weight control. The large-scale gravitation toward green tea isn't simply because it has a nice flavor when prepared; scientific data defends some astounding benefits when it's used as a supplement for immune system enhancement and fat burning. New evidence has demonstrated that green tea may help the body burn calories at a faster rate; that's why it shows up on the ingredient list of a growing number of fat-loss products.[2]

Green tea (specifically the polyphenols in the leaves) appear to stimulate the body's thermogenic mechanisms, thereby promoting the use of calories as energy. Polyphenols also seem to promote growth of natural viral killer immune cells, which scavenge and destroy bacteria and flush out toxins. This group of chemical substances may in addition protect our bodies from the free radicals that damage cells and weaken our immune systems. This function is especially important for active people because intense exercise has actual-

BELOW: The ancient Chinese may not have known that the active ingredient was polyphenols in the leaves, but green tea has been used for thousands of years as a therapeutic drink.

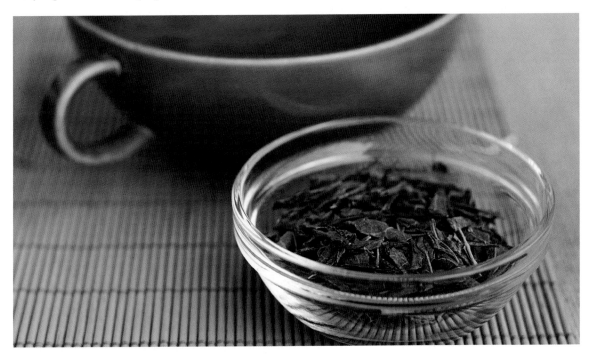

ly been linked to increased production of free radicals in the body.

Green tea also contains caffeine – a proven thermogenic compound. Unlike the older ephedrine-based products, green tea doesn't cause the same degree of nervous system stimulation – a feature that makes it an ideal fat-loss supplement alternative for those who are sensitive to thermogenic compounds with stimulant properties.

Most research on green tea suggests that maximal benefits are achieved by taking 300 to 600 milligrams each day with meals, and

201

that amount should contain up to 97% polyphenol concentrate. (Mathematically this works out to about four cups of tea per day.)

CHROMIUM

Chromium is another nutritional product that owes its origins to legitimate medical science, namely diabetes research. This essential trace mineral plays a vital role in the body to metabolize carbohydrates. Chromium seems to work by aiding insulin as it shuttles nutrients, especially sugar, from the blood into cells.

Certain reports suggest that nearly 25 million Americans may be borderline deficient in chromium. This number is frightening from a health perspective because not having enough of this mineral could be a main contributor to insulin resistance (diabetes), obesity and hypoglycemia (low blood sugar). Such medical conditions are reaching almost epidemic proportions in Western societies; it's for this reason that chromium has more recently become popular as a supplemental aid for bodyweight control and insulin regulation.

While scientists have yet to deconstruct exactly how chromium helps regulate blood sugar, a few theories have been presented. One hypothesizes that chromium binds both to the cell and the insulin molecule, thereby attracting blood sugar more efficiently. Under that framework of thinking, chromium essentially works as an insulin "helper."

Another theory suggests that chromium may decrease the extraction rate of insulin and improve glucose tolerance. This means the mineral helps insulin and glucose work together more efficiently. There is research to support that glucose tolerance can be restored in chromium-deficient patients when given a diet rich in chromium. In fact, millions of borderline diabetics avoid being dependent on insulin needles by supplementing their diets with chromium tablets.

With regards to chromium's specific ability to decrease bodyfat in healthy individuals, the efficacy is less clear. While anecdotal evidence among bodybuilders is generally favorable, the medical evidence is mixed. Some studies indicate that chromium users experience weight loss, while other investigations have observed just the opposite! Theoretically, a compound that helps regulate insulin should play a role in preventing new fat storage; such a function, however, is probably limited only to individuals who are chromium deficient to begin with. Healthy individuals with normal chromium and insulin levels likely won't experience much benefit from taking this mineral supplement.

For the purpose of supplementing, the suggested dosage is about 400 to 600 micrograms daily. To obtain the full benefits, chromium should be taken with meals, particularly those including carbohydrate-containing foods.

"It is one of the most vital substances in our food, yet even nutritionist-devised diets rarely include the minimum amounts, and the sugar we're so fond of depletes what little chromium we do get, contributing to fatigue, obesity and many diseases. Unfortunately chromium deficiency causes fatigue and excess fat production, and is also a major contributor to heart disease and diabetes."
– Dwayne Hines II, *Musclemag International* contributor

CLA - CONJUGATED LINOLEIC ACID

Though it may sound ironic, CLA is a member of the trans fat family used by millions of individuals for its fat-loss potential. Over two decades of research has shown that CLA may help to significantly reduce bodyfat. There's also good evidence in favor of its ability to increase muscle tissue synthesis. And it's not just the general public who are reaping its benefits – bodybuilders and athletes have recently begun supplementing with CLA because it can shift body composition to favor fat loss and muscle gain.

At a biochemical level, conjugated linoleic acid (CLA) is a naturally occurring free fatty acid primarily found in meat and dairy products such as milk, cheese, beef and lamb. It can also be found in certain processed foods, one example of which is Cheez Whiz (but of course, we wouldn't recommend eating spoonfuls just to get your CLA given the huge calorie penalty you'd pay).

Considering the importance of CLA to general health, you'd think food-processing companies would be taking every measure possible to ensure high levels were present in the foods we eat. Unfortunately, manufacturers don't share this thinking. Some sources, in fact, actually have less CLA than a few decades ago. The best example comes from the dairy industry: Grazing cattle and sheep have internal microorganisms that produce CLA, but because most cattle no longer graze, they consequently produce less of these acids. Studies at Utah State University have shown that grazing cattle have 500 percent more CLA in their milk and 300 to 400 percent more in their meat than non-grazing animals. And in general, cattle raised today have only about one-third the levels measured in 1960. That means in order to get the recommended amount from the meat and dairy products of non-grazing animals you'd have to consume three pounds of

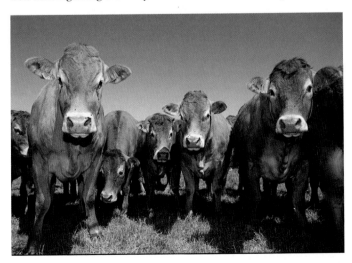

LEFT: Because so few cattle actually graze these days, they produce much less CLA – and thus we get less in the milk we drink.

hamburger, 25 slices of cheese, or a half-gallon of ice cream. While this may sound tantalizing to your taste buds, all that extra fat certainly wouldn't do your arteries and heart any favors.

Bodybuilding Benefits

Research on CLA has revealed its central function in the conversion of fat into lean muscle tissue. It's no wonder this supplement is so sought after by bodybuilders and other strength athletes. Other studies have found that while CLA doesn't appear to decrease the size of large fat cells already in existence, it does effectively inhibit the enlargement of small fat cells. CLA also seems to accelerate fat burning in skeletal muscle. All of these points seem to classify CLA as more of a lean muscle builder than solely a fat burner. Studies carried out by Dr. Michael Pariza at the University of Wisconsin Food Research Institute observed that individuals who stopped dieting and regained weight while supplementing with CLA experienced mostly muscle increases and not fat gains.

Research on the specific fat-burning relationship makes it worthy of a more in-depth discussion. Some scientists believe that CLA has the ability to modulate insulin sensitivity. Most readers are probably aware that insulin is one of the body's most anabolic hormones. Stabilized insulin levels facilitate the transport of fatty acids and glucose into muscle cells and away from fat tissue.

Other researchers have hypothesized that the properties of CLA specific to altering body composition are likely part and parcel of its ability to regulate fat metabolism. The process by which this occurs is complex and involves specific enzymes, namely lipoprotein lipase and hormone-sensitive lipase. CLA appears to not only block fat uptake but also speed up the rate of fat burning. In one study, 60 overweight people (who were not allowed to diet during the study period) were randomly assigned to take either a placebo of nine grams of olive oil or 1.7 grams, 3.4 grams, 5.1 grams, or 6.8 grams of CLA daily for 12 weeks. Their body compositions were measured at the start, midpoint and end of the study. The CLA groups lost a significant amount of bodyfat with the group who took 6.8 grams losing over two pounds of bodyfat in 12 weeks. These results are all the more interesting because the participants didn't alter their exercise or diet habits.

In another study, test subjects were measured for bodyfat and bodyweight over a three-month period. The first group took CLA at breakfast, lunch and dinner and the second group took a placebo, also at meal times. At the end of the study duration, the CLA group had lost an average of five pounds, which worked out to an impressive 15- to 20-percent decrease, whereas the placebo group experienced little quantifiable change.

A final notable investigation was one that compared the effects of CLA with CLA plus guarana (a natural source of caffeine). While the standard CLA group experienced a dramatic reduction in the size of

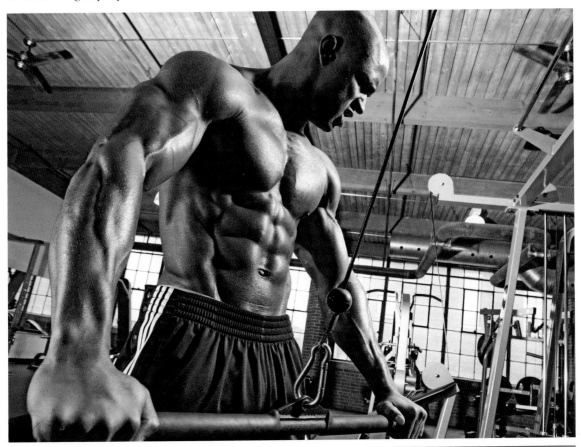

their fat cells, the CLA plus guarana group had a 50-percent decrease in total number of fat cells in just six weeks. It may seem logical then to combine CLA with straight coffee, but the researchers point out that the caffeine in most drinks only has a short-lived effect. Guarana on the other hand functions with extended release, thus providing benefits for many hours.

As there is no known toxicity with CLA, most researchers recommend about 3,000 milligrams (three grams) divided into three dosages per day with meals for fat reduction. However, a slightly higher range of 3,000 to 6,000 milligrams (three to six grams) split into three daily dosages with meals has recently been shown to help induce muscle-tissue growth. And we're not talking years of use here either – most of the data notes fat loss and muscle gains after four to eight weeks of CLA supplementing.

"This is incredible stuff, and it clearly warrants the superstar status given by the healthcare community. CLA supplementation is definitely a major step in the right direction to building a body you'd be proud to have."

– Dr. George Redmond, *Musclemag International* contributor

Photo by Paul Buceta
Model Reggie McKee

GUARANA

Guarana is an herb that's native to the Amazon rainforest in Brazil. Among its phytochemicals are guaranine, a compound that's virtually identical to caffeine. It has been used for centuries by various South American cultural groups to help reduce hunger, relieve fatigue and treat obesity. While it may be a valuable aid for promoting short bursts of energy (another reason that so many bodybuilders drink coffee before an intense workout), this herb has a specific aspect that makes it a "natural" choice for effective fat loss: Guarana possesses the ability to increase fatty acid levels in the bloodstream and break down and mobilize these fat cells for use as an energy source.

Similar to caffeine, guarana primarily works by stimulating the adrenal glands to release the hormones epinephrine, norepinephrine and dopamine. Once released these compounds increase the body's thermogenic mechanisms so fatty acids get used for energy production (not to mention increased endurance and cognitive abilities). Contrary to popular belief, these effects can be obtained without the often-cited negative side effects. Nevertheless, guarana does have mild diuretic properties, so increasing your water intake is very important when using this compound (yet another reason that caffeine and guarana are popular as pre-contest supplements).

One study involving 44 overweight individuals using guarana found that those taking the compound for 45 days lost an average of five kilograms (or about 11 pounds). This weight loss was considered significant as the placebo group only lost an average of 0.45 kilograms (approximately one pound). Also worth noting was that the guarana group experienced a delay in their gastric emptying by 20 minutes, meaning a longer feeling of fullness after eating a meal.

When you consider its reasonable price and almost identical action to caffeine, guarana could fairly easily be used in place of caffeine in the ECA stack. In fact, since the effects of this herb last a few

RIGHT: If you choose to include guarana in your fat-loss game plan, make sure to top up your water intake as it's a diuretic herb.

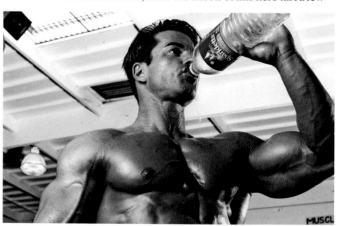

Photo by Irvin Gelb
Model Sagi Kalev

hours longer than that of caffeine, it may be a better option. Dosages are slightly higher with guarana as compared to caffeine – most reports suggest anywhere from 500 to 1,000 milligrams taken up to three times per day.

BITTER ORANGE

Citrus aurantium, commonly called bitter orange, has been used for thousands of years in traditional Chinese medicine to improve overall health. Over the past decade or so, scientists have discovered that compounds from the extract of these fruits appear to have powerful thermogenic properties. The most promising of these is synephrine, which is a substance that's gained a great deal of attention because of its similarity to ephedrine. But unlike ephedrine, synephrine increases the body's metabolic rate (or ability to burn calories), without producing the same degree of side effects on the central nervous and cardiovascular systems.

Synephrine also appears to reduce appetite much like ephedra, but again without the likelihood of side effects. This is because citrus aurantium also contains chemicals called amines, which do not cross the blood-brain barrier as easily as ephedra. Therefore, users of bitter orange will probably be spared from side effects such as the jitters, elevated heart rate or insomnia.

According to recent findings from McGill University (Montreal, Canada), another reason bitter orange causes a steady flow of energy without the jitters is because it stimulates beta-3 adrenergic receptors that help break down fat. Therefore, you're burning fat without stimulating beta-1, beta-2 or alpha-1 receptors, which play a prominent role in elevating heart rate and blood pressure. In contrast, ephedra stimulates virtually all such receptors, causing adverse symptoms as a result. These factors (and the fact that ephedrine is now banned) are the reason bitter orange is now used as a replacement for CNS stimulants in many thermogenic formulas.

Most research and anecdotal reports recommend 20 milligrams of synephrine per day, which usually provides 200 to 600 milligrams of a standardized citrus aurantium extract.

References

1) Badmaev V., *et al.* (2003). Standardization of Commiphora mukul extract in dislipidemia and cardiovascular disease. *Nutrafoods.* 2(2):45–51.
2) Dulloo A.G., Duret, C., Rohrer D., Girardier L., Mensi N., Fathi M., Chantre P., Vandermander J. (1999). Efficacy of a green tea extract rich in catechin polyphenols and caffeine in increasing 24-hour energy expenditure and fat oxidation in humans. *American Journal of Clinical Nutrition.* Dec:70(6):1040–5.

"Scientists have discovered that compounds from the extracts of bitter orange have powerful properties. The most promising of these is synephrine, which has gained a great deal of attention because of its similarity to ephedrine. But synephrine increases metabolism without the same degree of side effects on the central nervous and cardiovascular systems."

207

STIMULANTS

B4

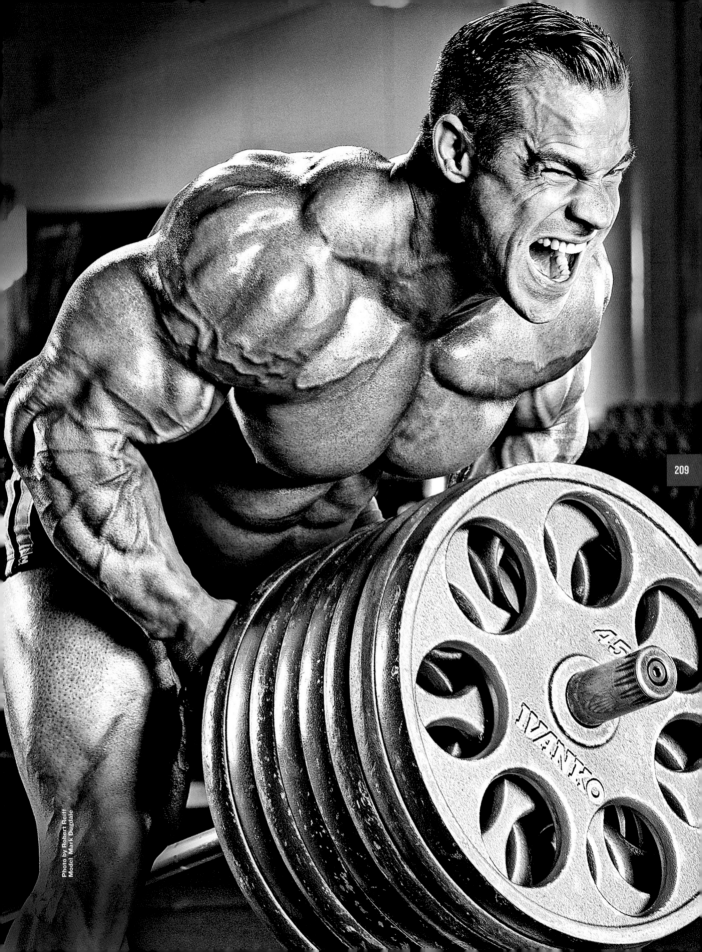

209

INTRODUCTION

Stimulants are one of the oldest types of performance-enhancing drugs, with use dating back thousands of years. Even athletes in the first Olympic Games held in Greece were known to have taken stimulants. More recent decades have seen these substances explode in popularity with everyone from bodybuilders and sprinters to truck drivers and college students choosing them as a pick-me-up method.

For bodybuilders, the extra cardio and strict dieting that characterize the pre-contest season can make getting to the gym and completing a workout a tiresome endeavor. Even with a dedicated training partner who's motivated to kick you in the ass, you'll still have days when even the thought of lifting a weight will make you tired. To combat this workout sluggishness many bodybuilders look to stimulants, of which a top choice is caffeine. Some individuals even consider caffeine to be a near-perfect stimulant: it's cheap, legal and relatively free of side effects (provided you don't abuse the drug). For every caffeine lover though, there's also a hater. Some athletes think caffeine is too "wimpy" and instead favor nothing but the granddaddy of all stimulants, amphetamines. And while this demographic is quite small, there are even a few questionable characters who hit the iron while under the influence of cocaine. When you factor in the legal status of these three stimulants, one might wonder why anyone would opt for anything other than caffeine – it's not banned, but amphetamines and cocaine will surely get you serious jail time. The latter two substances could also end up killing you if used improperly.

The next three chapters will focus on the more popular stimulants used by bodybuilders. Where applicable, the legal implications of these drugs will be discussed. Before you continue to Chapter 23, take a few minutes and read the eight commandments of stimulant use.

THE EIGHT COMMANDMENTS OF STIMULANT USE

1) Check the drug's legal status. Any discussion of a certain compound in this book doesn't automatically mean it's legal in your country. And

remember, a drug that is legal today might be reclassified tomorrow.

2) Try to buy stimulants from a reliable source. The further into a back alley you go, the greater your risks of buying counterfeit drugs. You also gamble with meeting some shady and dangerous dealers.

3) Limit your frequency of use. Stimulants are among the easiest drugs to become addicted to. The more you use the less effective these substances become. Before you know it that one ephedrine tablet grows to five or six, and the negative side effects start to kick in and magnify. If possible, cap your stimulant use at no more than two days in a row. At the first sign your body isn't coping, stop and seek help.

4) Stick to low dosages. The risk of addiction and side effects tends to be related to the amounts used.

5) Oral use is less risky. Smoking, injecting or snorting stimulants tends to cause a very rapid release of the drug into the bloodstream. This produces a faster "rush," but also predisposes a more severe crash later. And a vicious cycle is often created because some people try to avoid the crash by taking more of the drug.

6) Stay focused on your reasons for use. While occasionally using a stimulant to get through a tough workout is one thing, popping pills just to wake up or perform your daily activities is a short-cut to addiction. In fact, if you're using just to get through the day-to-day, you're probably already addicted.

7) Don't mix stimulants with drugs such as alcohol and other depressants. Some individuals start catering their lives to drugs, using certain ones as an "on switch" in the morning and others as an "off switch" at night. Elvis Presley was a classic example; John Belushi was also reported to have relied on some wonderful mixtures – their respective fates speak volumes about the dangers of stimulant abuse.

8) Be a bodybuilder, not an addict. Eat, train and sleep regularly. Aim for natural health and fitness as much as possible. Stimulants will only tax your body in the long run because your nervous system can only handle continuous stimulation for so long.

"The extra cardio and dieting that characterized the pre-contest season can make getting to the gym and completing a workout a tiresome endeavor. Even with a dedicated workout partner who's motivated to kick you in the ass, you'll still have days when even the thought of lifting a weight will make you tired."

211

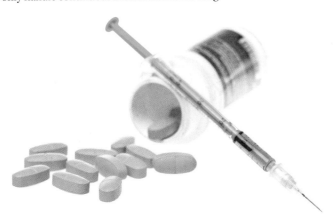

LEFT: Stimulants are popular among many bodybuilders, but there are numerous factors to consider depending on the types and forms.

CAFFEINE

With all due respect to the tea drinkers out there, coffee is one of the most popular beverages in the world. For many individuals, the day just can't begin until that first cup of java is brewing in the pot. Coffee has become so engrained in the lives of North Americans that most labor unions have mandatory coffee breaks written into their collective agreements.

It only makes sense that a drink so globally enjoyed has an equally as vibrant and colorful history. Although most historical data attributes the discovery of coffee to Ethiopian goat herders and its early promotion to trade with Muslims in Yemen, Egypt and North Africa, other theories of its origins exist. There is evidence to support that numerous cultural groups around the world were using coffee long before its introduction in the Muslim world.

The first European country to import coffee from the Muslims was Italy. Although coffee drinking was viewed as a Muslim and pagan practice at the end of the 1500s, the beverage was quick to be "baptized" by the Catholic Church after, as the legend goes, Pope Clement VIII supposedly got hooked on it.

During the first half of the 17th century, coffeehouses started to pop up across Europe in countries like Italy, England, France and Austria. These early coffee establishments quickly became popular meeting places for writers, scientists, philosophers and politicians. After Charles II (King of England) got word of serious anti-crown talk being conducted in coffeehouses, however, he immediately had them shut down. The English population didn't take too kindly to such actions, and with the threat of rioting in the air, the coffee pots were once again brewing just 11 days later.

The plants are grown throughout various regions of the world, but today, most coffee beans come from Latin America and the industry is worth billions of dollars to South American countries. Certain brands have become staple-like and such companies as Folgers, Maxwell House, Sanka and Nescafé have made themselves household names. But no matter what type of coffee you prefer, the main ingredient is the same across the board: caffeine. And while certain soft

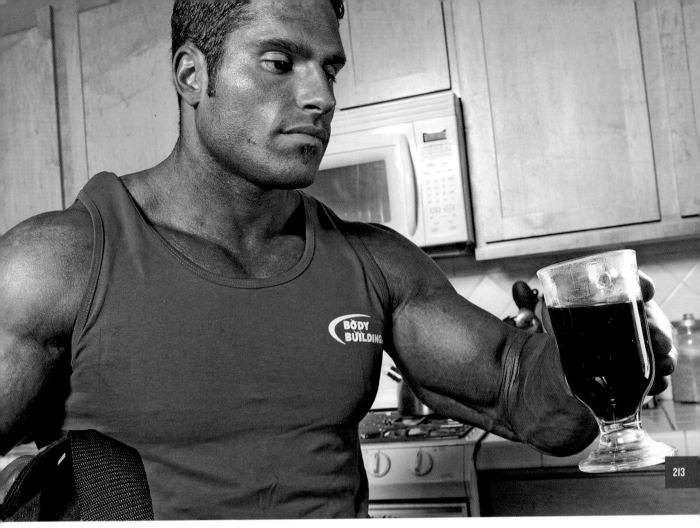

Photo by Robert Reiff
Model | David Hoffman

drinks and teas may be similar to java in caffeine content, the coffee bean is still the most popular source for that much-sought-after caffeine jolt.

ABOVE: For many, the day can't start without a steaming cup of coffee; for many bodybuilders, a workout just isn't the same with the stimulant effects of pre-training caffeine.

MECHANISM OF ACTION

Though you can find coffee on almost every street corner, caffeine is still a drug. It can cause a wide spectrum of effects that vary from one person to another. Some users will develop the jitters, anxiousness and insomnia after drinking just one cup of coffee (which contains about 150 milligrams of caffeine). Other java lovers need three or four cups to fully wake up in the morning, and can drink it right up to bedtime. When caffeine has such a mild effect on individuals, a combination of tolerance and drug insensitivity is probably explaining the situation.

Despite the occasional report of how "relaxing" coffee makes someone feel, caffeine is classified as a stimulant, and its primary action is to increase central nervous system activity. It does this by producing a number of physiological responses including elevated heart rate and blood pressure, increased stomach acid and dilated blood vessels. Caffeine also has thermogenic properties and can thus speed up the rate at which fat reserves are mobilized for use as an energy source. Since the government ban on ephedrine, caffeine has

> "Though you can find coffee on almost every street corner, caffeine is still a drug. It can cause a wide spectrum of effects that vary from one person to another. Some users develop jitters, anxiety and insomnia after just one cup. Other java lovers need three or four cups to fully wake up in the morning."

become one of the most popular ingredients in weight-loss products. Unfortunately for consumers, however, what supplement manufacturers fail to mention is that tolerance to caffeine develops quickly, making it a poor solution for long-term weight control.

BODYBUILDING APPLICATIONS

Of all the effects associated with caffeine use, the two considered most imperative by bodybuilders are the fat-burning and stimulant characteristics. It's rare these days to see even one hardcore bodybuilder arrive at the gym without a cup of coffee in hand. This observation is especially true in the weeks and months leading up to a contest, when regimented dieting and additional cardio can place enormous energy demands on the body. Sometimes that single cup of coffee is the only thing that gets the individual through the workout.

And while its stimulant effects are a key feature, bodybuilders have also gravitated toward caffeine for its diuretic properties. It's no secret that caffeine will increase urine output. Like many naturally occurring diuretics, caffeine interferes with the body's water-conserving systems. While endurance athletes will no doubt want to avoid coffee for this reason alone, bodybuilders find it particularly helpful when trying to shed those extra few pounds of water before a competition.

One of the least-touted effects of caffeine is increased strength levels. While the exact mechanism of action is unknown, it could be the stimulant properties of caffeine that cause strength improvements; theories also suggest that perhaps caffeine has some direct effect on muscle fiber contraction. Whatever the root cause, bodybuilders and strength athletes the world over take advantage of it, no questions asked.

In recent years, marketing campaigns have put a new spin on caffeine – as a thermogenic, or fat-loss, compound. This stimulant has always been part of the famous ECA stack (ephedrine, caffeine, aspirin), but with the crackdown on ephedrine in 2004, caffeine has jumped to the forefront of ingredients in fat-loss supplements. Unlike most of the questionable compounds manufacturers toss into products they claim will melt fat off your body, good evidence exists that caffeine does increase fat loss. Again the exact mechanism of action has not been scientifically determined, but the general belief is that caffeine stimulates the release of fats into the bloodstream where they're available as a fuel for energy.

ADDICTION

Admittedly, there are worse substances a person could become addicted to. Nevertheless, the risk of becoming hooked on caffeine is extremely high. This drug is cheap, legal, highly accessible and very effective – four of the top variables for predicting a drug's addictive properties. That one- or two-cup habit can quickly snowball into a 10-cup-a-day addiction. And because coffee drinking is such a mainstream practice, abuse of caffeine often isn't viewed as a true addiction per se. Bodybuilders are especially at risk given the "more is better" philosophy in the sport and tendency toward the overuse of supplements.

Further to the physically addictive properties of caffeine, a few words need to be said about the cognitive components of the drug. It's very common for university and college students to use caffeine as a sort of "brain-boosting" drug. This is especially true around exam times when pulling all-nighters to study becomes the norm. On top of the stimulant effects, there is both scientific and anecdotal evidence indicating that caffeine can increase a person's mental alertness and cognitive abilities (although there is still no consensus as to whether or not caffeine increases a person's ability to retain information). Unfortunately the post-caffeine crash is unavoidable, and the last thing a student wants to do is start the downward spiral right in the middle of an exam.

Specifically with respect to addiction among students, we concede that a few weeks of heavy caffeine use is probably not a big issue. However, you still need to be aware that many caffeine addictions begin during the college years. If you find yourself needing eight to 10 cups of java just to make it through the day, we strongly suggest you re-evaluate your entire daily routine and overall health.

CAFFEINE SOURCES

While coffee is by far the most popular delivery method for caffeine, there are other sources. The following section discusses some of the most popular forms.

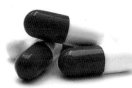

Pills

Caffeine tablets go by many brand names including Stay Alert, NoDoz and Wake-Up. If coffee has one disadvantage, it's that oftentimes it can be inconvenient. The beverage needs to be brewed (or mixed if it's instant coffee), and carrying it around can be awkward depending on what you're doing. Many bodybuilders are used to popping pills, so caffeine tablets are just another part of the iron pumper's arsenal.

However, the "convenience" advantage of caffeine tablets can at the same time be considered their primary disadvantage. Each tablet contains the caffeine equivalent of about one large cup of coffee. The physical act of drinking three or four coffees in a row can be difficult, but it's very easy to swallow three or four caffeine pills all at once. The downside of this is twofold: taking the tablets can more easily become

215

"It's rare these days to see even one hardcore body-builder arrive at the gym without a cup of coffee in hand. This is especially true in the weeks and months leading up to a contest. Sometimes that single cup of coffee is the only thing that gets the individual through the workout."

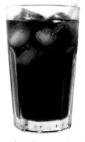

an addictive habit and they have the potential to be quite dangerous given the ease with which you could pump large doses into your body.

Soft Drinks

Although the high sugar content in soft drinks generally tends to receive the most attention from those in the nutrition field, many soft drinks are also loaded with huge amounts of caffeine. Some products are even specifically marketed as energy promoters. One main point to keep in mind is that if you are trying to quench your thirst by consuming a soft drink, you may actually be aggravating your dehydration given caffeine's diuretic effects.

Tea

Tea is believed to have originated in China and made its way to Europe courtesy of Dutch traders. It soon became a trademark of British culture, and during the reign of Queen Victoria, the Far East Tea Trade made up a large segment of the British Empire. From Britain, tea spread to the "colonies" including Canada and the United States. In fact, tea became entrenched in U.S. history when crates of it were dumped by colonists into Boston Harbor at the famous "Boston Tea Party," an event that helped initiate the American Revolution.

Contrary to popular belief, some teas contain nearly as much caffeine as coffee, but somehow the substance doesn't seem to provide the same kick when tea is the source. For those who find that coffee keeps them awake at night, switching to tea can often make a world of difference. As we discussed in the previous chapter, green tea is a top choice for fat loss since the banning of ephedrine, and many OTC fat-loss products include this specific form of tea as a main ingredient.

Cola Nuts

These seeds are from the cola tree and are very high in caffeine. In many countries, the seeds are chewed like candy for their stimulant effects. They haven't really caught on in North America, however, because of the taboos and certain state and municipal laws against spitting in public.

Chocolate

You won't find many individuals who will argue against chocolate's great taste, but one of the primary reasons why so many people love this treat is because it's high in caffeine. So the common statement, "I'm addicted to chocolate!" may actually have an element of truth to it. Chocolate is made by adding fat and sugar to roasted, ground cocoa beans. And while more recent studies have found certain benefits associated with dark chocolate (which contains high percentages of cocoa), given the sugar and fat content in most chocolate, we strongly suggest getting your caffeine fix from another source.

SIDE EFFECTS

The stimulant properties are a main reason that caffeine should not be used by anyone with pre-existing heart conditions. Those with kidney problems should also be wary of using the drug because of its diuretic effects. Caffeine abuse has also been linked to serious conditions such as heart disease and birth defects, but the conclusive evidence on this is sketchy at best. Some research indicates that caffeine can elevate cholesterol levels, but this observation is conflicted because other studies have found no such relationship.

For those who specifically train and participate in marathon events, caffeine's diuretic properties make it a drug to be avoided – especially during times of hot weather. Pregnant women should also refrain from heavy caffeine use as intake above 300 milligrams per day has been shown to increase the likelihood of miscarriages.[1] One or two cups of tea or coffee per day generally shouldn't be a cause for concern, but if you have any doubts, avoid caffeine products for the full pregnancy term. Finally, those who suffer from ulcers or other stomach ailments may want to avoid caffeine products because of the fact that it's acidic in nature (especially in concentrated forms such as tablets).

SPORTS CONCERNS

While caffeine is perfectly legal from a government standpoint, most sports organizations include it on their lists of banned substances. Of course, enforcing this ban does present certain problems. The IOC has set the upper limit cutoff at 900 to 1,000 milligrams, but this range is still subjective because individual tolerances differ – some individuals will experience a definite performance effect from a lesser dosage, while others may not derive any benefit despite taking more. On the flipside, many individuals run the risk of suffering performance impairment from taking huge amounts of caffeine because of the "crash" effect. Conversely, the "clean" athlete who properly times taking only one or two 100-milligram caffeine tablets may have his or her performance boosted considerably.

Reference
1) Mills J.L., *et al.* (1993). Moderate Caffeine Use and the Risk of Spontaneous Abortion and Intrauterine Growth Retardation. *JAMA*. 269:5.

"There are worse substances a person could become addicted to. But nevertheless, the risk of becoming hooked on caffeine is extremely high. This drug is cheap, legal, highly accessible and very effective – four of the top variables for predicting a drug's addictive properties."

AMPHETAMINES

Under the umbrella classification of stimulant drugs, amphetamines are among the most abused worldwide. During WWII they were heavily used by troops on both sides, and in the former Soviet Union these substances were even prescribed as "work enhancers." Amphetamines are the current drug of choice for many shift workers and those who put in long hours on uneven schedules – truck drivers statistically make up the largest demographic of users.

It's the powerful stimulant properties that attract those in the athletic world to amphetamines. And for those who accuse bodybuilders of being the biggest group of drug users, keep in mind that bodybuilding was among the last sports to see amphetamines make inroads – the 1950s marked the filtering of these drugs into the Olympics.

Similar to other stimulants, bodybuilders primarily use amphetamines to help get them through a tough workout. Most users report taking as little as 5 milligrams and achieving noticeable effects, but many users often up their dosages with the mindset that results will be magnified. And the potential for addiction is ever present, even more so than with some of the milder stimulants such as caffeine and ephedrine. Another reason amphetamines are used, particularly in the months leading up to a contest, is because they can suppress appetite.

Unfortunately for bodybuilders, this plus comes with a minus: the drugs are also catabolic in nature and can cause a loss of muscle tissue. This is one of the paradoxical characteristics of amphetamines – on one hand they can give you more energy during a workout, but on the other hand they may sabotage your hard-earned muscle mass. This pro-con seesaw has turned a lot of bodybuilders off of using amphetamines. After all, it's kind of difficult to justify them when milder stimulants such as caffeine and ephedrine are nearly as effective for stimulation purposes, and more beneficial for burning fat and preserving muscle tissue.

SIDE EFFECTS AND LEGAL ISSUES

Amphetamines rank among the most powerful of stimulants, and are thus more likely to cause serious side effects. The majority of reactions to this drug stem from the nervous and cardiovascular systems, the

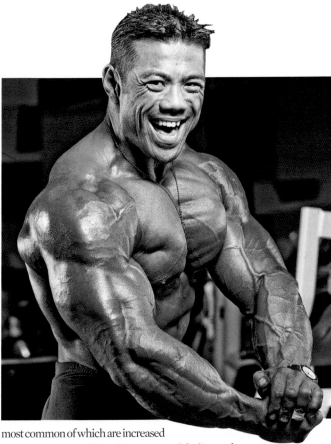

Photo by Kevin Horton
Model Ray Arde

LEFT: Amphetamines have highly powerful stimulant properties, and many bodybuilders also favor them for thier appetite-suppressing effects – a bonus when guys are trying to get ripped for a contest.

219

most common of which are increased heart rate, elevated blood pressure and feelings of anxiety. Amphetamines, when abused (or used by those with specific drug sensitivities), can cause an irregular heart beat, tremors, dizziness and in the most severe cases, even death.

In 1965 the U.S. Food and Drug Administration passed a group of amendments cracking down on the abuse of amphetamines. And while these substances continued to be over-prescribed into the '70s, newer drugs with fewer side effects gradually replaced them for most medical uses. Today amphetamines are used almost exclusively to treat narcolepsy (a sleeping disorder) and Attention Deficit Hyperactivity Disorder. Many people with ADHD have a paradoxical response to amphetamines – rather than becoming more jumpy and hyperactive, as most people would from taking amphetamines, these drugs tend to relax and sedate ADHD patients.

In the U.S., amphetamines are classified as Schedule II drugs: substances that have a high potential for abuse but a currently-accepted medical use. They are only available by prescription and must be used under severe restrictions. These drugs are also highly likely to cause severe psychological and physiological dependence.

When you factor in the potential dangers of amphetamines, and availability of safer and more effective drugs, leaving amphetamines out of your supplement plan is definitely a wise option.

"For those who accuse bodybuilders of being the biggest group of users, keep in mind that bodybuilding was among the last sports to see amphetamines make inroads – the 1950s marked the filtering of the drugs into the Olympics."

ALCOHOL

"Guzzling a 12-pack of beer backstage at a bodybuilding contest definitely won't increase your chances of winning. And you won't win any brownie points from the judges if, instead of hitting your poses onstage, you're floundering around in a drunken stupor."

Many individuals don't technically consider alcohol a drug, but it's one of the highest consumed drugs in society, not counting OTC cold medications. In small doses alcoholic beverages can relax you; in moderate amounts it can release your inhibitions to a point where you're more inclined to take risks and participate in activities you'd ordinarily avoid. When used in excess, alcohol can cause addiction and conditions such as liver disease — long-term abuse can even lead to death. Of all the mainstream substances, few are as prevalent, socially accepted and destructive.

Alcohol is widely considered a stimulant (which is why we included the discussion in this section), but it's actually classified as a depressant drug. The "downer" effects have less to do with the amount a person consumes and are instead more related to blood concentrations – a variation that exists because individuals metabolize alcohol at different rates. For a 200-pound healthy person, one or two drinks consumed over a period of one hour will generally produce a blood-alcohol reading of .02 to .06 percent. This amount of alcohol generates mild sedation, relaxation and often dismissal of personal inhibitions. The imbiber may also become more talkative, active and aggressive. For most bodybuilders, these would be welcomed attributes in the gym and especially in the nervous moments before and during a competition. This mildly tipsy state, however, can easily snowball with just a few more drinks, causing the individual's behavior to escalate to overly aggressive and hostile, even potentially reaching lethargic and unconscious.

Two other characteristics of alcohol make it notably popular among pre-contest bodybuilders. Certain beverages, especially wine, have the biochemical capacity to make the physique more vascular by drawing water from under the skin and making the veins more pronounced. Alcohol also functions as a diuretic (as most people who regularly drink a few beers can attest to), thus aiding pre-contest water shedding. Keep in mind that here again we're talking about small amounts – say one to two glasses of red wine. Guzzling a 12-pack of beer backstage at a bodybuilding contest definitely won't increase your chances of winning. Consuming such a large amount could also cause your already weak and dehydrated state to become that much more severe. Yet another factor to consider is that the effects will be heightened and you'll feel them set in earlier because you're at a lighter weight. Four months ago you'd probably shrug off a couple of drinks no problem, but a combination of lower bodyweight and calorie restriction has left you very susceptible to alcohol impairment. And you won't win any brownie points from the judges if, instead of hitting your poses onstage, you're floundering around in a drunken stupor.

No discussion of alcohol is complete without at least mentioning its connection to roid rage. Many in the legal field have used roid rage as a playing chip to get their clients excused from a potential conviction. The media industry has also placed much attention on roid rage in an effort to shed negative light on steroids. In a majority of legal cases of roid rage supposedly leading to violence, alcohol was present – and most often the individual already had a known history of violence when drinking. Whether the presence of steroids actually escalated the situation, no one will ever know. Indeed, the side effects of many drugs are magnified when alcohol is added to the mix, and it's possible that a drug such as anabolic steroids could increase aggression levels if the person is also using alcohol. The best advice we can offer to readers who tend to become aggressive when taking steroids or drinking alcohol is to refrain from both. If doing so isn't a feasible option, however, don't turn one problem into two by mixing these drugs.

221

BELOW: When you're working toward a contest-winning physique, an occasional drink or two is okay, but generally your intake should be limited.

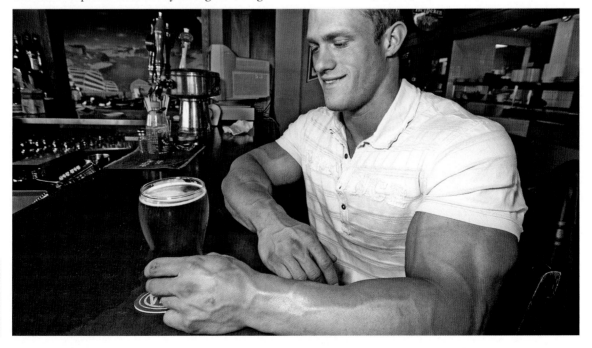

Photo by Rich Baker
Model Matthew Roberts

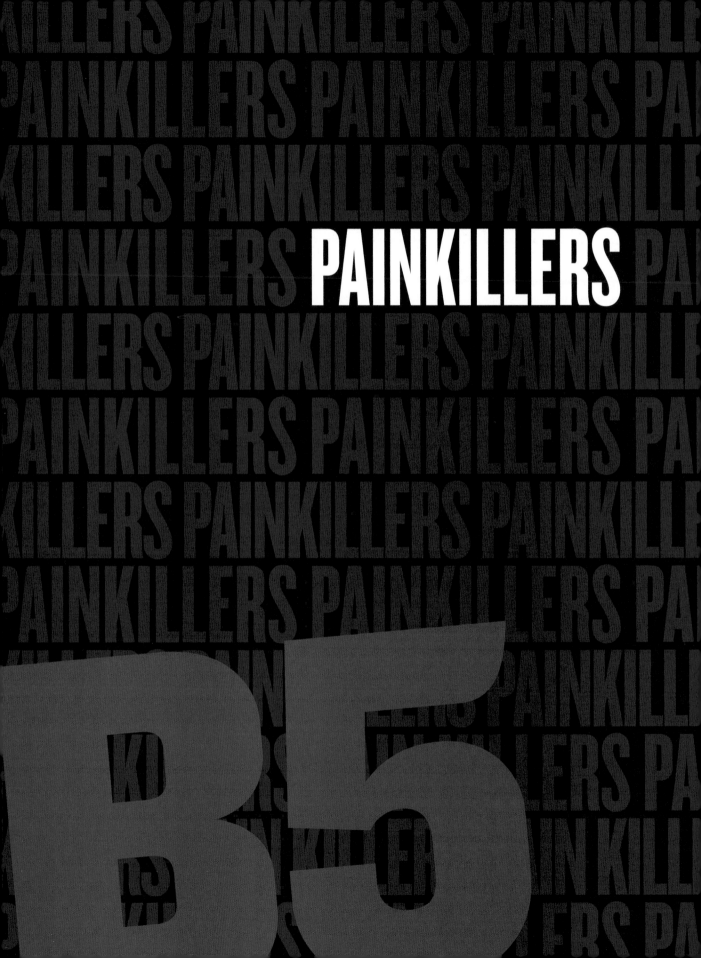

PAINKILLERS

B5

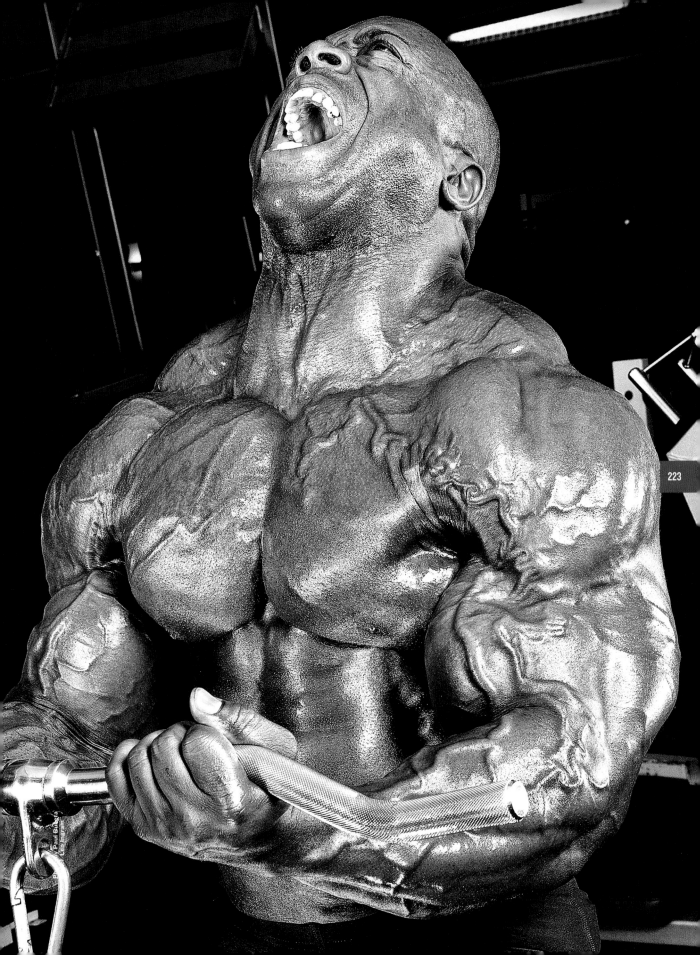

INTRODUCTION

> "Aspirin is generally taken for two primary reasons – pain relief and anti-inflammation. Bodybuilders and other athletes use it to treat the symptoms associated with sprains, strains and tears. This painkiller is also a favorite to treat the intense soreness that often follows an intense workout."

Few OTC drugs have become as rooted in modern society as painkillers. At the first sign of a headache many of us automatically reach for Aspirin. Cold symptoms – pop a Tylenol or two. Tough day at the gym or office – take two Anacin. Through trial and error, most people have discovered their favorite painkiller and preach its merits. Bodybuilders are no different in this regard. No matter how strict your exercise technique or attention to concentration, sooner or later you'll experience mild aches or even moderate pain as a result of training. While standardized pain relievers can be helpful, if you experience severe pain or moderate discomfort lasting more than a few days, you should get checked out by your doctor.

In the following five chapters we'll cover some of the more common painkillers. As you'll read in the various discussions, some were designed specifically for pain relief, while others were discovered by accident.

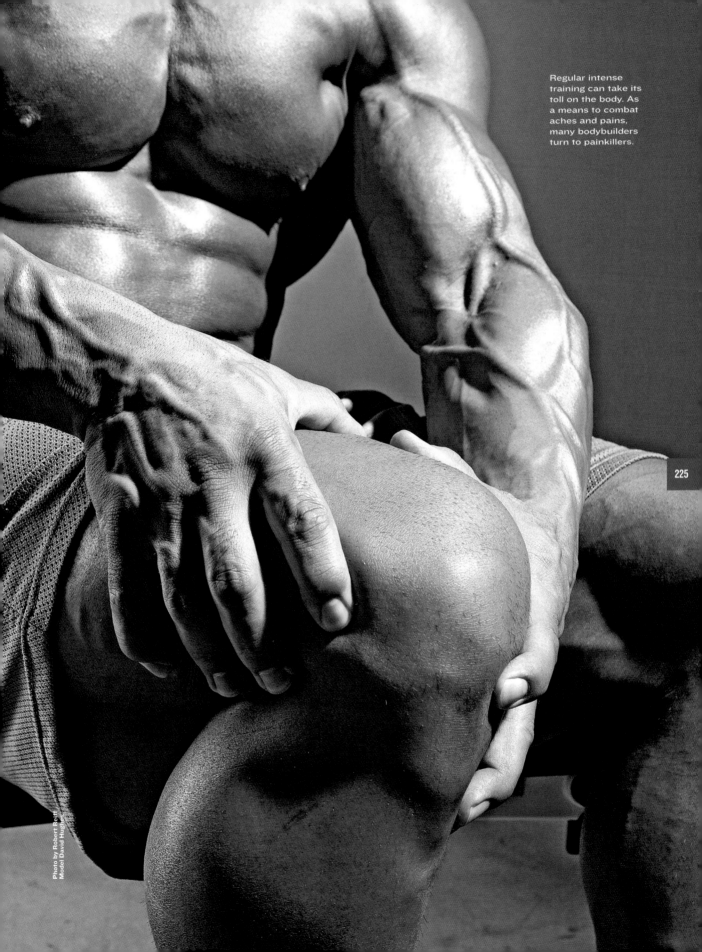

Regular intense training can take its toll on the body. As a means to combat aches and pains, many bodybuilders turn to painkillers.

225

ASPIRIN

The world's most widely used painkiller, Aspirin is the trade name for the compound ASA – acetylsalicylic acid. ASA is derived from willow bark, and while anyone can sell ASA and other medicines containing salicylic acid derivatives, Aspirin is a registered trademark of the Bayer corporation. As such, it can only be marketed with this product name (with the capital "A") when manufactured by Bayer. Most ASA products are labeled with the generic term aspirin – discussions in this chapter refer to the non-trademarked drug.

Aspirin is generally taken for two primary reasons – pain relief and anti-inflammation. Bodybuilders and other athletes use it to treat the symptoms associated with sprains, strains and tears. This painkiller is also a favorite to treat the intense soreness that often follows an intense workout.

Over the past 10 years or so, aspirin has been discovered to have a third main use: preventative medicine. Numerous studies have demonstrated that taking just one tablet a day can greatly reduce the risk of heart disease. The drug carries out this function by reducing the buildup of clotty deposits on arterial walls – one of the chief causes of cardiovascular disease. Specifically, the components of aspirin are believed to reduce clotting by interfering with platelet clustering (because of its biochemical effects, those with existing blood clotting problems should not use aspirin).

In terms of effectiveness, aspirin is one of the top OTC remedies currently available – the drug does what the advertisers claim, and in many cases, aspirin's painkilling and anti-inflammatory capabilities surpass those of some prescription drugs that cost exponentially more.

SIDE EFFECTS

There is only one regular side effect associated with aspirin: stomach upset. Because it's an acid, ASA can be somewhat harsh on the stomach and will often cause a burning sensation. Long-term use (often with higher dosages) may even damage the lining of the stomach. This

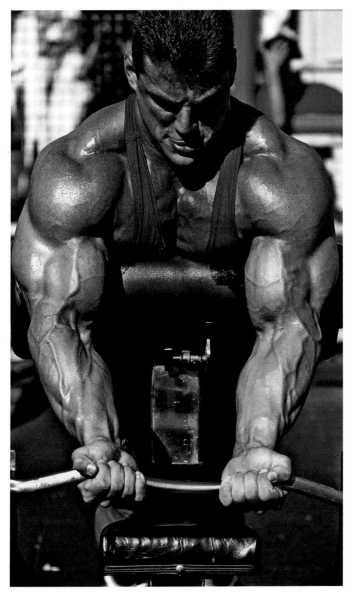

LEFT: The stresses of weightlifting make serious trainers prone to inflammation and muscle pain – two of the main symptoms aspirin is designed to treat.

227

adverse effect of aspirin was actually a driving force behind the development of the acetaminophen family of painkillers – manufacturers recognized that users who were susceptible to stomach pain with aspirin needed an alternative option for pain relief. In response, not wanting to lose a large segment of their market, Bayer introduced a coated version of aspirin that has been chemically engineered to pass through the stomach before breaking down and being absorbed, thus minimizing any stomach discomfort.

"Paul DeMayo's main addictions were painkillers like Percocet and Vicodin. Lately I've started hearing more about heroin in general in the USA. I know for a long time Nubain was a big problem in the bodybuilding world, but I don't hear much about it anymore."

– Ed Connors, former owner of Gold's Gym

ACETAMINOPHEN, NSAIDs, DLPA

228

ACETAMINOPHEN

In the painkiller marketing war, acetaminophen can be considered a rival to ASA. One of the main reasons acetaminophen was first developed was to offer an alternative for aspirin users who found the drug's negative stomach effects too uncomfortable. On drugstore shelves, the most popular trade name you'll see in the acetaminophen family is Tylenol. For many, acetaminophen provides the same degree of pain relief as aspirin. Where it does lag behind, however, is in its lack of anti-inflammatory properties.

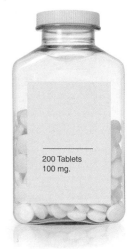

200 Tablets
100 mg.

When used as directed acetaminophen is considered the least likely of the common painkillers to cause side effects. Because this substance is metabolized by the liver though, heavy drinkers and those with liver problems should avoid taking it. And despite its relative safety, overdosing on Tylenol is possible and can be very dangerous – liver damage or failure is the most reported outcome of an overdose, but there have also been noted cases of death when extremely high dosages were ingested.

NSAIDs

NSAIDs is the acronym used for for non-steroidal anti-inflammatory drugs. The most common generic name in this substance category is ibuprofen, which can be found in certain well-known brands such as Advil and Motrin. Similar to aspirin (which itself is classified as a NSAID), ibuprofen is very effective for treating most forms of pain including common athletic conditions like sprains and muscle soreness. Another aspirin-like characteristic of ibuprofen is its powerful anti-inflammatory properties, which alone make it the OTC drug of choice among many bodybuilders and other athletes with complaints of inflammation. Most substances classified as NSAIDs can cause stomach irritation, but the majority of users report that the symptoms are nowhere near as troublesome as when taking aspirin. Ibuprofen also has a reputation for elevating liver enzymes in the body. The above-normal measure will show up on routine blood work, so make sure to mention ibuprofen use to your doctor if you're having blood tests done. You wouldn't want to be diagnosed with a liver condition when in fact it's simply the ibuprofen throwing off the readings.

DLPA (DL-PHENYLALANINE)

DLPA, or DL-phenylalanine, is an essential amino acid (phenylalanine) containing both the D and L form. For those who aren't familiar with the terminology, many compounds exist as mirror images of one another – the atoms are identical but arranged in reverse order around a central axis (just like your hands are the same but opposite). DLPA is structured in this manner: it's a mixture of LPA and its converse equal, DPA.

On the spectrum of painkiller potency DLPA falls at the mild end, but this substance is advantageous in that it's natural and doesn't cause the side effects some other painkillers are famous for. DLPA is believed to work by boosting endorphin and enkephalin levels – two compounds produced in the body that act as natural painkillers. As soon as an individual begins to experience pain, the body responds by increasing production of these two hormones. Unfortunately, the effects are short lived because both endorphins and enkephalins are rapidly metabolized by enzymes. DLPA, however, is thought to work by reducing the effectiveness of the enzymes, thus making the pain relief last longer in the body.

The benefits of DLPA aren't limited to pain relief – this substance also has a positive impact on mood, appetite and brain functioning. These secondary effects occur because phenylalanine is a precursor in the synthesis for many of the brain's neurotransmitters. In general, pain sensations are enhanced when levels of many transmitters are low.

DOSAGES AND LENGTH OF USE

Most anecdotal reports suggest 600 to 800 milligrams of DLPA taken 30 minutes before each meal to relieve most minor pain. This works out to about 3.5 to 5 grams per day. The specific dosage can vary among users and it's generally recommended to start with a lower amount (around 1 milligram per day) and gradually increase to a level that provides relief. This amino acid won't build up in your system right away, so you may need to take the supplement for approximately a week before noticing the initial pain-reduction effects. Unfortunately, this aspect of DLPA makes it a poor choice if you're looking for immediate pain relief. For some individuals though, the delay in initial efficacy is outweighed by its advantages as a natural compound with few, if any, side effects.

"In the painkiller marketing war, acetaminophen can be considered a rival to ASA. One of the main reasons acetaminophen was first developed was to offer an alternative for aspirin users who found the drug's negative stomach effects too uncomfortable."

229

DMSO

DMSO, or dimethyl sulfoxide, took the athletic world by storm during the early 1980s. The compound was promoted as a cure for numerous conditions ranging from arthritis to overtraining, but even with decades of athletic use, DMSO still has its share of doubters.

This chemical compound was first discovered in 1866 by Russian scientist Dr. Alexander Saytzeff. Despite his best efforts to popularize the colorless liquid, it would be nearly 100 years before DMSO found a practical application – in manufacturing as an industrial solvent. The primary source of most DMSO is as a byproduct from wood pulping (when trees are converted to paper). In industry it is used as antifreeze and as a solvent for a wide range of chemicals. DMSO also has many medical applications, of which its main uses are as an anti-inflammatory, a topical analgesic and an antioxidant.

One of DMSO's most remarkable properties is its capacity to rapidly cross the skin and get absorbed into the bloodstream. This compound has gained even more attention in the field of medicine because as a solvent, it can "piggyback" or carry other substances into the body's blood circulation. This characteristic, however, is a mixed blessing – DMSO on its own has a very low index of toxicity, but any dangerous chemicals and compounds that come in contact with it may also get transported across the skin and into the circulatory system.

While certain studies do cite adverse reactions to DMSO, this substance is relatively safe with few side effects (namely skin irritation and a garlic-like taste). Nevertheless, the FDA has approved it only for the treatment of a single condition, interstitial cystitis, noting little proof of its effectiveness for remedying other conditions.

Another strike against DMSO is that quantifiable medical research on this compound is scarce. This is largely because DMSO is not a substance that pharmaceutical companies can patent and make money on, so getting financial support for experiments is difficult. Researchers are also hard-pressed to find eager volunteers to participate in studies when DMSO can cause skin irritation and is known to have an unpleasant smell and garlic taste. As such, the lack of medical evidence to affirm any positive benefits of DMSO has influenced both the FDA and medical community to be reluctant about promoting it.

The exact mechanism of action for how DMSO relieves pain has yet to be pinpointed. One theory is that because DMSO has a strong affinity for water, it will rapidly draw the fluid from a swelled area, thus reducing inflammation. An equally plausible theory is that DMSO has good vasodilation properties and can thus cause the blood vessels to an injured area to dilate (become wider). Expanded blood vessels mean more blood gets transported to the area, and removal of waste products occurs at a faster rate. The end result of this chain of reactions is decreased swelling and pain.

Regardless of the specific biochemical actions, DMSO has found great acceptance worldwide by bodybuilders and athletes as a painkiller.

TYPES AND AVAILABILITY

There are three grades of DMSO on the market. Industrial grade often contains toxins and is *strictly* for use in manufacturing, not for human or animal consumption. This grade tends to be less than 50-percent pure. The toxins in this form can be absorbed into the body and many of the sealing and packaging materials can also be broken down by exposure to DMSO. For example, polyvinyl chloride can be converted

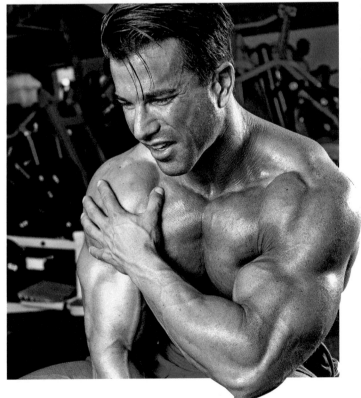

LEFT: DMSO is marketed to treat a wide spectrum of conditions from arthritis to pain from excessive training. Buyers beware, though – the compound isn't backed by solid medical research.

Photo by Irvin Gelb
Model Sagi Kalev

232

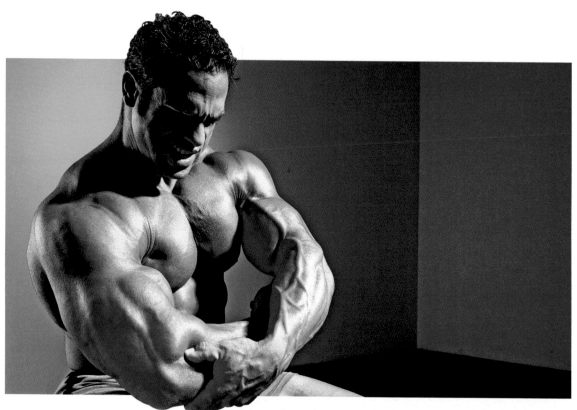

ABOVE: If you choose to use DMSO, you must thoroughly cleanse the injured area first, and then wait 20 minutes after application before covering it with any clothing.

into carcinogenic compounds when put in contact with DMSO. In the USA, DMSO products can only be sold legally in health-food stores and on the internet as an industrial solvent. There is no regulation in place to control how this form of DMSO is manufactured, making it potentially dangerous to use. Our advice: stay away from all industrial forms of DMSO.

Veterinary grade is widely used in animals, particularly race-horses. In most cases this type is a 50-50 mixture of water and DMSO. Your first inclination may be to shun any source that's vet-erinary in nature, but don't forget that most drugs manufactured for animals receive the same degree of scrutiny as drugs formulated for humans. Simply put, vets wouldn't give a potentially harmful drug to a million-dollar racehorse. If you're still not convinced, however, consider this fact: some of the most popular anabolic steroids, including Equipoise, are veterinary in origin and have been used for decades without problems.

The third type of DMSO is medical grade, which is classed as a prescription drug. This is your best source, provided you can get access to it. Odds are that you won't get your doctor to prescribe this compound, though; you'll instead probably have to take your chances by buying it on the black market.

When looking at DMSO, another important characteristic to account for, in addition to purity, is concentration. Any product

Photo by Robert Reiff
Model David Hughes

above 75 percent is considered too harsh and could burn the skin. Most health professionals generally recommend concentrations of 50- to- 70-percent DMSO.

METHODS OF USE

When applying DMSO to an injured limb or joint, make sure you first clean the area well. Doing so will remove any dirt or chemicals that may otherwise get absorbed into the body. Don't use soap or cleaning detergents, as they too can be transported across the skin. You may also want to shave the particular area if it's covered by a thick layer of body hair. Apply the solution evenly using a sterile gauze pad or cotton swab. Let the area dry for at least 20 minutes before allowing any clothing to come in contact with or cover it, since DMSO can break down and absorb the dyes in fabrics. Most health recommendations are to use DMSO two to three times a day for no more than seven to 10 days at a time. Treatment can be stopped if necessary for two or three days and then repeated. If the compound still has no effect, you're advised to seek medical advice.

We should note that like many painkillers, DMSO is beneficial for treating symptoms while you are trying to determine the underlying cause of the condition, but this substance is in no way a cure. For example, it will relieve the pain associated with tendinitis, but it will not cure the problem. DMSO will prevent herpes outbreaks and reduce the swelling and pain of arthritis, but with cessation of use, the symptoms of both health conditions will return. Don't fall into the trap of using DMSO to mask pain on a long-term basis. Use it only to null the symptoms until the condition has subsided (keeping in mind the upper limit for duration of use) or is being addressed by a medical professional.

"Your first inclination may be to shun any source that's veterinary in nature, but don't forget that most drugs manufactured for animals receive the same degree of scrutiny as drugs formulated for humans."

233

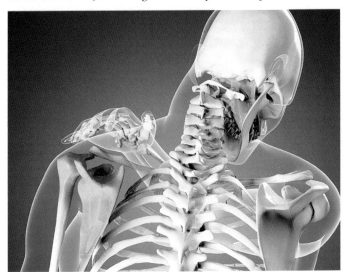

LEFT: Even with an acute injury to a limb or joint, your doctor likely won't prescribe DMSO because it's only FDA-approved for one condition: interstitial cystitis.

NUBAIN

The main focus of this section thus far has been on OTC painkillers. As many bodybuilders and athletes know, however, pain can often linger or become more severe, calling attention to an entirely different subset of drugs: prescription painkillers. When individuals seek something a little stronger to curb their pain, Nubain is a primary drug of choice. Nubain is the trade name for nalbuphine hydrochloride – a synthetic narcotic. Unlike most OTC painkillers, which come in tablet or capsule form, Nubain is usually administered by needle in 10- to 20-milligram per milliliter concentrations; this substance generally takes effect in as little as 15 to 20 minutes. Individual results will vary, but the pain relief typically lasts for six to eight hours.

SIDE EFFECTS

Nubain use can cause adverse reactions, although most people who use the drug never experience any severe side effects. The most common response symptom attributed to Nubain is sedation, which is due to the fact that this drug is a CNS depressant. Doctors will often prescribe a stimulant in combination with Nubain to counteract the depressive effects. When weighing the pros and cons associated with using this drug, keep in mind that working out (or any job that requires heavy lifting or demands high levels of concentration) is not recommended when in a state of sedation. While there's nothing like a good sleep to speed up the healing process, Nubain's sedative effects may do more harm than good to a bodybuilder trying to work out.

A second side effect occasionally reported with drugs containing nalbuphine is a slowing of the respiratory system. This reaction is also due to Nubain's depressive actions on the central nervous system. As with sedation, such symptoms are not welcomed by athletes who have higher oxygen demands than sedentary individuals.

Another red flag that potential users of Nubain need to be aware of is its addictive properties. Tolerance to this substance develops quickly, and like most narcotics, the risk of addiction is extremely high. Bodybuilders who become hooked on Nubain go through the same withdrawal

"Anyone who tells you he needed Nubain to get in shape is lying to you, himself or both. My suggestion would be to avoid this drug. I know far too many athletes in rehab centers because of the use of Nubain."

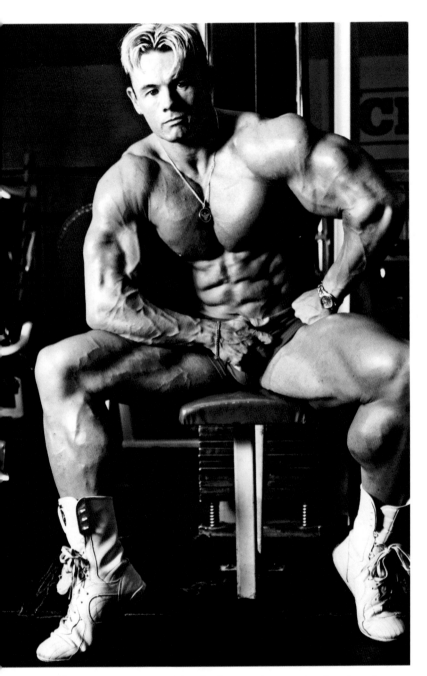

Model Guy Grundy

"I gradually cut back the dosage. Then I came to the point where I was almost out and needed another bottle. I knew getting a new bottle was a mistake so I quit cold turkey. After quitting I didn't sleep for seven nights. I was unable to sit still and shook uncontrollably. My legs were kicking and thrusting. The only way you can stop these symptoms is to get another bottle. On more than one occasion I had the phone in my hand to make the call. I stopped because I promised myself I would get off and I wasn't going to let it beat me."

– Guy Grundy, bodybuilder

235

symptoms as users of harder drugs such as cocaine, heroin and morphine. Unless your pain is severe enough to warrant a strong painkiller, or if you've been given a prescription by a physician, our advice is to pass on Nubain and stick to one of the safer OTC products.

LEFT: Advanced, serious, long-time trainers know severe or lingering pain all too well. To remedy such ailments, many bodybuilders step up to prescription painkillers.

CODEINE AND MORPHINE

CODEINE

Codeine (methylmorphine) is an alkaloid found in opium, and of all drugs that fall under the opiate classification it's by far the most globally used. According to numerous reports from organizations such as the World Health Organization, codeine is likely the most commonly used drug, period. It is also one of the top orally administered painkillers due to its safety margin and high level of effectiveness. In most people the strength of codeine is eight to 12 percent to that of morphine; metabolic differences, however, can change this figure as can the presence of other medications. In terms of its painkilling abilities, most users rank this drug above ASA/acetaminophen and below morphine (just as ephedrine ranks about halfway between caffeine and amphetamine on the stimulant scale).

Codeine was first isolated in 1830 in France by Jean-Pierre Robiquet. While the alkaloid can be extracted from opium, most codeine is synthesized from morphine through the process of O-methylation.

In most countries codeine is a regulated substance, meaning you can't buy it in pure form over the counter – instead it's only available in combination formulas with other drugs. The substances codeine is usually combined with are ASA, acetaminophen or muscle relaxants.

As a narcotic, the main side effects associated with codeine are depressive actions on the central nervous system. If not combined with a mild stimulant, most codeine users will experience some level of sedation. The body's cardiac and respiratory systems may also function suboptimally in the presence of this substance. In extreme cases users may note nausea, sweating and vomiting. Keep in mind, however, that healthy individuals who take the drug as directed (the usual adult dose is 15 to 60 milligrams every four hours) rarely experience severe side effects.

MORPHINE

Considered the king of painkillers, morphine is the standard against which all other opiates are tested. Stronger pain medications are out there, but none have quite reached the status held by this opiate-based

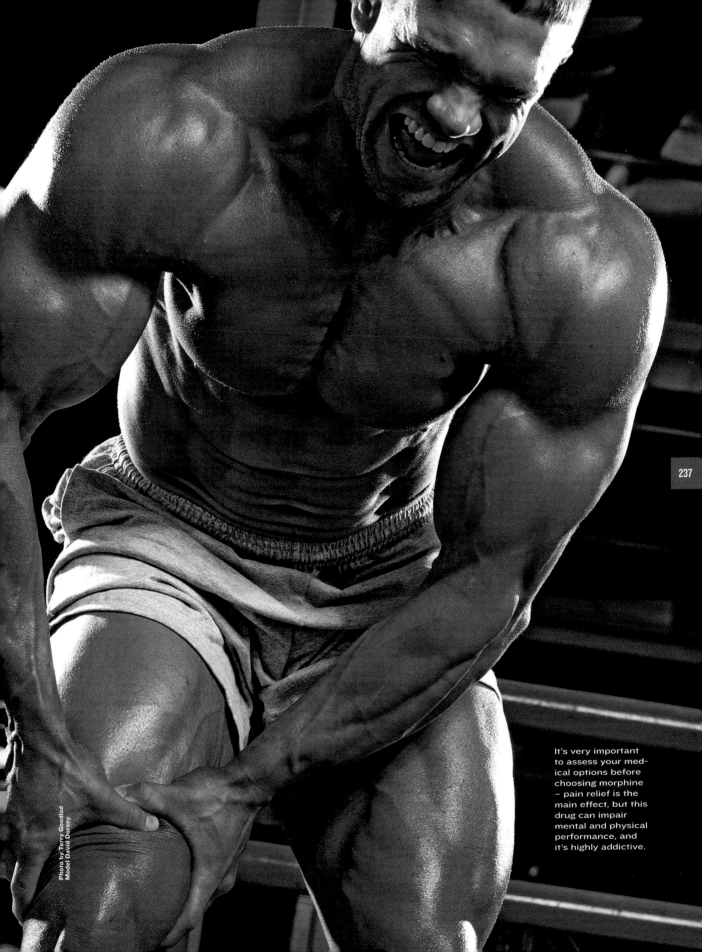

237

It's very important to assess your medical options before choosing morphine – pain relief is the main effect, but this drug can impair mental and physical performance, and it's highly addictive.

narcotic. Morphine was first isolated from opium in 1803 by German pharmacist Friedrich Wilhelm Sertürner who named it morphium, after Morpheus, the Greek god of dreams. Today morphine is still isolated from opium but in substantially larger quantities – over 1,000 tons per year. On the illicit market, opium gum is filtered into morphine base and then synthesized into heroin.

Morphine was first used medicinally as a painkiller, and ironically it was even adopted in the latter half of the 1800s as a treatment for opium addictions! In its early days, this drug was quick to supplant opium as a cure-all for most ailments and was readily available from drugstores or by mail order. Some physicians even recommended morphine as a substitute to treat alcohol addiction because alcohol was considered to be more destructive to the body and more likely to trigger antisocial behavior. It was later discovered, however, that morphine's addictive properties were even stronger. During the American Civil War morphine was used as a surgical anesthetic and injured soldiers were sent home with ample supplies for pain

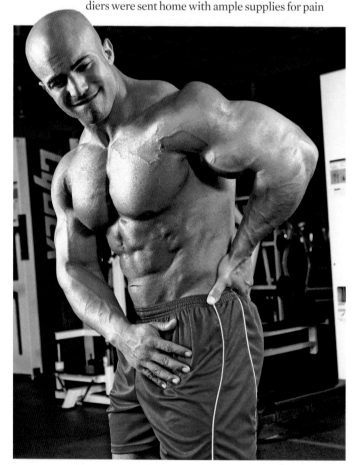

RIGHT: Every athlete who's suffered an injury knows that the body needs to be pain-free to function properly. To fight pain, many opt for codeine, a drug reported to be the most commonly used worldwide.

Photo by Jason Breeze
Model Lou Joseph

relief – they were the first generation of soldiers to demonstrate large-scale drug addiction. It's estimated that at the end of that war, over 400,000 people had what's been termed "soldier's disease" from becoming hooked on morphine.

Morphine is a powerful narcotic that exerts a direct impact on the central nervous system. While pain relief is the main effect sought by users, morphine can also impair mental and physical performance. This drug also relieves fear and anxiety, and it produces a heightened state of euphoria. Other secondary effects include decreasing hunger, inhibiting the cough reflex and reducing sex drive. Women who take morphine need to be aware that this drug may interfere with their menstrual cycle.

Morphine's ability to generate a feeling of euphoria is what led to its popularity as a recreational drug. Addictive drugs like this one primarily work by stimulating the brain's reward mechanisms. Once the body has experienced this sense of elation, the "promise" of reward becomes very intense in the brain, thus causing the individual to crave the drug. Unfortunately, tolerance builds quickly – a factor that opens the doors for addiction. Because morphine strongly activates brain reward mechanisms and chemically alters the normal functioning of these systems, a person's level of consciousness can also be reduced, sometimes making the user unaware of his or her surroundings while the drug is active in the body.

Self detoxification from morphine can be extremely dangerous and can cause severe physical trauma including stroke, heart attack and even death; psychological withdrawal symptoms are also quite common. Methadone (a synthetic opioid) is a choice drug used to help those with an addiction ease off the morphine. The value of methadone is questionable as treatment, however, as it often causes the individual to replace their morphine addiction with a dependency on methadone. Various studies and research have found that the most successful (but perhaps not easiest) way to get off and stay off morphine is to go cold-turkey in a safe and controlled environment such as an inpatient drug rehabilitation center. These medical facilities help to isolate the addict from the normal stresses of living and the surroundings that likely contributed to their addiction in the first place. The environment in which the treatment takes place is crucial, since there are so many factors that could inhibit the individual's ability to recover successfully.

With such severe side effects and given the drug's highly addictive properties, it's clear why morphine is a poor choice as a painkiller. Unless you're suffering from intense pain associated with a specific condition, disease or chronic ailment, there are far safer pain-relief drugs that will better manage the symptoms of most sports-related injuries – leave morphine to the doctors and hospitals.

"Considered the king of painkillers, morphine is the standard against which all other opiates are tested. Stronger pain medications are out there, but none have quite reached the status held by this opiate-based narcotic."

239

PROTEIN AND AMINO ACIDS

B6

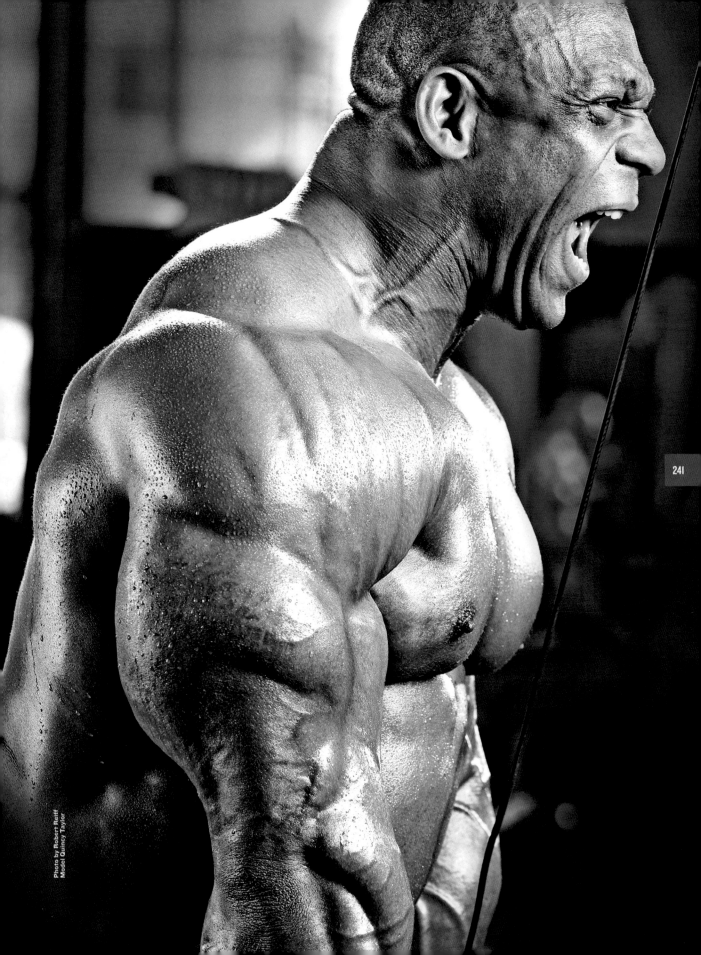

241

PROTEIN

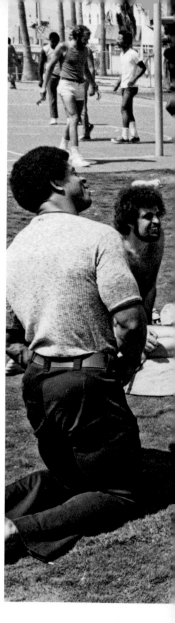

Of all the supplements used by bodybuilders, no other holds the same muscular value as protein. From the early days of bodybuilding over 50 years ago when tins of it were awarded as prizes to today's state-of-the-art whey isolates, protein is still the No. 1 supplement used by bodybuilders. The supplement industry is heavily driven by the demand for protein, and no true iron pumper feels complete without downing one or two protein shakes each day.

Now, high-protein diets were not an invention of Joe Weider's or the 1940s Muscle Beach gang. The heightened attention on this nutrient dates back to the ancient Greeks and Romans who were known to have eaten huge amounts of red meat, believing that doing so would produce superior soldiers and athletes.

MOLECULAR STRUCTURE

While bodybuilders focus on the relationship between protein and muscle tissue, protein is crucial to the body in numerous other ways: it's a major structural component of enzymes, hormones, organs, and tendons and ligaments. There are hundreds of different types of protein, but they all share one common element – nitrogen. When combined with such other chemical elements as carbon, hydrogen and oxygen, nitrogen gives protein an unparalleled place in human physiology. Since the body can't store ingested protein in its true form (as protein), foods containing this nutrient must be consumed on a daily basis. Any excess amounts will then be used for energy, stored as fat or excreted.

AMINO ACIDS

When an individual consumes a source of protein, the body's digestive system immediately begins to break it down into smaller sub-units called amino acids. Often called the body's "building blocks,"

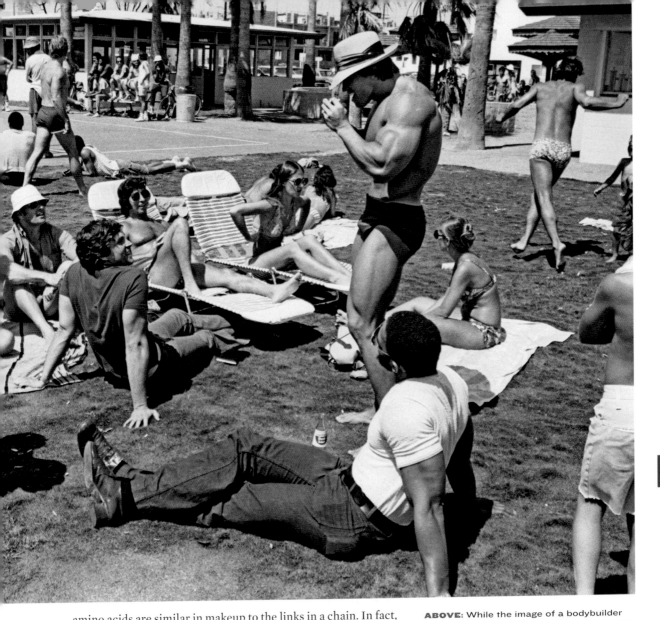

amino acids are similar in makeup to the links in a chain. In fact, strands of protein are called polypeptide chains and can be hundreds and sometimes thousands of amino acid molecules in length.

The molecular structure of a typical amino acid is a central carbon atom connected to four side chains or branches. At one end is an acid group, while at the other is an amine group (hence the name amino acid). The third chain is a single hydrogen atom. The fourth branch is what varies, giving each amino acid its unique properties.

ABOVE: While the image of a bodybuilder holding a tin of protein powder was popularized during the Muscle Beach era, the theory behind high-protein diets originated much, much earlier.

Here is the structure of a typical amino acid:

$$\text{Amine group} - \overset{\displaystyle \text{H}}{\underset{\displaystyle \text{R (fourth side group)}}{\text{C}}} - \text{Acid group}$$

243

In an earlier section we discussed L and D versions of molecules – amino acids are no different. While the illustration on the previous page is a two-dimensional representation, molecules are actually three dimensions. This means two versions of the exact same molecule can exist as mirror images of one another. Biochemists use the letters L and D to differentiate the two and indicate whether the molecule is arranged left or right around its central axis. Essentially, the atoms are in the same order, but they're completely reversed from the L to D version. Although the scientific evidence is not conclusive, it's believed that biological systems evolved to use only L versions of nutrients for metabolism. This is why many supplements you see on the market are labeled with the letter L in front of them (e.g., L-glutamine, L-tryptophan, L-arginine).

THE ALL-IMPORTANT 22

Despite the incredible complexity of many protein molecules, all proteins are derived from just 22 amino acids (though there is some debate on this number as scientists disagree about just what constitutes an amino acid – some experts suggest 20, while others argue there's anywhere from 24 to 28. We've chosen to use 22 since it's the most common number cited). The individual characteristics and

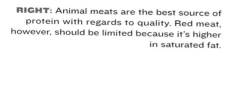

RIGHT: Animal meats are the best source of protein with regards to quality. Red meat, however, should be limited because it's higher in saturated fat.

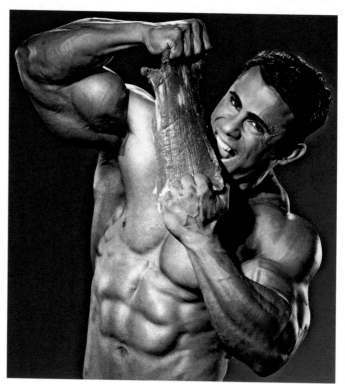

Photo by Robert Reiff
Model Moe El Moussawi

properties of each protein are determined by the order in which the amino acids are arranged. One sequence may produce insulin, while another denotes growth hormone. Of the entire group of amino acids, the body has the capacity to manufacture 13 from other amino acids. The other nine must be consumed in the diet and are hence called "essential" amino acids.

TRYING TO BE "COMPLETE"

When it comes to protein, not all sources are created equal. Biochemists and nutritionists use the terms complete and incomplete to describe the amino acid makeup of protein sources. Complete proteins are those that contain all nine essential amino acids in the correct proportions. The best sources of this type are meat, fish, chicken, eggs and milk.

Incomplete proteins are those in which one or more of the essential amino acids are missing or are only present in very low concentrations. Most vegetable proteins do contain all nine essential amino acids, but a few may only be trace amounts compared to most animal proteins. Beans, however, are rich sources of all the essential amino acids. Soy products likewise contain the full spectrum of aminos.

The old ideas that vegetarians needed to carefully combine different plant foods at every meal to ensure the correct supply of essential amino acids have for the most part been discarded these days. After observing populations of strict vegetarians who were just as healthy, if not healthier, and lived longer than meat-eaters, nutritionists now realize that the entire profile of essential amino acids can be obtained from a variety of vegetables or grains eaten over a one- or two-day period.

QUALITY OF SOURCES

While animal sources are far superior in terms of protein quality, animal meat – particularly red meat – tends to be high in artery-clogging saturated fat. Beef and pork are also loaded with protein, but can likewise contain whopping amounts of fat. Bodybuilders may be able to get away with eating these meats during the off-season, but come contest time, all extra fat must be eliminated from their diets (and midsections). Red meat is also not recommended for anyone with a family history of heart disease. And plant foods are crucial to maintain proper health – despite the fact that plant sources have an inferior amino acid profile, these foods do contain other nutrients that animal sources don't supply. This is why it's important to consume a well-rounded diet containing a wide range of both plant and animal foods.

Most bodybuilders who are conscious about their health, weight and appearance usually opt for lower-fat animal proteins such as poultry and fish sources rich in healthy fats. Many types of fish have very

"Eggs are the poster boys for bad eating yet they're perhaps the most anabolic substance on earth – so much so that training guru Vince Gironda advised his clients to eat up to a dozen eggs a day! This may be a case of extreme excess, but oddly enough no one suffered any side effects – other than a major boost in muscle growth. Egg consumption makes sense if you think about it: What is an egg but all the components of life itself? The cholesterol in eggs is a big deterrent for a lot of people, but it shouldn't be."

– Nelson Montana, *MuscleMag International* contributor

245

little if any saturated fat and the heartier varieties (herring, salmon, etc.) are loaded with omega-3 fatty acids. Particularly with respect to poultry, remember that the skin should always be removed. It may add taste to the meal, but most of the fat is contained in or just under the skin. Geese and duck are two other quality animal protein sources – just keep in mind that farm-raised birds are intentionally fattened for market sale. Wild game birds are another high-protein option; they're harder to get (and pricier), but their meat is much lower in fat.

Though not a meat source, eggs are one of the top protein foods. In many respects they are one of nature's perfect foods (even coming in their own container!). The one major downside of eggs is that they contain cholesterol. However, most nutritional experts now suggest there's far more involved in the development of cardiovascular disease than just dietary intake of cholesterol. And for those who are still worried about the artery-clogging part of eggs, it's simply a matter of separating the white from the yolk, because all of the cholesterol is contained in the yolk. Egg whites are a staple in numerous pre-contest diets and it's not unheard of for pro bodybuilders to scarf down two- or three-dozen egg whites a day in the weeks leading up to a contest.

DO BODYBUILDERS NEED MORE?

The requirements for protein is one of the most contentious issues in bodybuilding – few topics generate as much debate as whether or not bodybuilders and other athletes need extra amounts of this nutrient in their diets. Essentially there are two schools of thought on this topic: In one corner are the old-school nutritionists who stand by the belief that if individuals follow the RDIs (see "Protein Standards"), extra protein is not needed. The current RDI value for protein is about 1 gram of protein per *kilogram* (2.2 pounds) of bodyweight. Nutritionists who support this frame of thinking argue that any extra protein above this amount will either be excreted or converted and stored as fat. In the opposite corner are bodybuilders and other experts in this sport, and as expected, the supplement industry. Bodybuilders have been attesting for decades that they achieve their best results when they consume at least 1 gram of protein per *pound* (not kilogram) of bodyweight. Whether this mindset is strictly related to a placebo effect or the absolute belief in the qualities of extra protein for strength and size gains, or whether there is some physiological explanation for the improvement, no scientific data exists to prove or disprove either argument. Aside from the associated financial costs, bodybuilders don't really care as long as they see results.

The contention about protein requirements is central to supplement manufacturers. It shouldn't be very difficult to determine which side of the debate they back. Every year, the supplement industry generates billions of dollars, and protein products make up a huge slice of

"Although many conservative organizations still refuse to recognize the importance of high levels of protein in the athlete's diet, some of the more forward-thinking sports organizations such as the International Society of Sports Nutrition (ISSN) have let go of this myth. The ISSN recently concluded that vast research supports the contention that individuals engaged in regular exercise training require more dietary protein than sedentary individuals."

– Will Brink, bodybuilding and nutrition writer

that supplement pie. Therefore, it stands to reason that the supplement companies will whole-heartedly promote the concept that body-builders need extra protein – and promote they do. Beginning in the late 1940s, supplement companies have invested hundreds of millions of dollars in advertising alone. The typical ad of those times would feature a top bodybuilder of the day holding a tin of protein powder – complete with a couple of beautiful young babes hanging off each arm, or seductively wrapped around his legs. Such images of Arnold from the '60s and '70s made Joe Weider millions in protein sales. The fact that Arnold actually received most of his protein from whole foods was never mentioned. Instead, countless young males around the world looked at Arnold's body (and the babes), and envisioned taking their own steps on California's Venice Beach.

Before looking at the findings from the latest research, we first need to look at how protein requirements are measured and calculated.

BELOW: A clean muscle-building diet should be plentiful with fish – many types are very low in saturated fat and the heartier fish are packed with omega-3s.

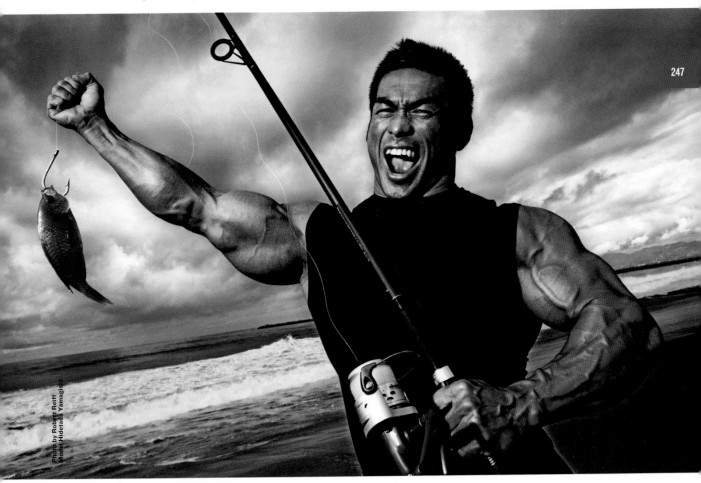

Photo by Robert Reiff
Model Hidetada Yamagishi

247

NITROGEN BALANCE

It may surprise many readers to learn that biochemists don't measure protein levels directly – they gauge an individual's nitrogen balance. This chemical element is used as the tool for measurement because it's common to all amino acids. By comparing the amount of nitrogen lost through waste products including sweat, urine and feces against the amount of nitrogen consumed in the diet, researchers can get a fairly accurate idea as to whether the person is in positive or negative nitrogen balance. A positive balance means the body is taking in more nitrogen than what's being emitted. A negative nitrogen balance is just the opposite – more of the element is being lost than consumed.

Although the balance of nitrogen impacts numerous metabolic functions, bodybuilders tend to focus on it specifically in relation to muscle building. In order to build new muscle tissue, the body must be in a state of positive nitrogen balance. When the individual is in the negative zone, not only will adding new muscle tissue be near impossible, but the body may even go into a catabolic state and break down existing muscle tissue to be used as fuel. If you're serious about building size and strength you have to be extremely conscious about avoiding a negative nitrogen balance.

PROTEIN STANDARDS

The RDIs (Reference Daily Intake) are nutrient guidelines set by the Food and Nutrition Board and various other government and health organizations. For convenience, biochemists specifically measure protein requirements in grams of protein per kilogram of bodyweight. For those who aren't familiar with using the metric system, 1 kilogram equals 2.2 pounds. The U.S. Food and Nutrition Board's recommendation is to consume 0.80 grams of protein per kilogram of bodyweight (for our Canadian readers the value is slightly higher at 0.86 grams per kilogram). For a 200-pound male this works out to about 72 grams of protein daily. The World Health Organization is more conservative and has set the guideline at 0.75 grams of protein per kilogram of weight.

You'd think such precise values would indicate that protein requirements are generally accepted across the board, but such is not the case. The controversy arises from the fact that the values were calculated based on the nutritional requirements for healthy but relatively sedentary individuals. Common sense should dictate that a 220-pound bodybuilder is going to have higher protein requirements than the typical couch potato. Just think of the muscle repair necessary after 3 or 4 sets of 10 to 12 reps using 500-plus pounds on the squat. All that muscle tissue needs to recover, and the only way to accomplish that is by providing the amino acid building blocks. If the required raw materials are not present in the body following such work, the end result could be muscle wasting.

"Common sense should dictate that a 220-pound bodybuilder is going to have higher protein requirements than the typical couch potato. Just think of the muscle repair necessary after 3 or 4 sets of 10 to 12 reps using 500-plus pounds on the squat. All that muscle tissue needs to recover, and the only way to accomplish that is by providing the amino acid building blocks. If the required raw materials are not present in the body following such work, the end result could be muscle wasting."

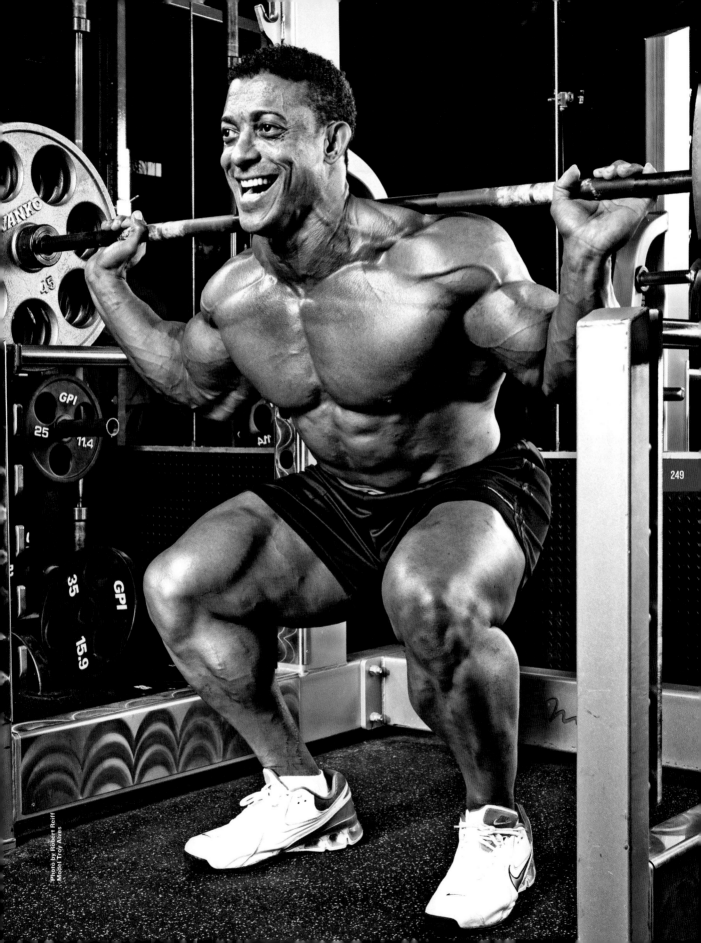

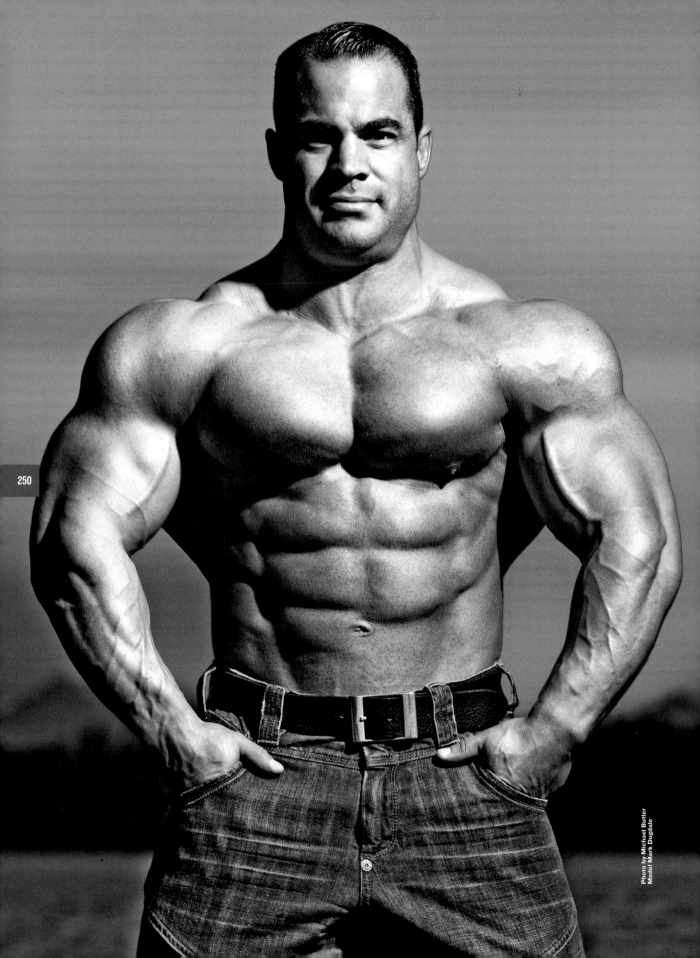

250

THE RESEARCH

For years a heated debate has raged between the conservative medical and scientific community and the protein pushers and athletes. Those in the medical and scientific field keep insisting that eating any amount above the RDI is a waste of money and could potentially be dangerous to one's health. At the other end of the spectrum, supplement companies and some die-hards in the sport insist that no less than 1.5 to 2 grams of protein per pound of bodyweight will suffice. So who is right? Is there an optimal quantity of protein that bodybuilders should consume?

It's difficult to offer a definitive answer, but the best range is likely somewhere between the two extremes. Because individual needs are different, the exact protein intake for bodybuilders will vary slightly. One thing, however, is for certain: The RDI value is not adequate enough to support the added requirements of intense bodybuilding training. The guidelines even include a warning that "No added allowance is made here for stresses encountered in daily living which can give rise to transient increases in urinary nitrogen output. It is assumed that the subjects of experiments forming the basis for the requirement estimates are usually exposed to the same stresses as the population generally." If bodybuilding isn't a form of stress above and beyond what most individuals encounter on a day-to-day basis, then you have to wonder, what exactly constitutes strenuous activity?

One of the leading researchers on protein requirements in athletics Dr. Peter Lemon wrote, "Recent data suggests that the recommended protein amount might actually be 100 percent higher for individuals who exercise on a regular basis. Optimal intakes, although unknown, may be even higher, especially for individuals attempting to increase muscle mass and strength."

In one of his more famous experiments Dr. Lemon found that strength athletes needed up to 1.8 grams of protein per kilogram of bodyweight to maintain a positive nitrogen balance. That's 0.8 grams per pound of bodyweight (almost 140 grams a day for someone who weighs 172 pounds). You'll notice that number is very close to the long-held belief of 1 gram per pound of bodyweight of most bodybuilders.

Another study involving sprinters and competitive bodybuilders revealed that both groups required 1.12 to 1.67 times more protein than the sedentary control groups.[2] A separate study using Romanian weightlifters also found that those given 4.4 times the RDI had much greater increases in size and strength.[3]

Similar studies have served to back up these outcomes, demonstrating that even higher protein intakes may be necessary in hard-training strength athletes. In one particular study, five of 10 Polish weightlifters demonstrated states of negative nitrogen balance even while consuming 250 percent of the RDI.[4]

"Recent data suggests that the recommended protein amount might actually be 100 percent higher for individuals who exercise on a regular basis. Optimal intakes, although unknown, may be even higher, especially for individuals attempting to increase muscle mass and strength."

251

References

1) *Nutrition Reviews*. (1996). 54:S169–175.
2) *Journal of Applied Physiology*. (1998). 64:1.
3) Proceedings of the International Congress on Milk Proteins, Wageningen, Netherlands, PUDOC, 1984.
4) *Nutr. Metabolism*. 12:259–274.

PROTEIN SUPPLEMENTS

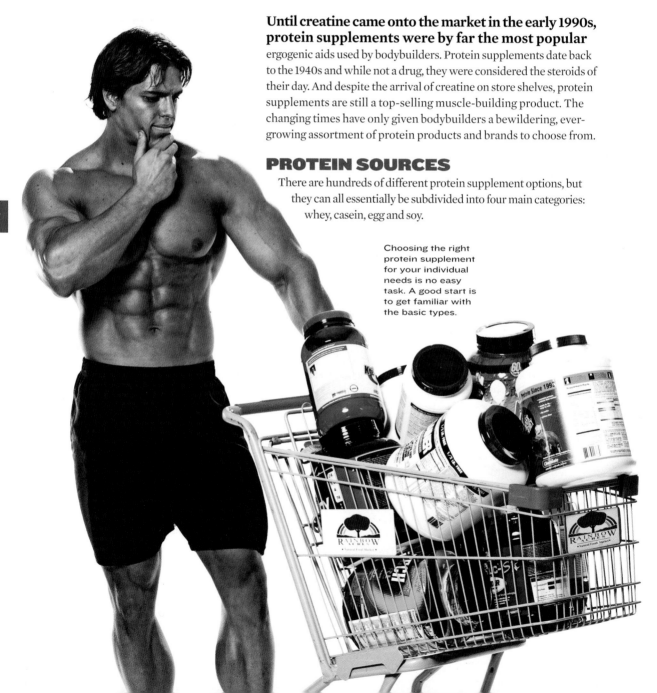

Until creatine came onto the market in the early 1990s, protein supplements were by far the most popular ergogenic aids used by bodybuilders. Protein supplements date back to the 1940s and while not a drug, they were considered the steroids of their day. And despite the arrival of creatine on store shelves, protein supplements are still a top-selling muscle-building product. The changing times have only given bodybuilders a bewildering, ever-growing assortment of protein products and brands to choose from.

PROTEIN SOURCES

There are hundreds of different protein supplement options, but they can all essentially be subdivided into four main categories: whey, casein, egg and soy.

Choosing the right protein supplement for your individual needs is no easy task. A good start is to get familiar with the basic types.

WHEY

Whey is one of the two major proteins found in cow's milk, the other being casein. Whey is a byproduct of cheese production. When cheese is manufactured, a thin layer of liquid is left over. That liquid is whey and in this form it's less than one percent protein. The substance is then concentrated and dried, a process that creates whey protein powder. This form of protein makes up about 20 percent of the total found in milk; whey is considered superior to most other sources because of its digestibility, bioavailability (amount absorbed versus amount utilized by the body) and high concentrations of proven muscle builders like branched chain amino acids and glutamine. From a practical point of view, this powder also mixes more easily than other sources and doesn't seem to cause the bloating and gastrointestinal discomfort that other protein products are known for.

Whey protein is considered a "fast-acting" protein, which refers to the amount of time it takes for the nutrient to be fully digested and absorbed into the blood. From the bloodstream it is taken up by body tissues, and ultimately gets utilized for a number of metabolic processes. The two dominant pathways by which protein functions are either the creation of a new protein from the individual amino acids or oxidation into urea and possibly glucose.

The elapsed time from when you eat protein until it's traveling in your blood is just 20 minutes. After about 20 to 40 minutes, the level of amino acids in your blood will have reached its high point. And within the hour it will have gone through the various metabolic processes, either protein synthesis or oxidation.

From a muscle-building perspective these actions are beneficial because muscle growth is dependent upon the relationship between protein synthesis and breakdown. If the synthesis of new muscle protein is greater than the breakdown, net gains in muscle mass will result. Conversely, if more protein gets broken down than synthesized, no gains in new muscle mass will occur. The individual could in fact lose muscle mass under these circumstances.

CASEIN

Despite the popularity points achieved by whey, in terms of protein content in milk, casein is the hands-down winner. This type makes up about 80 percent of the protein in cow's milk (remember, the remaining 20 percent is whey). The actual casein is extracted from milk through ultra-filtration processes without any use of chemicals. Such extraction techniques increase the amount of bioactive milk peptides, which not only enhance muscle growth but also boost immune function. Casein has an excellent amino acid profile and is considered an extremely slow-digesting protein.

> "Another shake you'd better be consuming on a regular basis if lean muscle gain is your goal is the post-workout shake. Your body is in a highly anabolic state immediately after a workout and in a unique position to suck up nutrients."
> – Ron Harris, *MuscleMag International* contributor

253

Photo by Robert Reiff
Model Bradley Castleberry

"You don't want your body to start breaking down hard-earned muscle while you sleep. With casein in your system, catabolism is staved off. If you were to instead take whey protein before bed, it would be absorbed within one hour and would thus do very little for your muscles. You might even still be awake by the time it's absorbed, peaked and utilized."

254

The reason the body digests casein slowly is because the protein forms a gel-like substance in the stomach, facilitating a steady release of amino acids into the bloodstream over time. Research indicates that when an individual consumes casein, he or she will reach a peak in blood amino acid levels and protein synthesis between three to four hours after ingestion. The complete release of amino acids into the bloodstream, however, can last as long as seven hours after consumption of this protein. This feature of casein is in marked contrast to that of whey, which reaches the bloodstream in as little as 20 minutes and then peaks within that first hour.

Since casein enters the bloodstream at a gradual rate, it has very little impact on protein synthesis. But what it lacks in that regard it makes up for with its powerful effect on suppressing protein breakdown. In other words, it's an awesome anti-catabolic (muscle-sparing) protein. As we noted, muscle growth is dependent on the ratio of protein synthesis to protein breakdown. In order to tip the balance in your favor, you want to increase protein synthesis and decrease protein breakdown. This can be achieved by supplementing with both whey protein (fast absorption/promotes protein synthesis) and casein protein (slow absorption/suppresses protein breakdown).

CASEIN FORMS

Supplement manufacturers have capitalized on the value of casein, offering different types and formulas. Casein protein can generally be separated into three categories: calcium caseinate, micellar casein and milk protein isolate. Of the three forms, calcium caseinate is the lowest in quality and is commonly used as a food ingredient. The other two, micellar and the casein in milk protein isolate are identical. While micellar casein is 100-percent pure, milk protein isolate contains both micellar and whey. As a result, milk protein isolate is the more economical choice of the two.

Like whey protein, not all milk protein isolates are created equal. Some supplement companies sell inferior products (with less casein and more whey protein). The best milk protein isolates have roughly 80 percent micellar casein and 20 percent whey. And just in case you're wondering, you can in fact get the same 80:20 casein-whey ratio found in the highest-quality milk protein isolates simply by enjoying a glass of milk. The difference, however, is in the protein quantities – one eight-ounce glass of milk has only 6.4 grams of casein, while one small scoop of a high-quality milk protein isolate has over 20 grams of casein.

TIMING

The different absorption rates of whey and casein are extremely beneficial – by using them at optimal times of day you can maximize your recovery abilities. Casein is the only protein you should be taking before going to bed at night. Remember, it's a slow-release protein. You'll be going six to eight hours without food, and you don't want your body to start breaking down hard-earned muscle while you sleep. With casein in your system, catabolism is staved off. If you were to instead take whey protein before bed, it would be absorbed within one hour and would thus do very little for your muscles. You might even still be awake by the time it's absorbed, peaked and utilized.

BELOW: No other protein can match casein when it comes to slow release. It's your best bedtime option to ensure aminos are steady while you sleep.

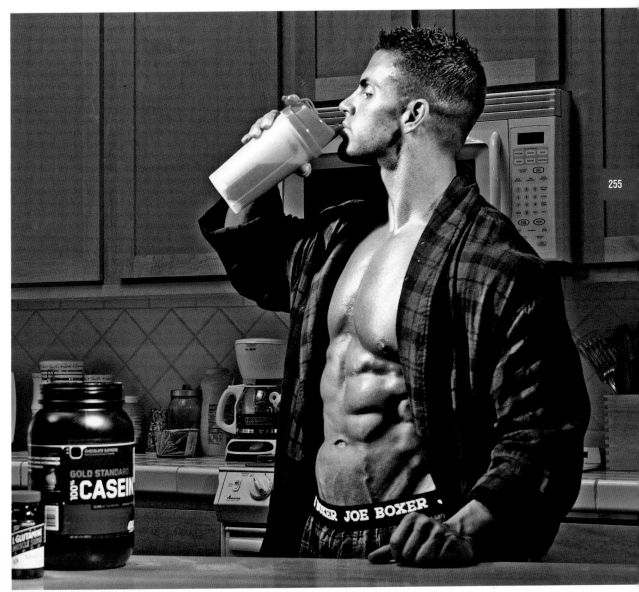

255

Photo by Robert Reiff
Model Chris Jalali

"Perhaps the biggest health benefit that soy has over other protein sources is its cholesterol-lowering abilities. The plant sterols have been shown to reduce amounts of cholesterol in the body."

The fast action of whey protein makes it the best option both as soon as you get up in the morning and after your workouts. These are the times when your body needs the rapid absorption of amino acids. At other points throughout the day, especially if you have to go more than three hours without food or are having a protein shake as a meal replacement, you should use a blend of whey and casein – about 50-50. This mixture will give you the benefits of both proteins: a quick shot and a sustained release to carry you through to your next meal. Finally, even if you are eating every two to three hours, you can still use whey on its own between meals as a protein snack.

EGG

A few years ago we would have said that egg sources were inferior to whey, but this is no longer the case, thanks to refinement techniques. These specific processes have closed the gap, so much so that you aren't missing out on much by opting for egg over whey. One key area, however, where egg protein doesn't stack up to whey is mixability. Despite better refinement procedures, most egg products still need to be mixed in a blender. Whey on the other hand is ready to drink with a few swirls of a spoon or a shake of your shaker cup. Egg proteins may also cause gastrointestinal problems for some individuals. Whey products are thus a good alternative because they most often have the lactose and other gastro-upsetting components removed. The few downsides notwithstanding, most people now consider the newer egg products to be just as effective as whey sources for bodybuilding and muscle-building needs.

SOY

Soy is another protein that's been revitalized in this sport. It's one of the few plant sources that contain the full profile of amino acids (most plants are deficient in one or more) and for this reason is a complete protein. No less an authority in the sport than Chad Nicholls (known in bodybuilding as the "Diet Doc") has stated that soy is comparable to egg- or milk-based protein – a claim that seems to be backed by medical science. In a study published in *Experimental Biology*, researchers found that subjects who ingested soy, a soy/whey blend or whey protein all experienced similar increases in muscle mass. A six-week study at Laurentian University (Sudbury, Ontario) found similar results when they compared the muscle-building effects of soy and whey. A third study in *Nutritional Journal* found that when test subjects ingested either soy or whey in the form of a protein bar, gains in lean muscle tissue were equal between the groups. Those who used the soy supplement also seemed to have better anti-catabolic abilities than the whey group (*MuscleMag International*, "Soy Good?," 2008, Issue 314).

RIGHT: While whole foods should make up the majority of your diet, a whey-casein shake is ideal when you have to go three-plus hours without food.

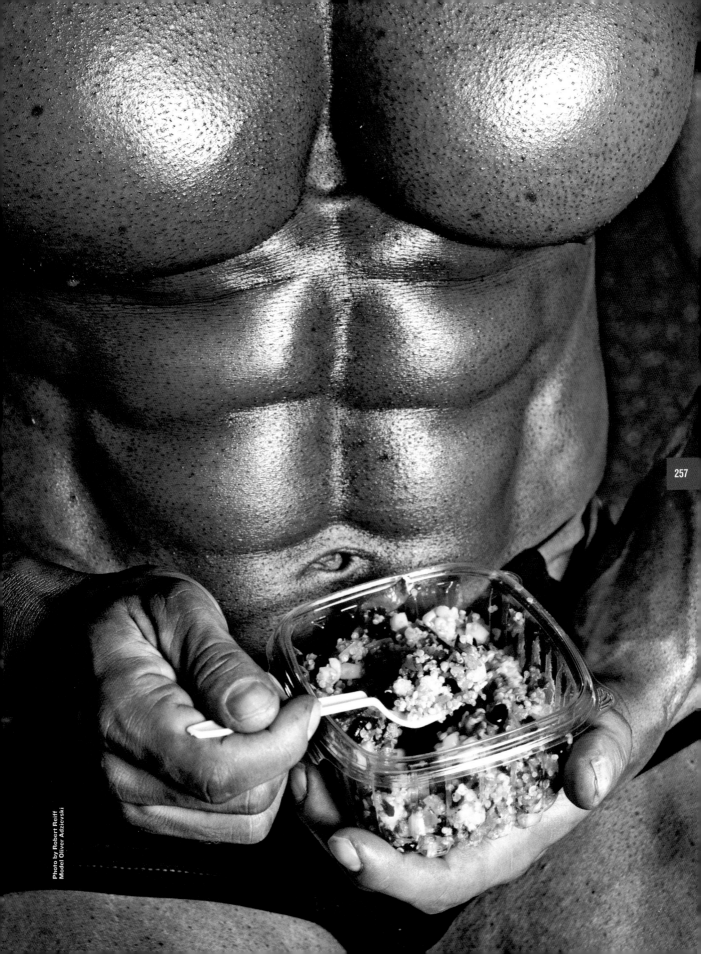

Photo by Robert Reiff
Model Oliver Adzievski

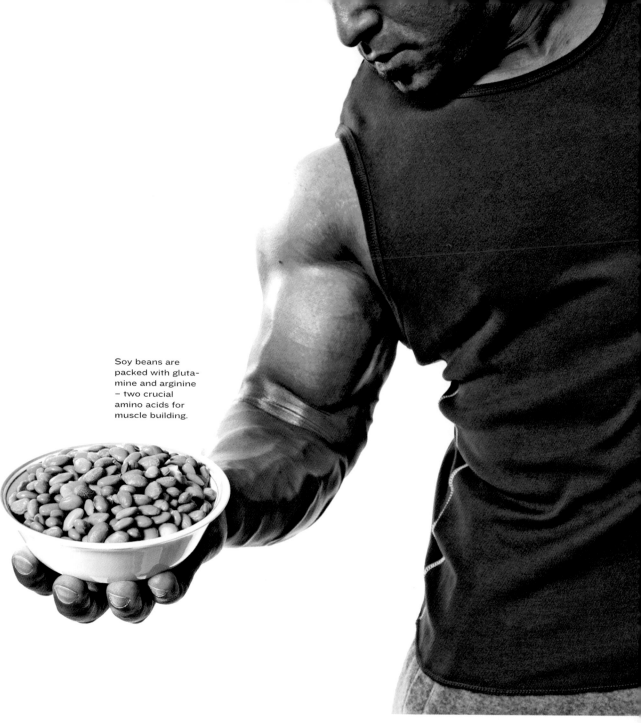

Soy beans are packed with gluta-mine and arginine – two crucial amino acids for muscle building.

Perhaps the biggest health benefit that soy has over other protein sources is its cholesterol-lowering abilities. The plant sterols contained in soy have been shown to reduce amounts of cholesterol in the body. And specifically from a muscle-building point of view, soy is loaded with two powerful amino acids, glutamine and arginine. These particular amino acids enhance recovery and boost the immune system, but it's their anabolic properties that make glutamine and arginine crucial for the bodybuilder.

Arginine has been shown to assist in boosting circulating levels of growth hormone. This amino acid also initiates the production of nitric oxide in the body. Nitric oxide increases blood flow to the muscles and transports oxygen, hormones and other nutrients to speed up the healing process and the rate at which protein synthesis occurs.

The many benefits of glutamine will be covered in detail in a later chapter (Chapter 35). The relationship between soy and glutamine is important to mention here, though: What most bodybuilders don't realize is that soy protein contains nearly double the glutamine content of whey protein sources.

"GIRLIE" PROTEIN

Considering the many positive aspects of soy, you'd think this type of protein would be a must-have for bodybuilders, but it's not. Soy has a feature that, although vastly exaggerated, causes many hardcore bodybuilders to shun it. Soy does get three big checkmarks in that it has arginine and glutamine and is also high in isoflavones, which help reduce soreness and improve recovery time. The downside, however, is that these compounds may have estrogen-like effects. Specifically, three of the isoflavones (genistein, glycitein and daidzein), are referred to as phytoestrogens and are very similar in makeup to the human hormone estrogen. For bodybuilders not familiar with isoflavones and how they function in the body, this would indeed sound detrimental; these components, however, are structurally very weak. In fact, the three are approximately 1,000 times weaker than the body's own natural estrogens. In other words, while isoflavones may slightly alter estrogen regulation in the body, an individual would need to consume enormous amounts before the trio of phytoestrogens would be able to compete with testosterone's anabolic effects. The numerous studies showing soy protein to be very effective at promoting muscle gains should be proof enough that estrogen-like isoflavones have no counterproductive effects on anabolism in the human body.

When you get right down to it, soy protein really isn't all that complicated. Just as whey, casein and egg proteins can help you build muscle mass, so too can soy. And when you factor in all of it's additional health benefits and low cost, soy is a worthwhile option for protein supplementation.

PROTEIN PREPARATION TECHNIQUES

Have you ever questioned the fancy jargon and catchphrases used by supplement advertisers and bodybuilding magazines to describe protein supplements? Terms like "concentrate," "isolate" and "microfiltration" are commonly printed on labels and ads to entice buyers to purchase their products. The wealth of supplement information and lingo can often be confusing, so we've devoted this section to explain some of the terms to help you become a more informed consumer.

259

"Soy is another protein that's been revitalized in this sport. It's one of the few plant sources that contain the full profile of amino acids. No less an authority in the sport than Chad Nicholls has stated that soy is comparable to egg- or milk-based protein."

SOY, WHEY OR EGG PROTEIN "CONCENTRATE"

This term usually refers to a protein supplement source, which has been concentrated through high-heat drying (dehydration), filtration or acid extraction to reduce the original content to a more concentrated protein source. This is the least expensive method of protein extraction. Unfortunately, other substances such as lactose, fat and certain other impurities also get concentrated with the actual protein. Products of this type are usually 60 to 70 percent protein by dry weight.

SOY OR WHEY PROTEIN "ISOLATE"

Protein isolates are created through various "washes" including alcohol, water or certain ionization concentration techniques. The objective of this process is to separate the protein from the carbohydrates and fats (hence the term "isolate"). The water method is the least expensive, while the ionization procedure is the most costly. Additional filtration techniques are then utilized to purify the protein isolate even further. Particularly in reference to soy protein isolates, alcohol is rarely used as an isolation method because the alcohol either destroys or removes the beneficial isoflavones. As such, most manufacturers alternatively use water separation to prepare soy protein isolates.

MICROFILTRATION AND CROSS MICROFILTRATION

These terms describe the type of filter used to further refine and separate unwanted substances from the concentrated protein. The words may sound complex, but there's nothing complicated about what they mean.

ION EXCHANGE

Most molecules possess either a negative or positive charge, and these traits can be manipulated to extract or separate the protein molecules from the other components in the source. This method is primarily used for manufacturing whey protein isolates.

HYDROLYZED PROTEIN

Hydrolyzed proteins have been put through a preparation technique involving the addition of water molecules to help break them down into smaller sub-units called peptides (lysis). These peptides are chains of two to five amino acids, which are thought to be absorbed faster by the body. The process itself is somewhat like a form of pre-digestion. Hydrolysis is the most expensive approach to concentrate proteins, and thus it rarely appears on supplement

"Have you ever questioned the fancy jargon and catch phrases used by supplement advertisers and bodybuilding magazines to describe protein supplements? Terms like 'concentrate,' 'isolate' and 'microfiltration' are commonly printed on labels and ads to entice buyers."

260

labels. For marketing purposes, some companies will add just enough of this type to get it on the label purely in an attempt to make their product look better. Remember though, unless you have digestive problems or another condition that interferes with protein breakdown and absorption, there is little benefit to forking out extra cash for hydrolyzed protein supplements.

MEASUREMENT METHODS

Biochemists spend quite a bit of time and effort classifying and measuring molecular compounds, and protein is a nutrient that's gotten a lot of attention in this regard. The following terms are some of the more popular ones you'll see in biochemistry and nutrition journals. These words (most often in acronym form) are also frequently used by supplement manufacturers as a strategy to generate hype around their protein products.

PER (PROTEIN EFFICIENCY RATIO)

This is an old (read: outdated) method for measuring the quality of protein based on the growth rate of young rats that were given various protein combinations. Egg protein with a PER of 2.5 was initially considered an excellent standard by which to compare other proteins. Casein (milk protein) with a PER of 3.0 later replaced egg as the base point for comparison. The drawback with the PER method is that it places too much emphasis on the importance of methionine (an essential amino acid). Methionine is known for the promotion of hair growth in rats – a cosmetic feature that most humans aren't usually too concerned about.

NPU (NET PROTEIN UTILIZATION)

This is another outdated and now seldom-used measurement that reflects the value of protein foods. Essentially, the NPU is the amount of protein that is made available to your body from a specific food based on digestibility and the amino acid composition. A value of 100 indicates that every gram of protein in the item would be utilized to produce lean tissue. The highest NPU is egg protein with a score of 94.

BV (BIOLOGICAL VALUE)

Although somewhat outdated, the BV scale is still used. This system evaluates protein based on the amount of nitrogen retained by the body after absorption from a given source. The highest value is 100, even though some supplement companies advertise that their products score 102 or 104. With this measurement scale, eggs are again the benchmark food.

"Hydrolysis is the most expensive approach to concentrate proteins, and thus it rarely appears on supplement labels. For marketing purposes some companies will add just enough of this type to get it on the label purely in an attempt to make their product look better."

261

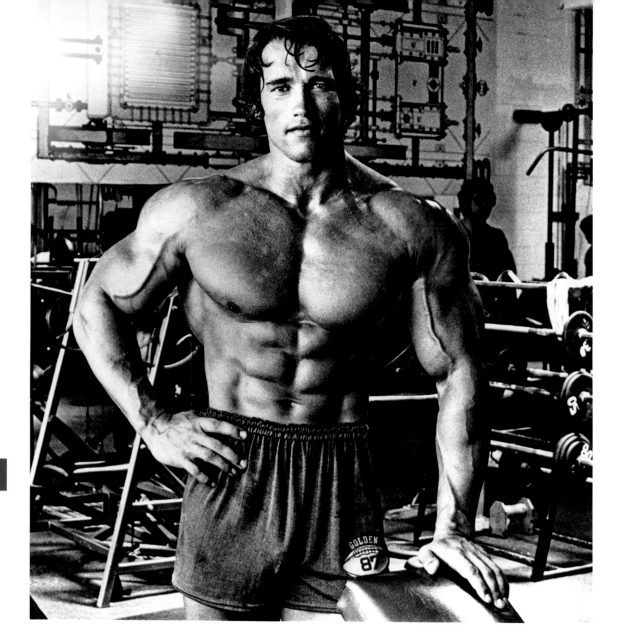

262

ABOVE: The success of the protein supplement industry is largely owed to the aspiring bodybuilders who idolized guys like Arnold and would buy whatever products necessary to help them achieve a physique such as his.

PDCAAS (PROTEIN DIGESTIBILITY CORRECTED AMINO ACID SCORE)

While the name is a mouthful to say, this evaluation system is considered the most reliable. The highest attainable score is 1.0, which means that after digestion, the protein provides 100 percent of the required amino acids. Soy protein isolates, egg white, whey protein isolates and casein protein supplements all score 1.0 on the PDCAAS. For comparison, foods such as beef and beans scored 0.92 and 0.68, respectively.

DO I NEED A PROTEIN SUPPLEMENT?

Supplement manufacturers have made billions of dollars from sales of protein to bodybuilders. In fact, much of the Weider empire was built from the profits made because aspiring Schwarzeneggers bought protein supplements. As we discussed earlier, critics have argued for

Photo by Art Zeller
Model Arnold Schwarzenegger

decades that excessive protein consumption is not only unnecessary but also potentially dangerous. These naysayers stand by their claims that bodybuilders and other strength athletes only need 0.80 grams of the nutrient per kilogram of bodyweight to make all the gains they want. Any surplus amount, they say, will simply be converted to fat. Some who support this thinking have even claimed that extra protein places stress on the kidneys. Conveniently for them, however, all the studies they use to support this assertion involve patients with pre-existing kidney problems. Few, if any, peer-reviewed studies linking high-protein diets to kidney issues in bodybuilders have been published to date.

SO, HOW MUCH?

Individual body chemistry prevents us from being able to tell you precisely how much protein to use; we are convinced, however, that the RDI of 0.8 grams per kilogram of bodyweight is too low (and just about every bodybuilder and bodybuilding expert will likely agree). Based on this value, an 80-kilogram man (approximately 176 pounds) would require about 64 grams of protein each day, which might be adequate if that 176-pounder lived a fairly sedentary lifestyle. If, however, this individual is performing four or five weight training sessions and three or four cardio sessions per week, he or she is simply going to need more. The amount that's quoted most often as a baseline among bodybuilders and in bodybuilding literature is 1 gram of protein per pound of bodyweight. Some supplement manufacturers, and 300-pound bodybuilders, suggest even higher – 2 to 3 grams per pound of bodyweight – but this is probably overkill. Once you've determined your optimal amount, our advice is to try and obtain most of your protein from whole-food sources such as meat, fish and chicken, and then supplement with one or two protein shakes per day.

MEAL REPLACEMENT POWDERS - MRPS

Meal replacement powders (MRPs) are nothing more than protein supplements fortified with extra nutrients. These products are often the go-to solution for nutrition nightmares among the general population. Most bodybuilders try to eat five to six times a day, with each meal ideally containing a balance of quality protein, moderate to high amounts of complex carbohydrates and a low proportion of healthy fats. But with the fast-paced lifestyle many of us lead, finding the time to prepare five or six daily meals can be problematic. The beauty of MRPs is that they contain all the good nutrients of a nutritionally correct meal and none of the bad such as saturated fat and simple sugar, all in a fast and easy-to-drink liquid. The best MRPs contain a precise balance of protein and complex carbohydrates, and most types have

"Critics have argued for decades that excessive protein consumption is not only unnecessary but also potentially dangerous. We are convinced, however, that the RDI of 0.8 grams per kilogram of bodyweight is too low (and just about every bodybuilder and bodybuilding expert will likely agree)."

263

"When you're using protein powder, the one essential piece of equipment you need is a blender. While most of the better protein powders can be mixed with just a spoon or in a shaker cup, a blender will allow you more variety and shake options by adding fruit, peanut butter, yogurt and other healthy (and tasty) ingredients."

264

less than 2 grams of fat. Also, most MRPs have less than 270 calories when mixed with water or slightly more when mixed with skim milk (the old weight gainers, which were really the first generation of MRPs, often contained 1,000-plus calories per serving!). Another benefit is that most of these products on the market include in excess of 100 percent of the U.S. RDI for virtually every essential vitamin and mineral.

Mixing these drinks involves the same process as protein powders: you simply pop one in a blender and it's ready to drink. You can even make one in advance, seal it in a container and bring it with you to drink on the go.

Some of the top choices for meal replacement powders are Met-Rx, RX Fuel by TwinLab, Myoplex from EAS and Meso Tech by MuscleTech.

MIXING PROCEDURES

Mixing a supplement drink sounds like an easy task to accomplish, but you'd be amazed how many people screw it up! The first point to understand is that you're trying to build quality lean muscle, not just body mass. Before you start conducting your own protein experiments, make sure to read the supplement labels carefully. Many less expensive brands are just loaded with sugar and inferior protein sources. You're best option is to stick with products from a reputable company such as MuscleTech, TwinLab, Optimum Nutrition or EAS.

When you're using protein powder, the one essential piece of equipment you need is a blender. While most of the better protein powders can be mixed with just a spoon or in a shaker cup, a blender will allow you more variety and shake options by adding fruit, peanut butter, yogurt and other healthy (and tasty) ingredients. If this will be your first blender, test it out first by using just water or a few simple ingredients. You'll probably be tempted to take double or triple the recommended amount of protein, but recall the earlier discussions about protein absorption: The human body can only use about 20 to 30 grams of protein at any given time (roughly the amount one scoop of protein mixed with a glass of milk will provide). Downing two or three scoops could give you gas, nausea or digestive problems. Furthermore, don't forget that the excess will likely end up deposited around your waistline.

When it comes to shake varieties, the options are almost endless. While juice and water make decent mixing mediums, most bodybuilders prefer to use milk. Unless you're lactose intolerant, milk is an excellent source of protein, carbohydrates and calcium. For extra nutrients and taste, you can add fruit like bananas or strawberries (or any other field berries), kiwi or other fruits you like. A tablespoon or two of peanut butter makes another great nutritional and flavor addition (natural peanut butter, not the commercial types that are loaded with sugars and hydrogenated vegetable oils). If you want to increase your fiber intake, add in a half to one cup of bran cereal. When making the shake, first blend on medium to slice the solid ingredients. Then blend again on high speed to really pulp the mixture.

If you can't digest lactose, yogurt is a great substitute. Yogurt is a milk product, but contains a very low amount of lactose (because special bacteria in yogurt breaks down much of this milk sugar) and can usually be tolerated by those who have problems digesting milk. One type of bacteria called lactobacillus acidophilus also implants in the intestine, producing some of the B-vitamins. Further to the protein content, yogurt is also an excellent source of minerals and carbohydrates. It has even been scientifically linked to lowered cholesterol levels and increased longevity.

We've included a few recipes to get you started and give you an idea of the countless shake options you can make. Some of the ingredients probably won't be readily stocked in your kitchen pantry or fridge, so you'll need to do some shopping. You may also consider buying certain ingredients in bulk to considerably cut the costs. For all shakes listed on the following two pages, simply add to the blender, mix and enjoy!

265

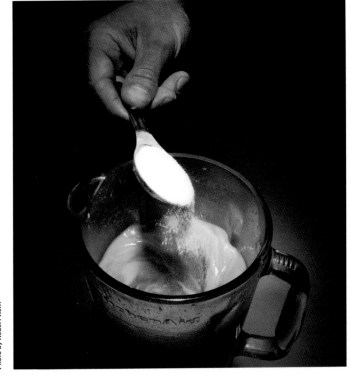

LEFT: It's important to read and follow supplement labels. The recommended measurements are listed for a reason, and mixing too much could interfere with your nutrition goals.

Photo by Robert Reiff

BASIC POWER SHAKE

- ½ cup nonfat cottage cheese
- ½ cup milk (skim, soy, almond, rice or goat's)
- 2 scoops whey protein powder (flavor of your choice)
- 1 orange, peeled and sectioned
- 1 tablespoon wheat germ
- 3–4 ice cubes

Nutrient Breakdown: Calories: 429, Protein: 73 g, Carbohydrates: 38 g, Total Fat: 5 g, Fiber: 6 g (Note: Totals are based on a shake made with skim milk.)

VITAMIN BOOSTER SHAKE

- ½ cup alfalfa sprouts
- ¼ cup frozen strawberries
- ¼ cup mixed berries
- 1 teaspoon flaxseed oil
- 2 scoops whey protein powder
- 1 tablespoon honey
- 1 cup cold water

Nutrient Breakdown: Calories: 381, Protein: 48 g, Carbohydrates: 31 g, Total Fat: 9 g, Fiber: 4 g

BLUEBERRY BUZZ SHAKE

- ½ cup milk (skim, soy, almond, rice or goat's)
- ½ cup water
- ½ cup blueberries
- 1 tablespoon flaxseed oil
- ½ cup unsweetened applesauce
- ½ cup plain nonfat yogurt
- 2 scoops whey protein powder
- 3–4 ice cubes

Nutrient Breakdown: Calories: 564, Protein: 58 g, Carbohydrates: 46 g, Total Fat: 18 g, Fiber: 5 g (Note: Totals are based on a shake made with skim milk.)

KIWI CITRUS SHAKE

- 1 kiwi, peeled
- 1 navel orange, peeled and sectioned
- 2 scoops whey protein powder
- ½ cup plain nonfat yogurt
- 1 teaspoon fresh lime juice
- ½ cup ice cubes

Nutrient Breakdown: Calories: 426, Protein: 55 g, Carbohydrates: 45 g, Total Fat: 5 g, Fiber: 7 g

"When it comes to shake varieties, the options are almost endless. For extra nutrients and taste, you can add fruit like bananas or strawberries. A tablespoon of peanut butter makes another great nutritional and flavor addition."

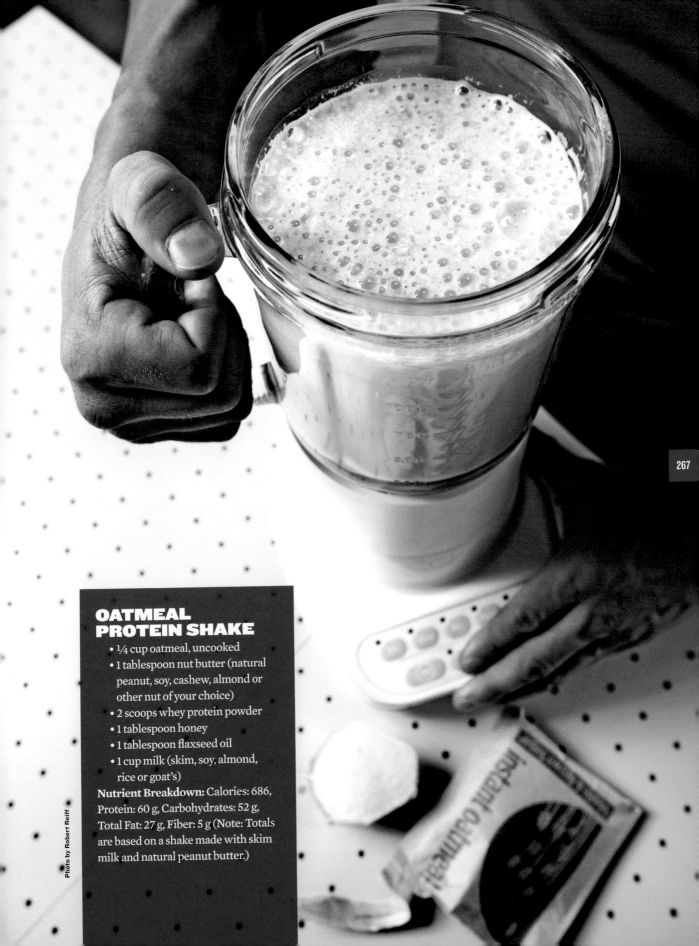

OATMEAL PROTEIN SHAKE

- ¼ cup oatmeal, uncooked
- 1 tablespoon nut butter (natural peanut, soy, cashew, almond or other nut of your choice)
- 2 scoops whey protein powder
- 1 tablespoon honey
- 1 tablespoon flaxseed oil
- 1 cup milk (skim, soy, almond, rice or goat's)

Nutrient Breakdown: Calories: 686, Protein: 60 g, Carbohydrates: 52 g, Total Fat: 27 g, Fiber: 5 g (Note: Totals are based on a shake made with skim milk and natural peanut butter.)

Photo by Robert Reiff

AMINO ACID SUPPLEMENTS

Over the years as food processing techniques improved, supplement manufacturers made more products for athletes – and amino acids were quick to be marketed in supplement form. As the building blocks of muscle tissue, it would indeed seem logical to consume amino acids instead of protein. Already in digested form and directly absorbed into the bloodstream, amino acids inflict less stress on the liver and kidneys, which would normally be involved to help break down and excrete the waste products of protein metabolism.

The process, however, isn't that simple. First, scientists are not exactly sure of the proportions in which amino acids should be consumed. Second, there are anywhere from 20 to 28 amino acids, meaning you'd have to consume this many different supplements. Third, amino acid supplements need to undergo a more extensive production process, making them much more expensive for consumers. Finally, both scientific and anecdotal evidence suggests that large amounts of certain amino acids may be harmful when taken separately or combined with other amino acids or supplements.

These risk factors are the reason many health experts argue that eating enough high-quality protein from whole foods negates the need for amino acid supplements, making them simply a waste of money. The growing tendency to use pills as a "quick fix" is also a topic of concern – it seems that members of today's society are becoming increasingly dependent on medication or supplements as a fast solution to every health issue. This trend has the potential to become extremely dangerous because many individuals incorrectly assume more is better. Specifically with regards to amino acids, ingesting too much could cause serious bodily harm. The human body evolved to remove the amino acids it needs from food in a slow and controlled manner – a digestive process that can be called selective absorption. The body breaks down food at its own pace and removes the amounts it requires on an as-needed basis. Trying to bypass much of the digestive process by taking a supplement does not necessarily mean you're making things more efficient. Doing so may in fact overload your system and disrupt the balance needed for crucial metabolic reactions to occur.

Those who argue against amino acid supplements aren't without opposition, though. Some individuals claim there is enough research to prove that bodybuilders can use these supplements without worry-

> "The growing tendency to use pills as a 'quick fix' is also a topic of concern – it seems that members of today's society are becoming increasingly dependent on medication or supplements as a fast solution to every health issue. This trend has the potential to become extremely dangerous because many individuals incorrectly assume more is better. Specifically with regards to amino acids, ingesting too much could cause serious bodily harm."

268

ing about health issues or injury. In fact, certain experts even go as far as to suggest that aminos are an absolute must to maximize strength and size gains. The theory here is that since muscle growth is heavily dependent on a positive nitrogen balance, nitrogen-based compounds such as amino acids will have a beneficial impact. As we discussed in Chapter 31, biochemists use nitrogen balance as a tool to measure, among other things, muscle growth potential. Positive nitrogen balance indicates that the amount of nitrogen being taken in from protein and amino acids is greater than the amount of nitrogen being excreted. This is the necessary state for amino acids and protein to be converted into new muscle tissue. Conversely, a negative balance indicates that more nitrogen is being wasted from the body than is absorbed. When this is the case, the body will have difficulty building new muscle tissue – it may even start burning existing tissue as a fuel source. And when hard-earned muscle is at stake, you can see why some bodybuilders would opt for amino acid supplements despite the known risks and extra costs.

BELOW: To gain serious muscle, the body must be in a positive nitrogen balance – some bodybuilders opt for amino acid supplements for this very reason.

269

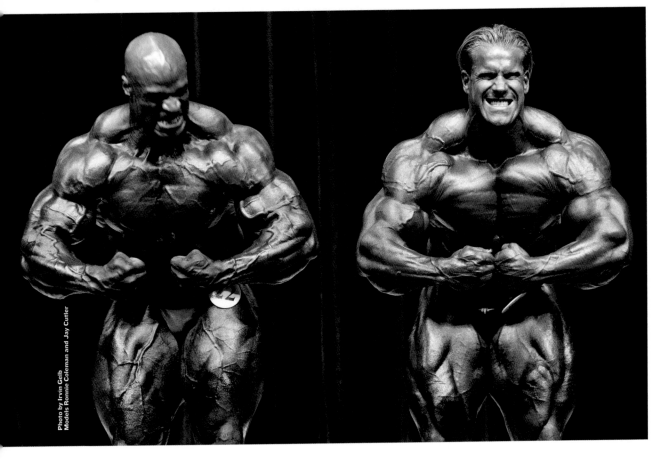

Photo by Irvin Gelb
Models Ronnie Coleman and Jay Cutler

ARE AMINO ACIDS DRUGS?

Some researchers are convinced that when certain amino acids are taken in dosages of 2 to 3 grams or more, a drug-like effect is achieved. If symptoms similar to those caused by other drugs really do occur, then shouldn't these amino acids be classified as such and be regulated under drug laws (i.e., prescription only)? Unfortunately, the answer is not clearly defined as there's an equally valid counter argument: as natural food substances, some health experts believe amino acids should remain in the food supplement category.

The argument, however, may be somewhat of a moot point because the practice of taking high dosages of individual amino acids has become less popular over the past decade or so. Most bodybuilders simply can't justify the costs when results aren't major.

BELOW: With all the advertising out there, it's difficult to decipher the good from the bad when it comes to supplements.

270

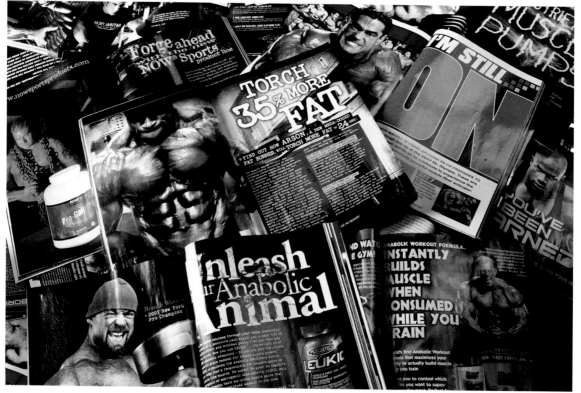

Photo by Rich Baker

The following are some of the amino acids and the effects associated with each:

AMINO ACID	EFFECT
Serine	Energy production
Alanine	Improved glycogen storage
Arginine	Growth hormone release
Proline	Tissue repair
Leucine	Manufactures other components in the body
Taurine	Counters the effects of aging
Glutamine	Increased nitrogen retention; boosts immune system
Histidine	Protein synthesis
Tryptophan	Induces sleep

Before discussing a few of the individual amino acids in more detail, we offer a few words of caution. Don't assume you can just go to the nearest health-food store and fork out $20 for the latest amino acid supplement. There will likely be hundreds of different brands for you to choose from. To the uninformed, a trip to the supplement store can be bewildering. So here are some basics about what you need to know before you go strolling down the store aisles.

There are two basic types of amino acid supplements: pure crystalline and peptide bond. Crystalline incites the greatest biological activity in the body and this type is the most effective for obtaining specific effects from individual amino acids. Peptide bond products are probably fine as a protein source, but if you're just looking for extra protein, your better option is to buy a straight protein supplement. The only real advantage to peptide bond amino acid supplements is the price.

You should also be looking for L-form amino acids. As we noted earlier, the human body evolved to use L-form amino acids as a primary source – not D-form. The D-forms for the most part are useless and may in fact interfere with the metabolism of L-forms.

Finally, for readers who live in areas with limited access to good-quality supplements, remember that most of the legitimate big players in the supplement industry advertise in *MuscleMag International* and other bodybuilding magazines. Most of these companies offer various methods to order their products (online, over the phone), so if you're willing to spend a few extra dollars for shipping, you can buy just about any amino acid supplement available.

"Some researchers are convinced that when certain amino acids are taken in dosages of 2 to 3 grams or more, a drug-like effect is achieved. If symptoms similar to those caused by other drugs really do occur, then shouldn't these amino acids be classified as such and be regulated under drug laws (i.e., prescription only)?"

L-GLUTAMINE

Of all the amino acids that can be taken separately, none have the biochemical potential of glutamine.

This amino acid is classified as "conditionally essential" – under normal circumstances the body can synthesize sufficient amounts of glutamine to meet physiological demands from other amino acids. But there are also times when the body cannot do so, such as conditions of high metabolic stress. Recently, L-glutamine has come to be regarded as one of the most important amino acids when the body is subjected to physical stress such as trauma (including surgical trauma), cancer, burns, and yes – intense exercise and/or dieting! Under these circumstances, L-glutamine becomes essential, and it is therefore very important to ensure consumption of this amino acid is sufficient to meet the increased physiological demands.

L-glutamine is primarily synthesized and stored in skeletal muscle. Glutamine can also be manufactured from a closely related nonessential amino acid, L-glutamate, which gets converted into L-glutamine through a reaction catalyzed by the enzyme glutamine synthase. This specific chemical process requires ammonia, ATP and magnesium.

L-glutamine is a very versatile amino acid and is the main source for a number of bodily processes and reactions. It serves an important role in the regulation of acid-base balance and allows the kidneys to excrete high acid urine, thus protecting the body from acidosis.

For bodybuilders, glutamine is particularly beneficial for helping to keep the body's nitrogen balance in a positive range. With ample amounts of this amino acid in your system, you'll retain more nitrogen and thus maintain an anabolic (muscle-building) state. Without enough glutamine, you risk muscle tissue breakdown due to a shortage of nitrogen. A simple way to determine whether your body is experiencing a negative nitrogen balance is to use your nose – that's right, take a good sniff! When the body is breaking down muscle tissue for fuel, one of the byproducts is ammonia; and there is no mistaking the smell of ammonia. Triathlon athletes and marathon runners are among the best examples of this biochemical occurrence. Next time you see an athlete from either of these sports at the gym, walk by and inhale. Chances are you'll detect the distinct odor of ammonia from their sweat. Pre-contest bodybuilders can also often emit this smell if they are in a depleted, catabolic (muscle-wasting) state.

272

"Glutamine's positive impact on immune function ensures that chronic training won't result in having to take days off due to sickness. These benefits are especially advantageous for competitive bodybuilders. Anything that acts as an anti-catabolic agent is critical to achieving your bodybuilding goals."

– Dwayne N. Jackson, *MuscleMag International* contributor

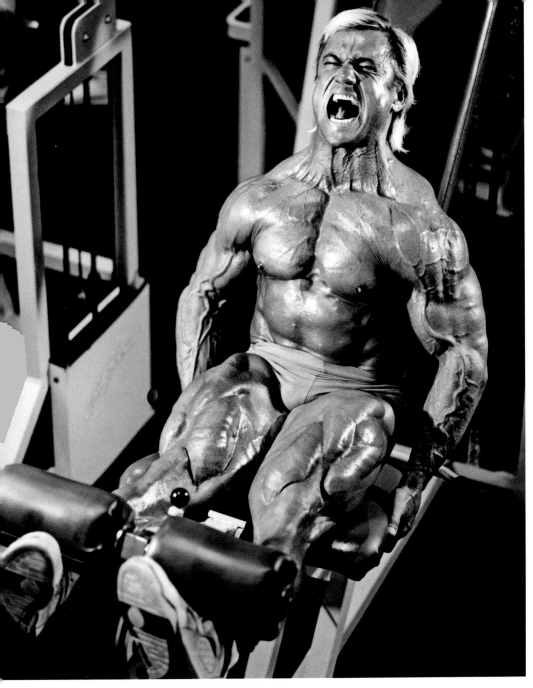

Bodybuilder or not, everyone wants to remain healthy. Further to being a powerful muscle builder, glutamine is also a primary ingredient in many of the immune system's potent germ fighters. These particular cells such as monocytes, lymphocytes and neutrophils, are enhanced by glutamine supplementation. And since long periods of intense exercise can depress the body's immune system, athletes are thus wise to supplement with glutamine. By taking this amino acid, you'll also reap the added benefit of boosting muscle tissue synthesis.

The standard dosage of glutamine used by bodybuilders and other athletes is 5 to 10 grams per day. It's also recommended that you split the dose over the course of the day, taking smaller amounts more frequently.

ABOVE: When the body is put into a state of high physical stress – like a Tom Platz leg workout – glutamine is essential to prevent muscle tissue breakdown.

ARGININE

274

> "When amateur body-builders heard that some of their pro idols were stacking growth hormone with steroids and other perform-ance-enhancing drugs, some (those who could afford it) were quick to follow suit. Recognizing the potential for a product that could natu-rally stimulate growth hor-mone levels, supplement manufacturers began look-ing for an alternative to $1,000 injections. And med-ical science came to their rescue with key findings from a number of studies."

Arginine has gained the reputation for being a stimulator for growth hormone release. And despite the liberty that supplement manufacturers have taken with the research, this amino acid is still a popular seller.

One of the primary reasons that individuals lose muscle size and strength and gain fat with age is because growth hormone levels decrease in the body. Drops in this hormone are also partially responsible for the slower rate at which skin cells regenerate – the end result being thinner and less-taught skin that we all recognize as wrinkles. As we discussed in Chapter 14, regular injections of growth hormone can help to counteract these problems. But despite the price of growth hormone having come down over the past decade, relatively speaking this supplement is still very costly.

When amateur bodybuilders heard that some of their pro idols were stacking growth hormone with steroids and other performance-enhancing drugs, some (those who could afford it) were quick to follow suit. Recognizing the potential for a product that could naturally stimulate growth hormone levels, supplement manufacturers began looking for an alternative to $1,000 injections. And medical science came to their rescue with key findings from a number of studies.

One of the first examined the effect of arginine and lysine on GH and insulin levels. A group of 15 test subjects were given one oral dose of 2.4 grams of arginine and lysine; blood tests were then conducted after 60, 90 and 120 minutes. The experiment was repeated at 10 and 20 days. The results indicated that plasma levels of both GH and insulin were elevated by arginine/lysine administration.[1]

Another study investigated sleep-related GH release after oral administration of arginine in concentrations of 250 milligrams per kilogram of bodyweight. While the research sample size was small (five individuals), all subjects showed a 60-percent increase in GH following ingestion.[2]

The initial results of these low-dose studies seemed promising, but unfortunately further research revealed that concentrations of 10 to 30 grams or more were needed to elevate arginine levels. And keep in mind these studies also used intravenous infusion of arginine – not small amounts administered orally. Popping a few single-gram capsules of arginine seems to have no effect on growth hormone levels in adults.

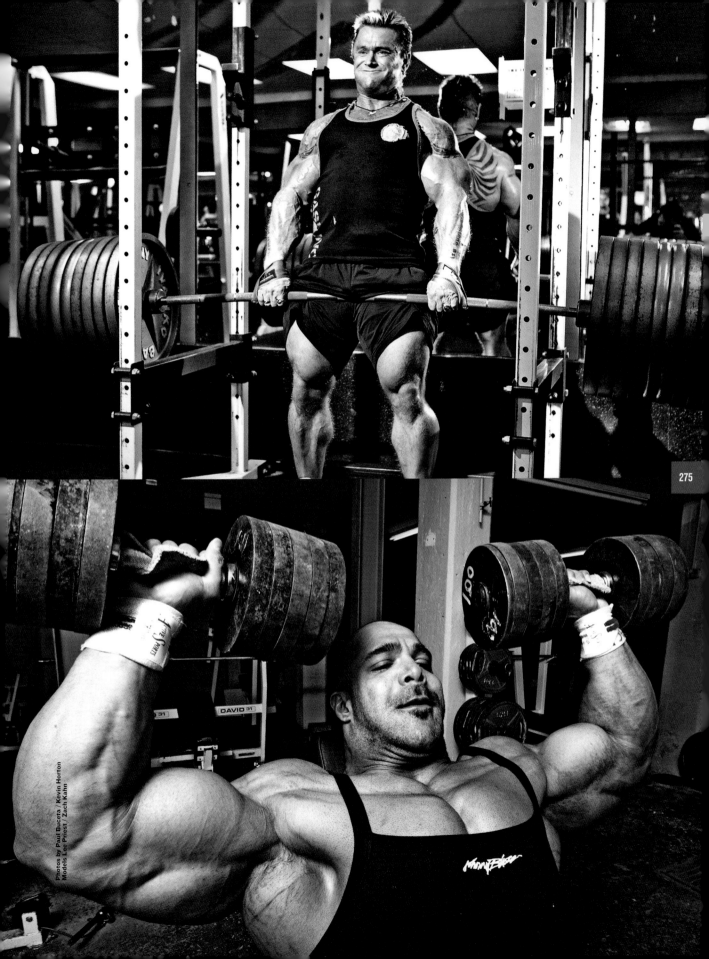

275

Photos by Paul Buceta / Kevin Horton
Models Lee Priest / Zach Kahn

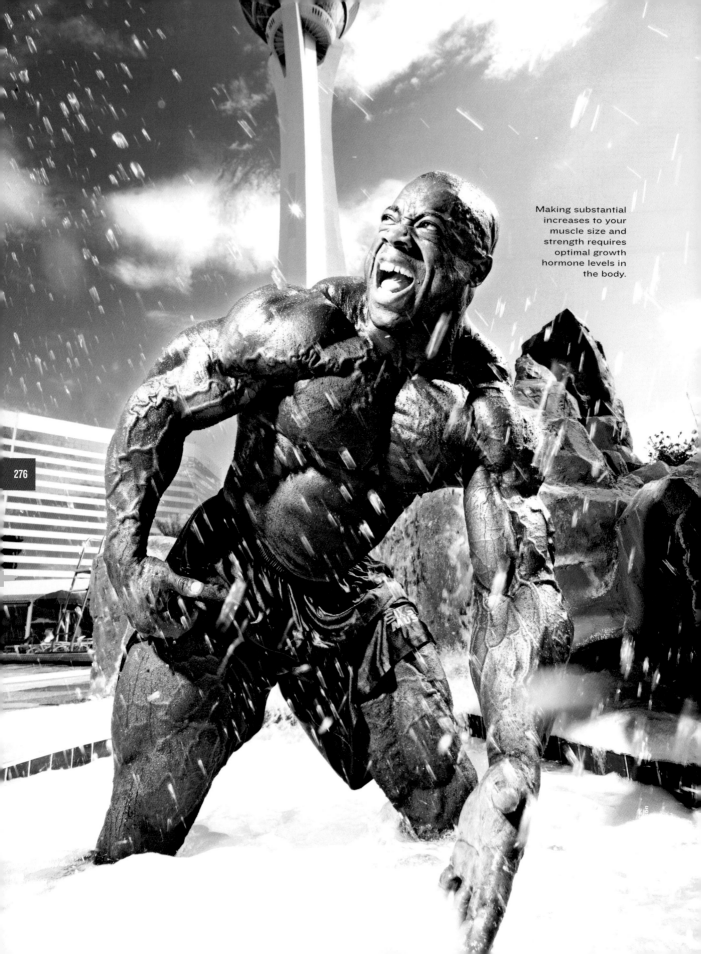

Making substantial increases to your muscle size and strength requires optimal growth hormone levels in the body.

One of the best studies verifying this information was carried out by former *MuscleMag International* contributor Don Kelly. As part of his post-graduate degree research, he used a sample of nine bodybuilders and gave them various amino acid preparations including 1.2 grams of lysine and 1.2 grams of arginine, 5 grams of ornithine, 4 grams of tyrosine, 3.5 grams of argine and 2.5 grams of lysine, or a placebo (inert) pill. These substances were administered on Saturdays and the test subjects had no idea which mixture they were taking. Blood samples were analyzed immediately upon ingestion and then after 30, 60, 90, 120 and 150 minutes. To eliminate the possibility of skewed results due to exercise-induced GH release (short bursts of high-intensity exercise such as weight training is known to promote GH release), Kelly had the entire test group refrain from working out. After collecting all the data and making a careful analysis, Kelly concluded that none of the four amino acid preparations significantly elevated GH levels.

No doubt many readers have already been sold on the product because of supplement manufacturer's claims about arginine's GH-boosting properties. Before actually taking it, you first have to ask yourself whether the expense alone is worthwhile. Keep in mind the study findings we've just discussed – a couple of 500-milligram capsules will most likely have no beneficial impact on your GH levels. You'd essentially need to take 20 just to get the minimum dosage used in most of the cited research studies. And seeing as the majority of arginine products are sold in bottles of 60 to 90 capsules, you'd end up going through a bottle every three to four days. If you do the math at $20 to $30 each, the cost could get extremely substantial.

With regards to health and safety, you probably have little to worry about with low dosages. If, however, you attempt to take a dosage high enough to elevate GH levels, you may run the risk of destroying your social life! While the specific results are not conclusive, some evidence does indicate that arginine may increase the replication rate of the herpes virus – both the genital and cold sore versions. For those readers who already have this condition, we strongly suggest checking with your physician before using any product containing 1 gram or more of arginine.

> "A couple of 500-milligram capsules will most likely have no beneficial impact on your GH levels. You'd essentially need to take 20 just to get the minimum dosage used in most of the cited research studies. And seeing as the majority of arginine products are sold in bottles of 60 to 90 capsules, you'd end up going through a bottle every three to four days."

277

References
1) Isidori A., A study of growth hormone release in man after oral administration of amino acids. *Current Medical Research and Medical Opinions.* 7:7, 1981.
2) Besset A., *et. al.*, Increase in sleep-related GH secretion after chronic arginine aspartate administration in man. *Acta Endo.* 99, 1982.

TRYPTOPHAN

For those who have never suffered through a bout of insomnia, the frustration of hitting the sack and not falling asleep will seem foreign. Yet millions of individuals spend their entire six- to eight-hour sleep cycle tossing and turning or staring at the ceiling. And for some people, the ongoing and sometimes nightly episodes can become physiologically and psychologically damaging.

Individuals facing insomnia symptoms essentially have two basic choices – tough out the sleeplessness or try sleep-inducing medications. Struggling through the experience may be manageable for one or two nights, but humans generally need to get anywhere from six to eight hours of rest just to function properly in everyday activities. For readers fortunate enough to have normal sleeping patterns for the most part, just take notice of how cranky and irritated you get the next time you don't get your regular 40 winks. Now multiply those feelings by 10 or 20 – not such a pleasant thought is it? While popping sleeping pills may do the trick and knock you out, they often

BELOW: Insomnia is a frustrating condition for anyone who experiences it. But losing sleep is even more detrimental to bodybuilders because the muscles aren't able to recuperate.

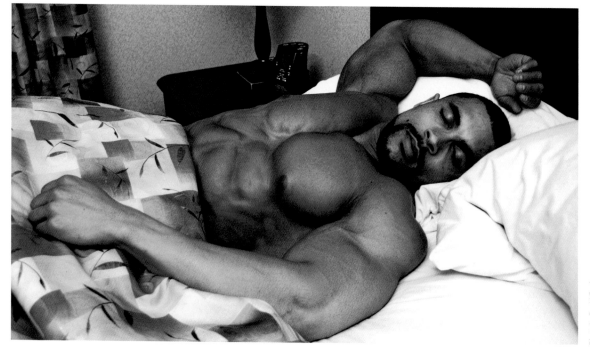

Photo by David Ford
Model Tim Liggins

interfere with a user's ability to fully wake up the next morning, leaving such individuals groggy and lacking concentration. So unfortunately for sufferers, neither of these two options truly offers a happy medium to relieve insomnia.

For the average person, dealing with a lack of quality shut-eye is difficult enough, but for hard-training bodybuilders, not getting adequate sleep ranks right up there with missing meals and skipping workouts – it can seriously impact progress and detract you from reaching your training goals. Achieving proper rest is more than just getting in the eight hours – besides the restorative powers, humans also need to enter the phase known as deep sleep in order for growth hormone to be released.

When the functional potential of individual amino acids became vogue in the late 1970s and early 1980s, it was discovered that one of them, tryptophan, held great promise as a sleep inducer. And despite the bad press it received during the late 1980s, this amino acid is still regularly endorsed as a natural sleeping aid.

MECHANISM OF ACTION

An essential amino acid, tryptophan can't be manufactured by the body and thus must be consumed in the diet. While it's an important part of protein structures, tryptophan is also a precursor of the brain transmitter serotonin, which serves two main functions: to induce sleep and to modify mental activity.

Serotonin prompts sleep by decreasing blood pressure, alertness and appetite. It was originally thought that neurotransmitters were immune to eating habits since they were supposedly "safe" behind the blood-brain barrier – a layer of specialized cells that filter out substances before they can reach brain cells. Without this protective barrier, waste products and toxins could damage and kill cells in the brain. Over time, however, researchers discovered that certain substances including amino acids could cross this barrier. Specifically with regards to tryptophan, once inside the brain it combines with other molecules to produce serotonin.

Research carried out in the 1980s determined that 3 to 5 grams of tryptophan not only promoted sleep, but also increased total sleep time and generated feelings of well-being when test subjects were awake.

Tryptophan's effects on sleep are a factor for why this amino is considered an indirect GH releaser. In general, maximum GH is freed during the deepest phases of slow-wave sleep. As such, individuals who have trouble getting to sleep, or achieving a deep state of sleep, produce less GH. By increasing the time an individual spends in the slow-wave phase, tryptophan is more able to create an optimal environment for GH release.

"Individuals facing insomnia symptoms essentially have two basic choices – tough out the sleeplessness or try sleep-inducing medications. Achieving proper rest is more than just getting in the eight hours – besides the restorative powers, humans also need to enter the phase known as deep sleep in order for growth hormone to be released."

279

A final benefit of tryptophan concerns its effects on carbohydrate cravings. Experiments have shown that individuals given tryptophan supplements seem to consume less carbohydrate snacks between meals. Although the exact mechanism of action hasn't been isolated, it is believed that increased serotonin levels heighten the brain's sensitivity to certain food constituents. For example, animals given tryptophan demonstrated decreased carbohydrate but not protein intake. Although most bodybuilders who use tryptophan take it primarily for its sleep-inducing properties, the supplement's ability to curb sugar cravings is an added bonus.

RIGHT: Every hard-training bodybuilder knows how tough it is to stay on track with their diets. Carb cravings are a common challenge, but tryptophan may be a helpful supplement in this regard.

280

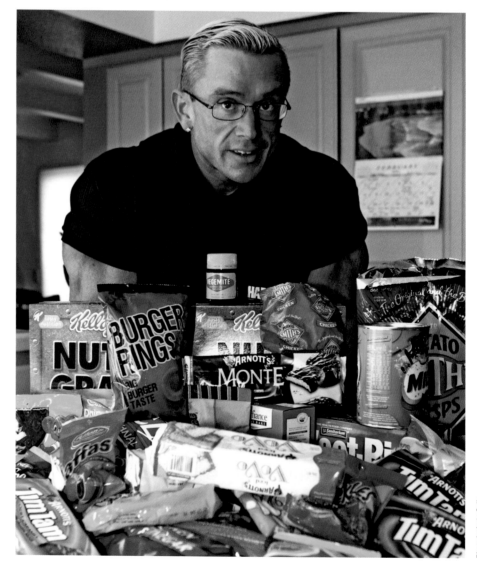

Photo by Irvin Gelb
Model Lee Priest

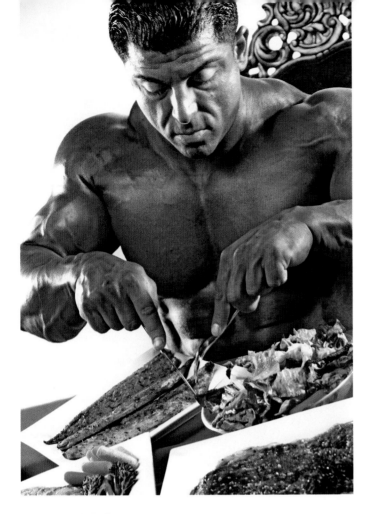

LEFT: Bodybuilders eat fish largely for the protein and healthy omega-3 fatty acids, but fish is also rich in tryptophan.

SOURCES

Tryptophan is found naturally in such foods as milk, fish and turkey. This is why many people drink a glass of warm milk before bed – because it serves as a great natural sleep aid. The increased temperature of the liquid promotes absorption of the amino acids, particularly tryptophan. And, have you ever wondered why so many people like to flake out on the couch and snooze after feasting on Thanksgiving Day turkey? You guessed it – tryptophan! Despite the amounts in whole sources though, it's far more convenient to take tryptophan in supplement form to get the 3- to 5-gram amount considered most beneficial for inducing sleep.

The conversion of tryptophan to serotonin is heavily dependent on vitamin C and B6, so it's recommended to take the amino acid with both vitamins. Absorption of tryptophan also seems to be primed when taken on an empty stomach and followed with a carbohydrate meal. Carbohydrates stimulate the release of insulin, which as you'll recall, facilitates transport of amino acids and sugar. Keep in mind though that like many supplements and most drugs, the body can build tolerance to tryptophan. Within a few weeks of use, those 3 grams won't be as effective as when you first started taking the amino acid. For this reason, it's suggested that you cycle tryptophan; exact lengths vary, but most users find a one-week-off/two-weeks-on cycle works best for optimizing tryptophan's sleep-aid properties.

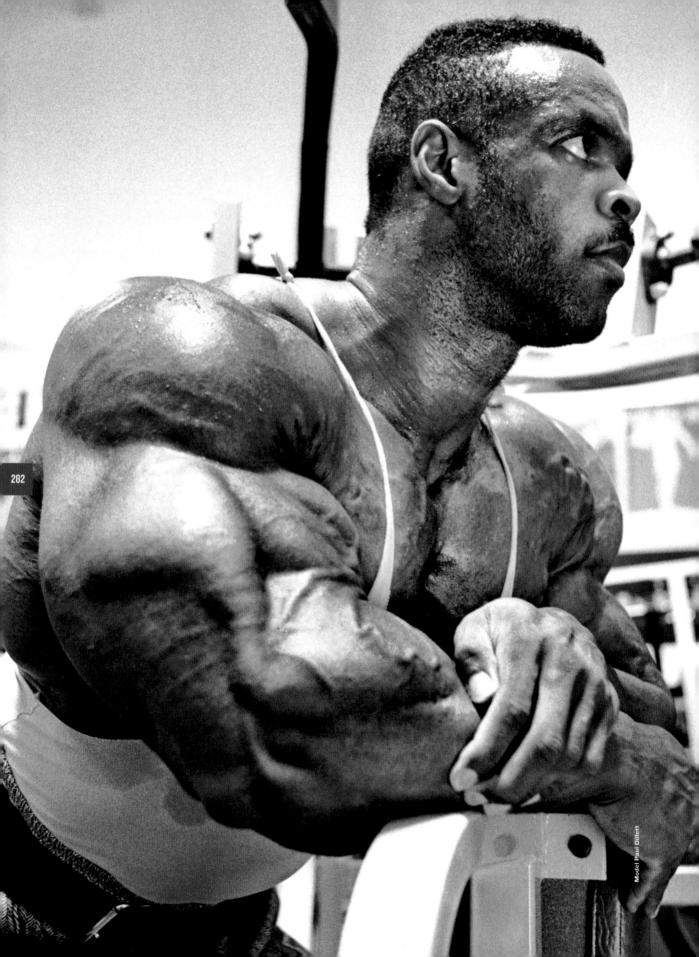

282

SIDE EFFECTS AND "THE GREAT TRYPTOPHAN SCARE" OF 1989

On the grand scale of supplements, tryptophan is regarded as a relatively safe compound. Some evidence, however, does indicate that tryptophan may cause bronchial constriction in some users, so asthma sufferers will want to check with their physicians before taking this supplement. (Pollack, 1986) Animal experiments have also found that high dosages of tryptophan may cause cataracts, but no such evidence has been confirmed in humans. As with any substance taken in large amounts, liver or kidney problems can result but usually don't present themselves until 20 or more years down the road. Those being treated for depression should also be cautioned to avoid tryptophan as many anti-depressive drugs work similarly by increasing serotonin levels. Taking tryptophan under such circumstances could push your serotonin levels through the roof.

This discussion of side effects would not be complete without briefly touching on "the great tryptophan scare" of 1989. Toward the end of the 1980s, over 1,500 cases (and 37 deaths) of EMS (eosinophilia-myalgia syndrome) were reported and linked with tryptophan use. The most prominent instance of this mass affliction was goalie Mark Fitzpatrick who played for the National Hockey League's New York Islanders.

EMS is a painful, flu-like neurological condition that affects the white blood cells along with the muscular and nervous systems. After the scare in 1989, the U.S. FDA banned all tryptophan sales at a speed seldom seen by any governmental department. This decision turned out to be quite a jump of the gun, as it was later determined the amino acid wasn't at fault but rather contamination at one Japanese manufacturing plant. Not content to stop there, however, the FDA began using this case in an attempt to get legislation passed for a ban on most OTC sales of food supplements. It was only an organized effort on the part of millions of individuals including *MuscleMag*'s own Robert Kennedy that managed to stop any such laws from being passed.

The implications of such Draconian laws would have been nothing short of enormous. Individuals would have been legally able to buy alcohol and tobacco – drugs that kill millions of people every year – but need a prescription to purchase vitamin C or protein powder!

While we've discussed the potential negative aspects and bad press associated with tryptophan, rest assured that it's generally no more dangerous than any other amino acid supplement. A few individuals may be sensitive to high dosages, but the odds of developing severe side effects are extremely low. In fact, toward the end of 2001 and into 2002 the FDA loosened the restrictions on tryptophan and it's once again available in health-food stores.

283

"The implications of such Draconian laws would have been nothing short of enormous. Individuals would have been legally able to buy alcohol and tobacco – drugs that kill millions of people every year – but need a prescription to purchase vitamin C or protein powder!"

BRANCHED-CHAIN AMINO ACIDS – BCAAs

284

"During exercise BCAAs are broken down into their basic components and eventually get used as a fuel source. This fact alone justifies BCAAs as a valuable supplement for anyone engaged in intense exercise. If you don't have sufficient quantity on hand, the body will find this powerful trio somewhere – in many cases from protein chains that are being used to repair or build new muscle tissue."

One group of amino acids deserves specific discussion because of its popularity among athletes. The branched-chain amino acids (leucine, isoleucine and valine) are named as such because of their molecular structure, with side groups or "branches" attached. BCAAs are among the fastest absorbed amino acids. It is believed that upward of 70 percent of amino acids processed by the liver and released into the bloodstream are BCAAs. Within about three hours of eating a high-protein meal, anywhere from 50 to 90 percent of the amino acids taken in by muscle tissue are BCAAs. The reason this group is so highly utilized is that muscle cells have an affinity for BCAAs. Many physiologists postulate that after muscle cells take in this trio, the body kick-starts its absorption of other amino acids to keep systems in balance. With leucine being a stimulator of insulin release, the end result is an elevation in amino acid transport and muscle-tissue synthesis – this is the reason many promoters of BCAAs consider them to be anabolic compounds.

Of the three BCAAs, leucine seems to have the greatest anabolic effect in humans. It's truly a rate-limiting BCAA for protein synthesis (i.e., if you don't get enough of it, you're really hurting yourself in terms of promoting muscle growth). However, the anabolic drive with leucine supplementation is dependent on adequate calorie consumption, so those who are in a calorie deficit will not reap the muscle-building properties of leucine. Studies have demonstrated that leucine supplementation on its own can actually deplete the body's stores of BCAAs. You should therefore always supplement with all three BCAAs together to ensure maximum results.

MUSCLE SPARING

Although they make up a large percentage of skeletal muscle, BCAAs also play a role in energy production. During exercise BCAAs are broken down into their basic components and eventually get used as a fuel source. This fact alone justifies BCAAs as a valuable supplement for anyone engaged in intense exercise. If you don't have sufficient quantity on hand, the body will find this powerful trio somewhere – in many cases from protein chains that are being used to repair or build new muscle tissue. BCAA supplementation helps prevent such muscle atrophy and wasting that can often accompany overtraining.

AN ANABOLIC SWITCH?

Certain research has indicated that BCAAs may serve a function further to being a component of muscle tissue. These studies demonstrated that BCAAs may initiate anabolic signaling pathways to speed up the body's muscle-recovery mechanisms. This property in effect makes the amino group what could be termed an anabolic "switch" to turn on protein synthesis.

FATIGUE FIGHTERS?

There's general acceptance in the health field that exercise increases release of the brain transmitter serotonin, which influences such behaviors as mood, arousal and sleep. The synthesis of serotonin is very sensitive to tryptophan changes because that amino is one of the major structural components of the neurotransmitter. Ingestion of BCAAs before exercise is believed to decrease the transport of tryptophan across the blood-brain barrier, thus decreasing serotonin synthesis. And since feelings of fatigue are activated by high serotonin levels, BCAAs thus play an important part in combating exercise-induced fatigue.

BELOW: It appears as though BCAAs may function as somewhat of an anabolic switch – opening pathways to improve muscle recovery.

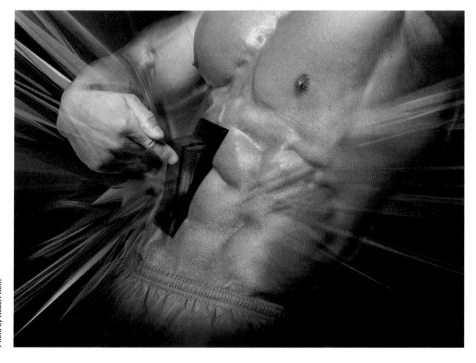

Photo by Robert Reiff

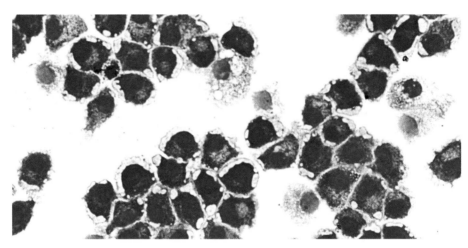

RIGHT: The benefits of BCAAs don't stop at the energy levels – these aminos also promote immune system health.

Test subjects supplementing with BCAAs have reported significantly lower ratings of perceived exertion and mental fatigue from training. Those who regularly ingest BCAAs before exercise also find their overall mood and mental capacity to be enhanced.

IMMUNE POWER

In addition to fighting both fatigue and muscle wasting, evidence does exist to support BCAAs as a central player for boosting the immune system. The body's white blood cells such as lymphocytes rely on BCAAs to help them synthesize proteins, DNA and RNA. Animal experiments with rats have found that BCAA restriction increases susceptibility to germs, leading to a greater frequency of infection. If you consider these findings, in combination with knowing that intense exercise can decrease BCAA levels, it stands to reason that BCAA supplementation would help you fight sickness, especially during times of intense training or overtraining.

DAILY DOSAGE

Most experts recommend taking 0.1 grams of BCAAs per pound of bodyweight. For example, a 200-pound male would consume 20 grams of BCAAs daily.

FREQUENCY

In general, dosages should be split into smaller amounts to be taken throughout the course of the day. Try starting with three to four 5- to 7-gram servings and see how your body responds.

TIMING

You should ingest one serving before breakfast, one before and after your workout, and one just before bed.

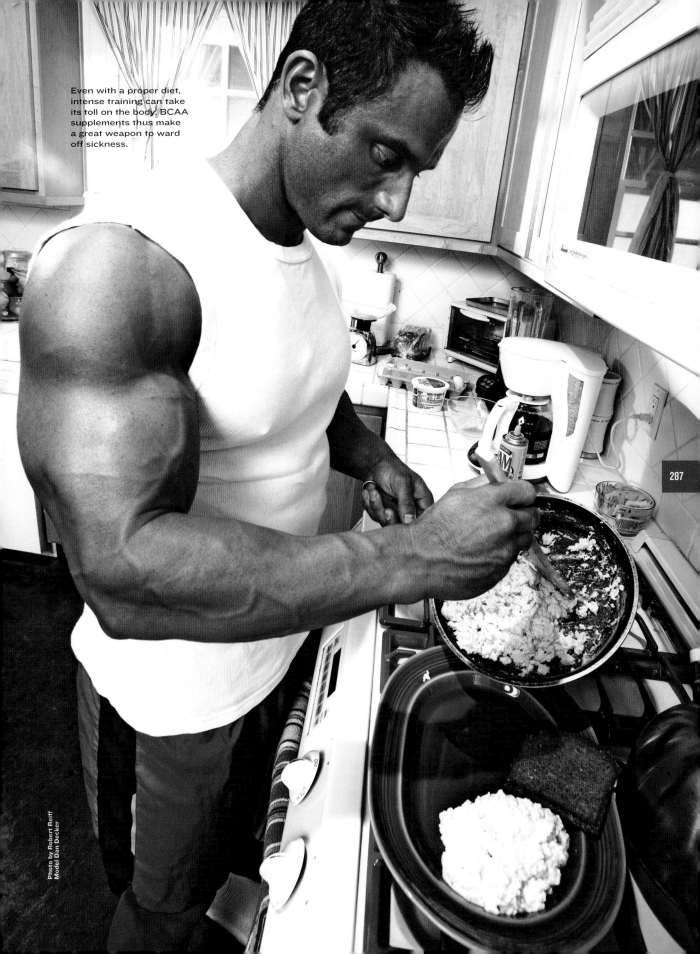

Even with a proper diet, intense training can take its toll on the body. BCAA supplements thus make a great weapon to ward off sickness.

287

CARNOSINE

288

Carnosine is not a single amino acid but a dipeptide made from beta-alanine and histidine. The body manufactures carnosine, which is found in many tissues including the heart, brain, nerves and skeletal muscles, using the enzyme carnosine synthetase. Specifically in relation to skeletal muscle, this dipeptide seems to be most concentrated in Type II (fast-twitch) muscle fibers – the ones responsible for short bursts of explosive power.

THE MANY BENEFITS

Carnosine is similar to glutamine in that it offers bodybuilders a wide range of benefits:

Anti-Catabolic Properties

Most readers are by now aware that avoiding catabolism should be a primary training goal. A number of studies now suggest that carnosine increases the production of certain anti-catabolic compounds such as growth hormone, insulin-like growth factor 1 (IGF-1) and insulin – and the fact that each of the three also increase anabolic reactions doesn't hurt either.

A Natural Buffering Agent

Scientific research has generally confirmed that it's the hydrogen ions from lactic acid that cause muscles to fatigue. These particular ions make the surrounding environment more acidic and interfere with muscle contractions. Carnosine gets used by muscles to slow down the production of hydrogen ions by neutralizing both lactic acid and ammonia, thus stabilizing the pH levels (the ratio of acid to base compounds).

Antioxidant Power

Research conducted by Dr. Marios Kyriazis in the U.K. has determined that, while many antioxidants can block damaging free radicals from entering cells, carnosine has the ability to neutralize free radicals after they enter cells. Similarly, carnosine also plays a vital role in neutralizing MDA – malondialdehyde – a byproduct of fat metabolism. If left unchecked MDA can damage cell DNA and proteins, and accelerate the plaque buildup of atherosclerosis.

"Research conducted by Dr. Marios Kyriazis in the U.K. has determined that, while many antioxidants can block damaging free radicals from entering cells, carnosine has the ability to neutralize free radicals after they enter cells."

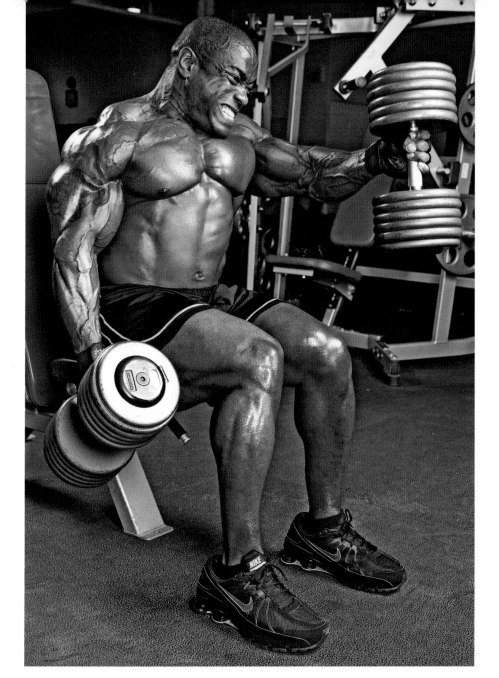

Photo by Paul Buceta
Model Leo Ingram

Nitric Oxide Booster

Nitric oxide supplements have become very popular in the bodybuild-ing community because of their ability to increase vasodilation and thus speed up blood flow to muscles. When blood flows faster throughout the body, the transport of nutrients to muscles is improved. This in turn increases the body's recovery abilities and stimulates new growth and repair. Although not conclusive, certain research suggests that carnosine can increase nitric oxide production at a faster rate than the compound's arginine precursor.

Dosage

The general consensus on the daily dose of carnosine is 3 to 3.2 grams to bring about the full spectrum of benefits discussed in this chapter.

ABOVE: Short, explosive bursts of power are generated by fast-twitch muscle fibers – where carnosine is most concentrated.

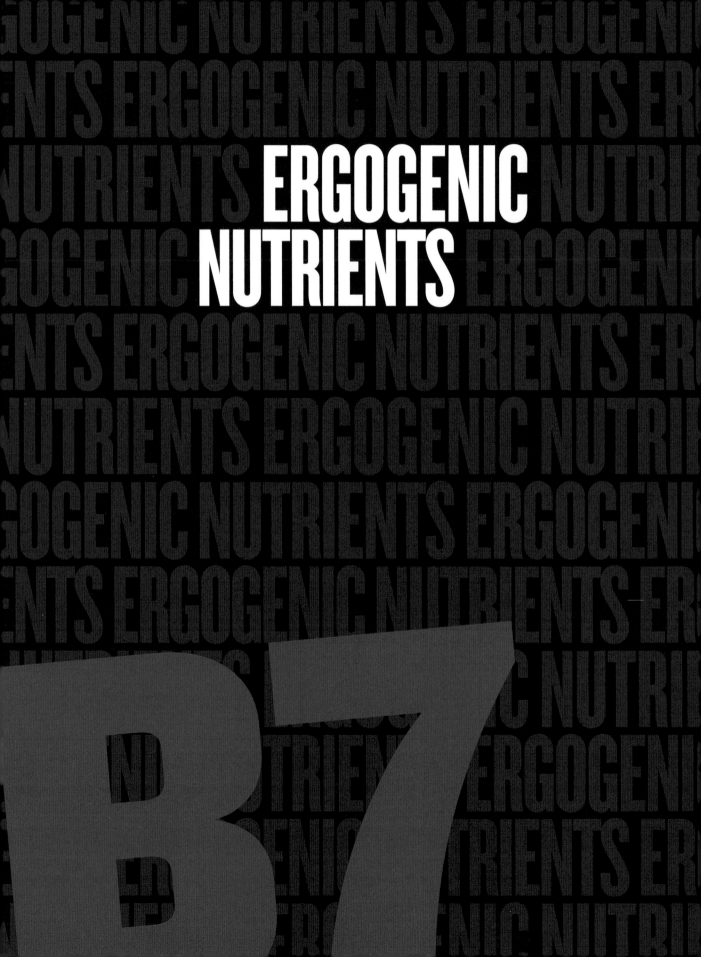

ERGOGENIC NUTRIENTS

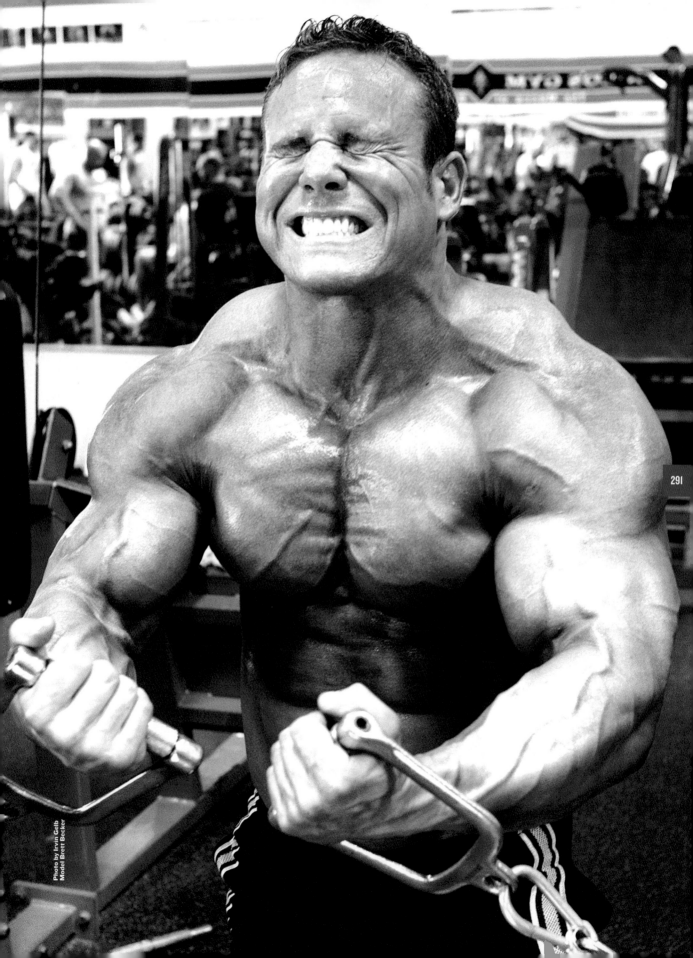

291

FAT – THE MUCH-MALIGNED NUTRIENT

292

Few nutrient groups have seen the dramatic turn around as fats. The human body has always depended on certain fats for optimum health, but the media prosecution has tarnished the reputation of this vital compound in the eyes of the public – ironic given that fats are just as important for health as protein and carbohydrates. Also, despite what their name implies, fats actually play a role in fat loss.

Biochemically, fats are concentrated sources of energy that contain nine calories per gram versus four calories per gram for both protein and carbohydrates. Fats can be divided into a number of different categories with saturated and unsaturated being the two primary types. Without going into too much biochemistry, the terms saturated and unsaturated refer to the number of hydrogen atoms connected (bonded) to the central carbon atoms. Saturated fats have the full compliment of hydrogen atoms while unsaturated are lacking. Given that hydrogen is nature's simplest atom you wouldn't think that a few less or more of them would make much of a difference, but it makes a huge difference especially as it applies to human health.

Saturated fats are commonly called "bad" fats, but the word evil is more appropriate! Saturated fats tend to be solid at room temperature. Because the body doesn't digest them that readily, they tend to get deposited along arterial walls. It's saturated fat that causes heart disease, stroke and certain cancers. Your goal should be to keep saturated fat to a minimum. Closely related to saturated fats are trans and hydrogenated fats. If saturated fat should be kept to a minimum, trans and hydrogenated fats should be entirely avoided. Both these fat mutations are the result of 20th century food processing. As they rarely occur in nature, the human body doesn't have the enzymes necessary to break them down. As evil as saturated fat is for increasing the risk of heart disease and stroke, trans and hydrogenated fats are among the greatest health destroyers. Do everything in your power to eliminate them from your diet.

Unsaturated fats are commonly called "good" fats and can be divided into monounsaturated and polyunsaturated. Unlike their saturated

"Cholesterol is the building block of every cell in our body. Without it we die. We also need cholesterol to make hormones, including the bodybuilder's best buddy – testosterone. Low cholesterol equals low testosterone production, which in turn equals low muscle growth. Using the same math we see that increasing cholesterol equals increased testosterone, which adds up to more muscle growth. Not bad."

– Nelson Montana, *Musclemag International* contributor

cousins, these fats are vital to life. Unsaturated fats are usually in liquid form when at room temperature and are used for important metabolic processes such as transporting vitamins A, D, E and K, lowering cholesterol levels, and serving as a source of energy. They are also used in the manufacture of some hormones.

FAT SUPPLEMENTS

One of the groups of polyunsaturated fats receiving a lot of press these days are called essential fatty acids (EFAs). Essential fatty acids are polyunsaturated fatty acids that the human body requires for optimum health. Like essential amino acids, they cannot be synthesized by the body and therefore must be acquired in the diet. The two most important EFAs are omega-3 and omega-6. Omega-3 fatty acids have a special bond called a "double bond" in the third carbon position from the naming end (hence the use of "3" in their name). Omega-6 fatty acids have their first double bond in the sixth carbon position from the naming end (hence the "6" designation).

Foods containing high amounts of omega-3 fatty acids include salmon, halibut, sardines, albacore, trout, herring, walnuts, flaxseed oil and canola oil. Other foods that contain omega-3 fatty acids include shrimp, clams, light chunk tuna, catfish, cod and spinach. Examples of foods rich in omega-6 fatty acids include corn, safflower, sunflower, soybean and cottonseed oil.

EFAs offer numerous health benefits for the human body and help control and regulate an amazing number of metabolic processes. Essential fatty acids help regulate the fluidity of cell membranes and improve their "gatekeeping" abilities by helping to keep toxins out and bring nutrients in. Essential fatty acids also influence the activation of cell genes, and help produce eicosanoids. These hormone-like compounds play a role in helping reduce inflammation in the body. They also help prevent blood from clotting internally, and help keep the blood vessels dilated (open). Finally, a diet rich in EFAs can be helpful in warding off many diseases including cancer and heart disease.

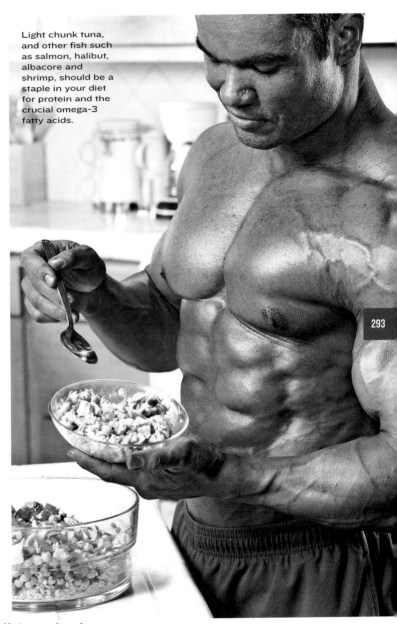

Light chunk tuna, and other fish such as salmon, halibut, albacore and shrimp, should be a staple in your diet for protein and the crucial omega-3 fatty acids.

293

Photo by Robert Reiff
Model Troy Tate

CARBOHYDRATES

The true energy generators of the human body are carbohydrates, or "carbs." Next to protein, few other nutrients receive as much press (both good and bad) as carbs. Unlike protein, however, where the general consensus is that hard-training bodybuilders need more than sedentary individuals, opinions on carbs are mixed. Some experts suggest that 70 to 80 percent of a person's caloric intake should be in the form of carbohydrates. Others recommend no more than 40 to 50 percent should come from carbohydrate sources. As with the various types of fats there are "good" and "bad" forms of carbohydrates.

Carbs get their name from their chemical makeup of just carbon (C), hydrogen (H) and oxygen (O). The most familiar carbs are sugars, starches and cellulose. The most common sugar molecule in the human body is glucose. In fact, the liver converts most other simple sugars into glucose.

There are two major types of carbohydrates: simple and complex. Simple carbohydrates are also called simple sugars and are represented by foods such as candies, chocolate bars and cakes. In fact, just about any food that contains refined sugars (such as the white sugar you'd find in a sugar dish) can be considered a simple sugar food. Of course, you'll also find simple sugars in more nutritious foods such as milk, fruit and some vegetables. Hopefully, most readers are aware that it makes far more sense to obtain simple sugars from fruits and vegetables than chocolate bars and candies! The fruits and vegetables will provide you with more than sugar – they give you vitamins, minerals and fiber. That extra-large slice of cake does not provide these nutrients!

Starches are one source of complex carbohyrates. This group includes vegetables and grain products such as bread, crackers, pasta and rice. Refined grains such as white flour and white rice have been processed. This unfortunately removes much of the nutrient and fiber content. These are no longer considered complex carbs. Unrefined grains, however, are loaded with valuable nutrients such as vitamins, minerals and fiber (which helps your digestive system work better and promotes fullness, making you less likely to

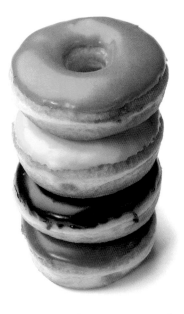
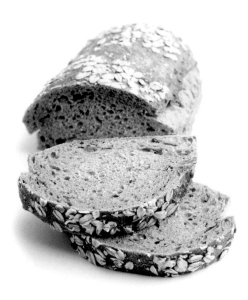

LEFT: While the doughnuts may look tasty, they offer very little nutritional value. Complex carbs like whole-grain bread will provide your body many more nutrients and energy.

295

overeat). This is one reason why a bowl of oatmeal makes you feel fuller than a sugary cereal, even if the cereal had the same or more calories than the oatmeal.

As soon as you eat carbohydrates, the body starts breaking them down into simple sugars. These sugars are then absorbed into the bloodstream. As the sugar level rises in your body, the pancreas releases a hormone called insulin. Insulin transports the sugar from the blood into the cells, where it's used as a source of energy. If this process moves fast – as it usually does with simple sugars – you're more likely to feel hungry sooner. Complex carbs (i.e., whole-grain foods), however, take much longer to break down and you won't experience those hunger cravings as quickly. Complex carbohydrates give you energy over a longer period of time.

Besides their relationship to energy, complex carbs are healthier. Simple sugars cause a rapid rise in insulin (called an insulin spike). Over time, this extra stress on the pancreas can lead to diabetes. Diabetes is caused by an insufficient production of insulin or an inability of the body's insulin receptors to interact with the hormone. In either case, the end result could be multiple medical problems including obesity, cardiovascular disease, reduced circulation in the extremities (often leading to amputation) and blindness. Even though the primary focus of this chapter is on eating for bodybuilding purposes, you're also improving your overall health by restricting your intake of simple sugars. Eating complex carbohydrates like whole-wheat breads and pastas, brown rice, fruits and vegetables, and whole-grain cereals are guaranteed to have you looking and feeling great.

"It makes far more sense to obtain simple sugars from fruits and vegetables versus chocolate bars and candies! The fruits and vegetables will provide you with more than sugar – they give you vitamins, minerals and fiber. That extra-large slice of cake does not provide these nutrients!"

> "Although fruit is one of the healthy foods that we should be eating on a regular basis, there are a couple of groups of individuals who may want to limit consumption – competitive bodybuilders and those trying to maximize fat loss. As ironic as it may sound, fruit has one major drawback – the majority of carbohydrates in most fruit gets stored as fat. This is because about 80 to 90 percent of the calories in fruit come from such simple sugars as fructose and glucose."

THE GLYCEMIC INDEX SCALE

Besides the complex and simple categories another popular way to classify carbohydrates is by their glycemic index. The glycemic index (GI) was first proposed in 1981 by David Jenkins and Thomas Wolever of the University of Toronto. It classifies carbohydrate-containing foods according to how fast they raise blood glucose levels inside the body. In simple terms, a food with a higher glycemic index value raises blood glucose faster and is less beneficial to blood-sugar control than a food which scores lower. Not only do low GI foods raise your blood glucose more slowly and to a less dramatic peak than higher GI foods, but most low GI foods are all-around healthier choices. Low GI foods are usually lower in calories and fat, while also being high in fiber, nutrients and antioxidants. Choosing low GI foods more often may help you increase levels of HDL ("good") cholesterol in your blood and might help you control your appetite, since these sources tend to keep you feeling fuller for longer periods of time.

Here are some examples of low, medium and high GI foods:

Low Glycemic GI Foods (55 or less)
Skim milk
Plain yogurt
Soy beverage
Apple/plum/orange
Sweet potato
Oat bran bread
All-Bran™
Converted or parboiled rice
Pumpernickel bread
Al dente (firm) pasta
Lentils/kidney/baked beans
Chickpeas

Medium GI Foods (56–69)
Banana
Pineapple
Raisins
New potatoes
Oatmeal
Popcorn
Split pea or green pea soup
Brown rice
Couscous
Basmati rice
Shredded wheat cereal
Whole-wheat bread
Rye bread

High GI Foods (70 or more)

Watermelon
Dried dates
Instant mashed potatoes
Baked white potato
Parsnips
Instant rice
Corn Flakes™
Rice Krispies™
Cheerios™
Bagel, white
Soda crackers
Jellybeans
French fries

A NOTE ON FRUIT

Although fruit is one of the healthy foods that we should be eating on a regular basis, there are a couple of groups of individuals who may want to limit consumption – competitive bodybuilders and those trying to maximize fat loss. As ironic as it may sound, fruit has one major drawback – the majority of carbohydrates in most fruit gets stored as fat. This is because about 80 to 90 percent of the calories in fruit come from such simple sugars as fructose and glucose.

Fructose deserves special mention as unlike most carbs, which are usually converted to glycogen, fructose is rapidly converted by the liver into fat. The reason is that fructose skips one of the steps in normal carbohydrate metabolism. The average human can store about 300 to 400 grams of glycogen, depending on the amount of skeletal muscle mass. This may sound significant but at 4 calories to the gram we're really only talking 1,200 to 1,600 calories. One good weight-training and cardio workout would expend most of this. Given the body's low storage capacity for glycogen, it's easy to see how excess carbohydrate could get stored as fat.

When carbohydrates are consumed in the diet the body uses them for many different purposes. Some are lost in the form of heat – one of the end products of basal metabolism. Other carb calories are used to provide energy for day-to-day living. Any leftover carb calories are then stored as glycogen. Once the primary glycogen storage areas are full (the liver and skeletal muscles) the rest is converted to fat by the liver. The enzyme responsible for converting most carbohydrate to glycogen or fat is called PFK-1 or phosphofructokinases-1.

Unlike most other sugars, fructose is not influenced by PFK-1, and therefore excess amounts tend to be stored as fat rather than glycogen. Hopefully now you are beginning to see why those trying to lose weight or pre-contest bodybuilders trying to harden up for a show

RIGHT: Watermelon is a tasty, hydrating fruit, but it's a high GI food so it will raise your blood glucose faster.

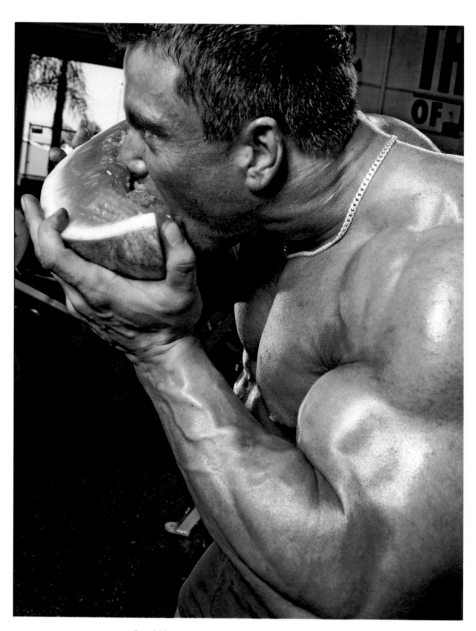

should limit their fruit intake. Better choices for these individuals are brown rice, oatmeal and vegetables.

One Last Fruity Comment

Before the nutritionists jump all over us, we must add that the previous recommendations are aimed specifically at pre-contest bodybuilders and those having trouble losing bodyfat. In the case of

Photo by Robert Reiff
Model Mark Erpelding

bodybuilding, bodyfat percentages of two to four percent are the desired goal. Eating large amounts of fructose-loaded fruit will make achieving such low levels extremely difficult. For the aspiring body-builders trying to gain muscular bodyweight, and for most of the pop-ulation, fruit should be a regular part of the diet as it's loaded with vitamins, minerals, fiber and a whole host of much-needed nutrients. It's just when maximizing fat loss becomes the No. 1 priority that fruit should be reduced.

DAILY CARBOHYDRATE RECOMMENDATIONS

Before we give our recommendations for total carbohydrate intake, we need to point out that nutritionists and experts have various opin-ions on the issue. Even within the bodybuilding community there is widespread debate. The problem comes down to individuality. No two bodybuilders will respond exactly the same, and what works for one may not work for another. It often takes a couple of years of trial and error to find the best nutrient ratios for achieving optimum competi-tive shape. The following suggestions play more of a role in showing you how to do the math rather than giving you precise values for your carbohydrate needs.

Generally speaking bodybuilders should consume about 50 to 60 percent of their calories in the form of carbohydrates. If you were eat-ing 4,000 calories per day this would work out to 2,000 to 2,400 calo-ries in the form of carbohydrates (.5 X 4,000 = 2,000 and .6 X 4,000 = 2,400). To find the number of grams, simply divide these two values by four (there are four calories per gram of carbohydrate). Doing the math, we have a range of 500 to 600 grams of carbohydrate per day.

As with protein consumption it makes more sense to spread the 500 to 600 grams out over five to six meals rather than one or two huge portions. Not only does this make it easier for the body to utilize, but there's far less chance that the body would store it as fat.

CARBOHYDRATE SUPPLEMENTS

As you might expect supplement manufacturers have made available to bodybuilders and other athletes a variety of carb supplements. Whether you use them is a personal decision. The evidence suggests that it makes little difference whether your carbs come from natural or supplement sources. Those involved in sports requiring sustained energy over long periods of time (triathlons, marathons or cycling) would probably benefit from carb supplementing. Those in sports of short duration (bodybuilding, judo or wrestling) may or may not ben-efit from ingesting extra carbs. As discussed earlier, natural stores will last for approximately 60 to 90 minutes – the maximum length of most weight and cardio sessions. Taking in supplementary carbs may

> "Those involved in sports requiring sustained energy over long periods of time (triathlons, marathons or cycling) would probably benefit from carb supple-menting. Those in sports of short duration (bodybuild-ing, judo or wrestling) may or may not benefit from in-gesting extra carbs. As dis-cussed earlier, natural stores will last for approxi-mately 60 to 90 minutes – the maximum length of most weight and cardio sessions."

299

allow you to extend the duration of your workouts, but the question becomes, why would you want to? It's pretty much accepted by most bodybuilding experts that short, 45- to 60-minute high-intensity workouts are far more productive than extended low-intensity workouts.

You also have to understand that most carb supplements are primarily simple sugar in nature. Odds are you're getting enough of that in your diet as it is. Like salt, you probably don't need to make a conscious effort to consume more. With the possible exception of the post-workout snack or meal, most of your carb sources should be complex in nature; and this means natural sources, not supplements. For people intent on taking carbohydrate supplements, they generally fall into three categories – powder, liquid and solid, commonly sold as sports bars.

Powders

Powdered forms of carbs are similar to protein powders except that they're usually far easier to mix. Instead of a blender you can simply toss a few spoonfuls in a glass of your favorite beverage and mix it with a spoon. Powdered forms of carbs can be simple or complex, or a mixture of both. One of the most popular is maltodextrin. Although maltodextrin is a form of sugar, it's actually a hydrolysate of starch, and is used in many energy-boosting products, meal replacements, weight gainers and often in liquid sports drinks. Despite being a sugar derivative it's actually a complex molecule, and has a much slower release than typical sugar into the bloodstream. This makes it a perfect choice for sustained energy. Typically a slow-releasing carbohydrate such as maltodextrin can sustain energy release for a number of hours. This is why maltodextrin is clearly a better choice for the majority of good sports supplements rather than fast-releasing high-glycemic sugars often found in cheap weight gainers and sports drinks.

Liquids

For those looking for a quick and convenient way to get some simple sugar into their systems, liquid carb drinks are the way to go. Most are sold as sports drinks and owe their existence to the works of Dr. Robert Cade in 1967. Through experiments conducted on university football players, Dr. Cade came up with a drink containing carbs and electrolytes. To honor the university where most of the experiments were carried out – the University of Florida – Dr. Cade called his drink Gatorade after the university's nickname – The Gators. It wasn't long before a commercial product was available and nowadays the all-familiar big green barrel is as much a part of college football as the cheerleaders. And it's also become somewhat of a tradition to dump the remaining contents of a Gatorade cooler over the winning coach at the end of a game. Despite the success of rival products,

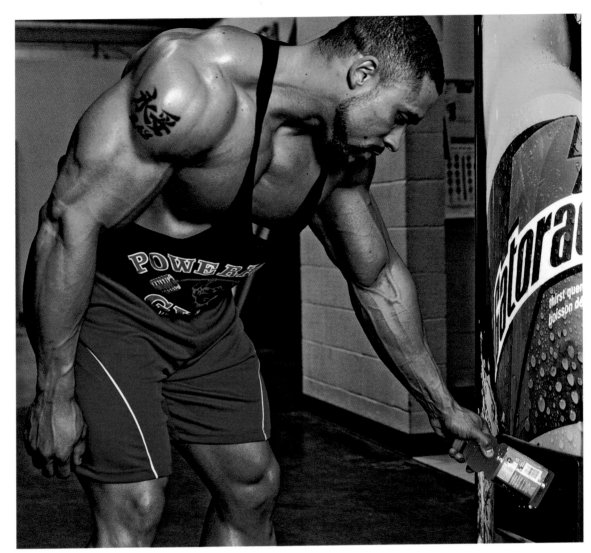

ABOVE: When you say sports drink, most people immediately think Gatorade – the pioneer liquid carb-electrolyte drink.

Photo by Jason Breeze
Model Tim Ligglins

Gatorade is still the largest-selling sports drink in North America.

The first versions of Gatorade had limited appeal, as they were very sweet and syrupy in texture and taste. But over the years, Gatorade and its "ade" rivals have released a whole spectrum of products to suit just about everyone's tastes.

Most sports drinks are marketed with such fancy terms as "carbo," "energize" and "fuel." Don't be misled, however, as all contain the same primary ingredients – varying degrees of sucrose, glucose and fructose. The biggest advantage of carb drinks is their convenience. No mixing or blending. Just unscrew the bottlecap and start drinking. The fact that these drinks are also an excellent source of fresh water doesn't hurt either.

Although it varies among individuals, generally speaking you should start drinking the beverage about 10 to 15 minutes into your workout. If you start too early when there is no demand for the sugar, your body will respond by increasing insulin levels, which in turn could lead to hypoglycemia-induced drowsiness. Exercise, on the other hand, tends to slow down insulin release.

Don't drink the whole bottle in one or two chugs either. This is not a fraternity house bash. You want to sip the drink slowly throughout the remainder of your workout and the drive or walk home. This not only increases utilization but also reduces the risk of developing stomach cramps.

Sports Bars

Sports bars are probably one of the cleverest forms of marketing ever carried out by supplement manufacturers. The first sports bars – both protein and carbohydrate – were decently healthful but tasted, as many bodybuilders discovered, like dried-out chalk! After the initial fanfare died down and sales dropped, manufacturers decided to take a different approach. Instead of trying to improve the taste of an otherwise healthy product, they loaded in copious amounts of fat and sugar. Other than some extra protein and maybe some complex carbohydrates, the vast majority of sports bars are no better than a typical chocolate or candy bar. In many cases they contain more calories. To justify the extra sugar, supplement manufacturers use such marketing terms as "energize" and "power" to target unsuspecting athletes. Most sports bars are loaded with simple sugar like fructose as this keeps manufacturing costs down and gives the bar a great taste, but as we discussed earlier, fructose is a poor carb source for bodybuilders because of its tendency to be stored as fat. The best bars are those that contain maltodextrin and other complex carbs. Of course you'll pay extra for this (anywhere from $2 to $3 per bar), but at least you'll be getting a product that is somewhat healthy and less likely to put a spare tire around your waist.

Side Effects

Some readers may question a section on side effects in a chapter on a natural substance like carbohydrates, but there's a good reason for doing so. Excess carbohydrates can lead to such serious health issues as heart disease and diabetes. If those don't qualify as side effects we don't know what does. Excess carbohydrates – both simple and complex or high and low glycemic index – will be stored as fat. It's that simple. Not only will excess fat derail any chance you have of building an attractive-looking physique, but remember that by the time fat has built up on the outside of the body it has already become deposited in and around your organs. Excess bodyfat in turn leads to cardiovascular disease and diabetes. So not only will you look unhealthy – you'll also be physically unhealthy.

If any nutrient needs to be eaten in moderation it's carbohydrates. Unless you're a triathlete or marathon runner there's no reason for you to be eating 70 to 80 percent of your calories in the form of carbohydrates – 50 to 60 percent is more than adequate.

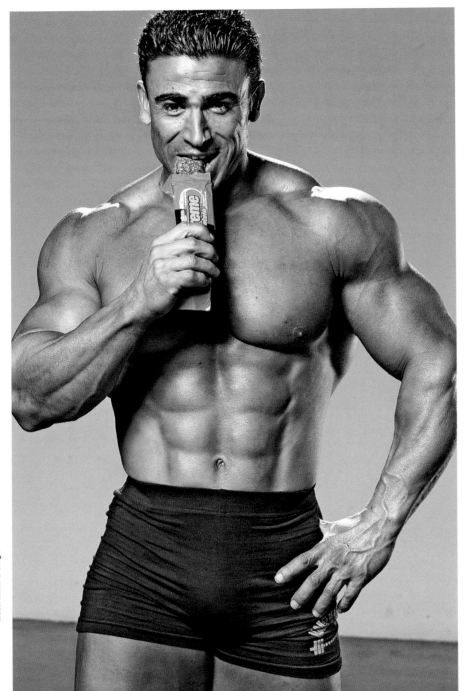

Photo by Robert Reiff
Model Kamal El Gargni

LEFT: Sports bars have come a long way since the chalky, dry versions. Buyers beware, though. Many of these bars are now loaded with fat and sugar.

CARBOHYDRATE LOADING

When you start attending bodybuilding contests on a regular basis you'll notice that some competitors look small and flat at the prejudging but full and vascular at the evening show. Others look pathetic for the full contest day, but would easily win the overall on Sunday or Monday. This even happens at the pro level and you'll hear such explanations as "I missed my peak," or "I left it too late," at the Sunday or Monday photo shoot when they're displaying the physique that they should have brought to the stage on Saturday. So what is it that explains the dramatic change in a bodybuilder's physique in as little as 12 or 24 hours?

The biological explanation lies in a unique interplay between water and glycogen (stored carbohydrate). By depleting and then ingesting (called "loading") carbohydrates, bodybuilders can show up on contest day as big as a house and ripped to shreds. Get the timing wrong and they'll appear small, flat and smooth. It's that simple and here's how it works.

The stored form of sugar is glycogen – each gram of which holds three to four grams of water. Competitive bodybuilders make use of this fact by depleting their carbohydrate levels starting about a week before the contest. They also restrict their water intake as well. After a couple of days of depleting (usually Sunday to Tuesday) they then switch to a carb-loading phase (usually Wednesday to Friday evening) to greatly increase glycogen levels. In fact, muscles will store more glycogen after a period of depletion than under normal circumstances. In addition, with each gram of glycogen holding three to four grams of water, the muscles start drawing water from under the skin. The end result is muscles filled with glycogen and therefore much larger and fuller. As well, by drawing water from under the skin the individual's vascularity will be that much more visible and pronounced. The whole process can take as little as eight hours or as long as 72. This is why bodybuilders who look flat and smooth at the prejudging can look so much fuller and harder at the evening show. The reason so many bodybuilders look so good the day after the show is that traditionally there is a post-show pig-out. Most promoters rent a

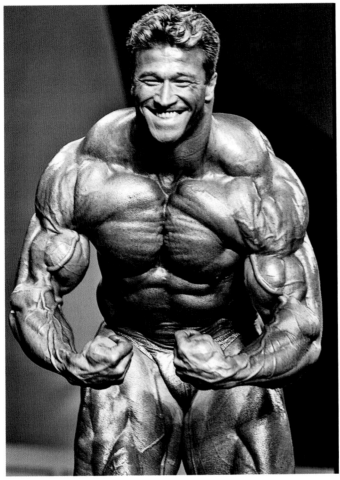

LEFT: Every competitive bodybuilder has a slightly different pre-contest plan. Diet, water intake and training need to be customized by each individual to bring forth the best physique onstage.

305

nightclub or restaurant and after a couple of months of strict pre-contest eating, most bodybuilders let loose in a feast of nutritional debauchery. The next morning they wake up fully glycogen loaded and hard as nails. Of course by then it's too late. If you keep detailed notes about what you eat and how you look, you'll know how far in advance to start your preparations for the next contest. If you looked your best at the evening show then start your loading a half-day earlier next time. If you're in top form on Sunday then shift everything forward a full day for future contests. A Friday peak means you'll need to start things a day later the next time.

Of course, there is a limit to how much glycogen the muscles can hold and once they are saturated excess glycogen may be stored in the body's tissues. This can lead to a buildup of water under the skin leading to that dreaded "smooth" or "holding water" look. The worst scenario for this is appearing smooth at the prejudging and then arriving

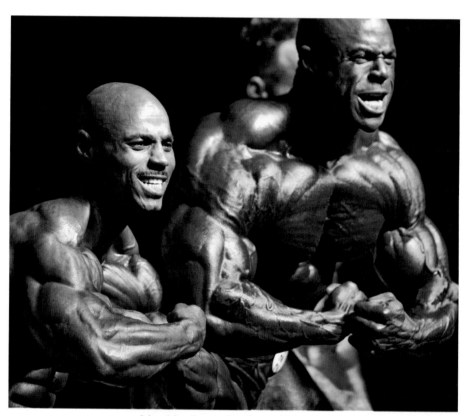

306

ABOVE: Competitors even need to account for the exess water they'll sweat out under the stage lights during a contest.

rock hard for the evening show. All the posing during the prejudging under the hot lights sweats out the excess water, allowing the person's true muscularity to show through. The problem is that the effect won't be seen until the evening show. Since most of the placings are decided at the prejudging, the competitor probably won't place as high as he could have. This often puzzles the audience, as they can't understand how the best-looking physique didn't win. Those who attended the prejudging would realize what had happened, but the majority of those watching the evening show have no prior reference point. All they see is a great-looking physique placing lower than expected.

BEST SOURCES

As you might expect, complex carbs seem to do a much better job of replenishing carb levels during the loading phase than simple carbs. Most bodybuilders rely on those two staples of pre-contest nutrition – brown rice and yams. Both are loaded with complex carbs and release slowly into the bloodstream. They promote a steady release of insulin (rather than the huge spike seen with simple sugars), which in turn promotes maximum glycogen synthesis. Simple sugars are either burned as energy or stored as fat. They make poor choices for carb loading.

STEP BY STEP

To start you off we present a step-by-step program. Our advice is to follow it to the letter for your first contest. Then depending on how you look on contest day, you may need to modify it the next time around. There's only one person who can determine how your body will respond to a given set of circumstances and that's you. You may need as little as 12 hours to fully carb-load or it may take three or four days. The odds are good to excellent that you won't nail it dead on the first time. It may take two or three contests of experimentation to get it right, but when you do the results are worth it and undeniable.

Step 1 – Increase Sodium Intake from Day 13 (13 days out) to Day Two (Two days out)

Put salt on every food item and use regular soy sauce (not the low-sodium type). Doing this ensures that the body's levels of aldosterone will be kept low. As we explained earlier, this hormone controls the body's water and electrolyte levels. When your sodium restriction starts on Day Two, your aldosterone levels will start increasing. By commencing sodium restriction late, the aldosterone level would not have been able to increase much, thus setting up an ideal condition for excreting water later on and water removal from the right areas of the body. When carb loading, water and sodium are necessary for getting glucose into the muscle cells and increasing glycogen levels.

Step 2 – Drink Plenty of Water Up to Day One

To achieve the full benefit of carb loading, you need to drink copious amounts of water right up until one day from the contest. Glucose is co-transported with sodium into the muscle cells, and with this transport follows water. Drinking large amounts of water also causes the body to shed water that is stored under the skin. This gives the muscles a harder, more vascular appearance.

Step 3 – Start Your Carb Depletion on Day Seven

On Days Seven and Six, reduce your carb intake by 50 percent. From Days Five to Three, reduce your carbs to between 100 and 150 grams per day. Try to obtain all your carbs from such complex carbs as brown rice and sweet potatoes.

Step 4 – Increase Protein Consumption

During the carb-depleting phase you should increase your protein intake from the recommended one gram per pound of bodyweight to 1.25 grams per pound of bodyweight. If carb depletion results in too severe a calorie restriction, increase your fat consumption. One excellent way to do this is to eat peanuts or natural peanut butter before bedtime. Other suggestions are salmon and red meat.

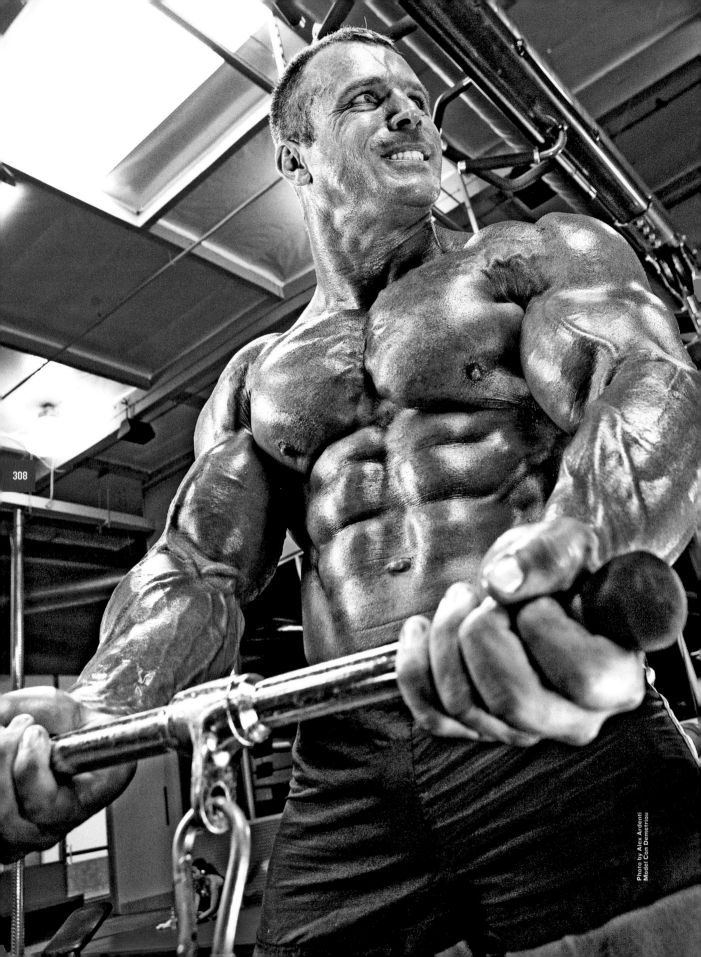

Photo by Alex Ardenti
Model Con Demetriou

Step 5 – Increase Your Training Volume

This is one of the toughest parts, as you'll be taking in fewer carbs and calories and your energy levels will be low. The goal here is to deplete all your muscle glycogen reserves. Some experts suggest high-rep training, but others feel this is a good way to lose muscle density. Instead they recommend lifting as heavy as possible but increase the training volume (i.e., add on extra sets). You'll also need to be doing extra cardio work.

Step 6 – Reduce Sodium Intake on Day Two (Two days out)

This is not as easy as it sounds, given that there's salt in just about everything. Even chicken breasts may have been soaked in a salt broth before packaging – both fresh and frozen.

Step 7 – Start Carbing Up on Day Two

This is probably the hardest step to be precise on. By starting your carb up on Day Two and continuing until the morning before the contest (in most cases this will mean carbing up on Thursday and Friday and then Saturday morning before the prejudging), it gives you over two full days to restock your glycogen levels. Some bodybuilders may need to start on Wednesday while others could get away with leaving it until Friday. It may take you a couple of contests to find out how your body reacts. You should also aim for starchy carbs. Unlike the rest of the year when you go brown, now it is time to go white (i.e., white bread, white rice, regular potatoes, etc.).

Step 8 – Decrease Protein Intake During the Loading Phase

To ensure that you don't go over your calorie limit and encourage fat storage, start reducing your protein intake on the same day you begin carb loading. With only a few days to go before the show you won't have to worry about losing muscle mass.

Step 9 – (One day out) Reduce Water Intake

On Day One (one day out) you should decrease your water intake to one quart or three pints. On contest day just sip lightly throughout. Try to keep it to less than one quart.

Step 10 – Easy on the Training

This is another debated step in the whole process. Some experts recommend giving up all training three to four days out from the contest (i.e., Tuesday or Wednesday), while others say you can train right up until Friday as long as it's light and low volume. Our advice is to go by how you feel. Odds are the calorie restriction and all the posing practice will leave you with little left for much training.

> "The biological explanation lies within a unique interplay between water and glycogen. By depleting and then loading carbohydrates, bodybuilders can show up on contest day as big as a house and ripped to shreds. Get the timing wrong and they'll appear small, flat and smooth."

309

DESICCATED LIVER

Desiccated liver lost its biggest fan in 1997 when the Iron Guru, Vince Gironda, died just short of his 80th birthday. Even as more popular state-of-the-art supplements arrived on the scene, Vince continued to proclaim the benefits of this humble but potent bodybuilding supplement.

Desiccated liver is animal liver (usually beef) that is concentrated by vacuum drying at low temperatures. As most supplement manufacturers use defatted liver, desiccated liver supplements are much lower in fat than what you'd get eating regular animal liver. As Vince was fond of saying, "Desiccated liver is four times as potent as whole liver and has more going for it than any other bodybuilding supplement."

WHAT IT CONTAINS

Because of the way it's manufactured, desiccated liver products contain all the enzymes and nutrients of the original source – including high amounts of the B-complex vitamins – without the high levels of fat. Liver is also a great source of amino acids and heme iron – something few other protein supplements provide.

The importance of iron in the diet cannot be overstated. Heme iron is probably the best source as it's the most readily absorbed of all iron sources. The primary function of iron is to bind oxygen to red blood cells. It does this by forming a heme complex, which in turn forms a major component of the binding protein hemoglobin. It's the heme complex that gives blood its distinct red color.

Besides hemoglobin, iron is a major component of myoglobin – an oxygen-binding protein found inside muscle cells. Without adequate levels of iron, both oxygen transport systems in the body would be seriously impaired.

Other functions of iron include facilitating the enzymes involved in the electron transport chain used in the cell's utilization of oxygen, the transport of oxygen from the lungs to muscle cells, the transport of oxygen across cell membranes and the modulation of oxygen burning by cells.

USING DESICCATED LIVER TABLETS

As you might expect there's no precise dosage recommended for desiccated liver tablets. Vince had his beginners start with six tablets daily and then add a tablet a week for six weeks. He routinely had his advanced bodybuilders taking 50 to 100 tablets a day for a couple of weeks and then going off for a few weeks. The advantage of such dosages is that you can take in a lot of extra protein and nutrients without having to eat a huge amount of high-calorie meat.

Although desiccated liver tablets have been overshadowed in recent years by more modern and expensive supplements, they remain one of the cheapest yet potent sources of nutrients available. For less than $20 you'll be getting protein, iron, vitamins, enzymes and a whole host of other high-quality nutrients. Few supplements offer such a wide spectrum.

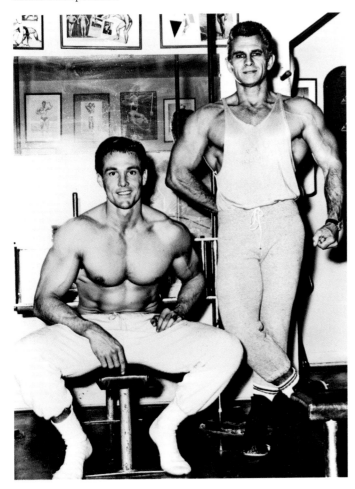

LEFT: Vince Gironda was an advocate for desiccated liver supplements – he was a strong believer in its potency for bodybuilders.

OILS

"One of the ironic aspects of modern food-processing techniques is that while the shelf life has been extended, the same cannot be said for what such foods are doing to human health. The typical vegetable oil has been heated, bleached and mixed with various chemicals."

Although there is overlap with fats, and some of the information on conjugated linoleic acid (CLA) was discussed in the chapter on fat burners, oils deserve their own separate chapter given their popularity and importance in bodybuilding.

WHY THEY ARE IMPORTANT

Fats are the most concentrated forms of energy with each gram of fat supplying nine calories while one gram of protein and carbohydrate supplies just four calories. During sleep about 70 percent of the body's energy needs are met by fat (not counting the brain which burns carbohydrates). Fat is also used for the absorption of such vitamins as A, D, E and K. Fat plays a crucial role in the synthesis of hormones, prostoglandins and bile. Structurally, fat helps insulate the internal organs, provide warmth to the body, and from a cosmetic point of view, give the female form its characteristic shape. It's hard to believe that something as vilified as fat plays such an important role in human health.

TYPES OF FATS AND OILS

The primary types of fats found in foods are called triglycerides because they contain one glycerol molecule attached to three fatty acid groups. As with protein and amino acids, the length and molecular makeup of each fatty acid determines each fat's characteristics. The glycerol molecule contains three hydroxyl groups (OH), whereas the fatty acid molecule contains a carboxyl group (COOH) and a long carbon chain.

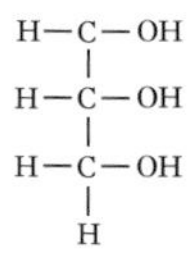

Glycerol

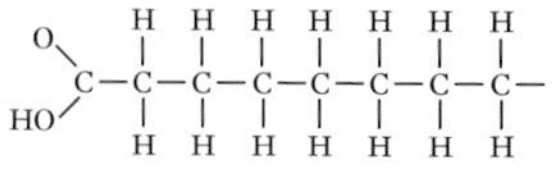

Saturated

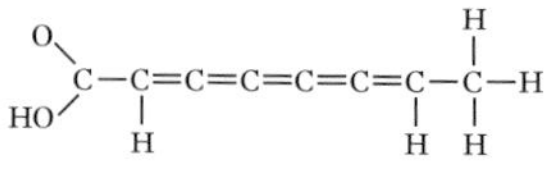

Unsaturated

SATURATED AND UNSATURATED

Chemists are similar to office secretaries in that they like to use short-hand wherever possible. In the previous diagrams the single lines joining the atoms together are called single bonds while the double lines are called double bonds. A fat is said to be saturated if there are no double bonds present between the carbon atoms. Saturated fats tend to be solid at room temperature. If there are double bonds present the fat is said to be unsaturated. As the number of double bonds increases the fat becomes more "oily," hence the reason for vegetable oils being referred to as polyunsaturated oils. Animal products tend to contain more saturated fats than plant materials and are potentially more dangerous in the long run since saturated fats greatly contribute to heart disease.

MEDIUM vs. LONG-CHAIN TRIGLYCERIDES

Besides classifying fats according to the presence or absence of double bonds, fats may be categorized by the number of carbon atoms in their chains. Fats containing eight to 12 carbon atoms are termed medium-chain triglycerides (MCTs). Fats containing more than 12 carbon atoms are called long-chain triglycerides (LCTs).

LCTs are more difficult to digest than MCTs and may need six to eight hours to be fully broken down. From a health (and competitive bodybuilding) perspective, LCTs are more harmful since there is a greater tendency for them to be stored as fat.

CIS AND TRANS – A HUGE WORLD OF DIFFERENCE

One of the ironic aspects of modern food-processing techniques is that while the shelf life has been extended, the same cannot be said for what such foods are doing to human health. The typical vegetable oil

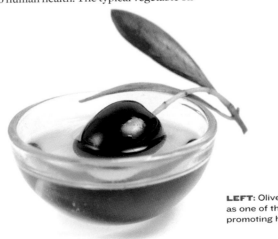

LEFT: Olive oil is touted as one of the top oils for promoting health.

has been heated, bleached and mixed with various chemicals. The end result often bears no resemblance to what exists in nature. Unfortunately human enzyme systems evolved to process what exists in natural food – not what scientists cook up in the lab. In the case of oils the food-processing industry has created a whole new class of fats called trans fatty acids that play havoc with human health. For illustration purposes we'll use the following simple molecule (at right):

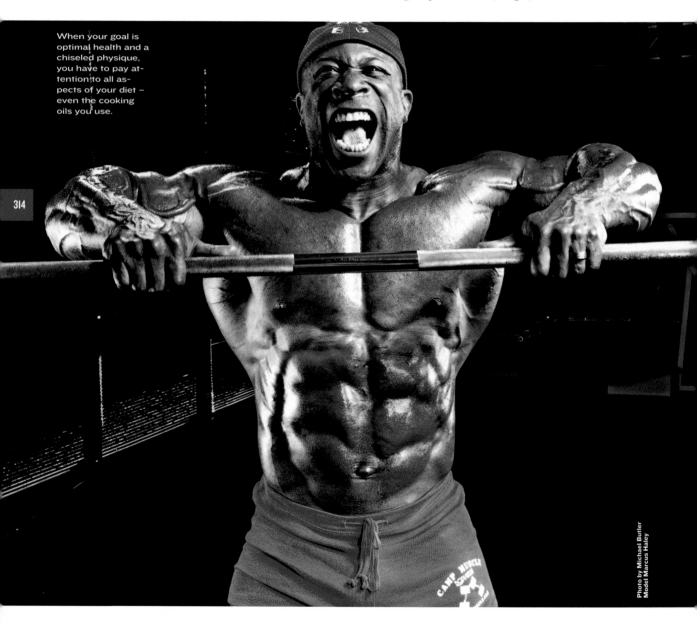

When your goal is optimal health and a chiseled physique, you have to pay attention to all aspects of your diet – even the cooking oils you use.

314

Photo by Michael Butler
Model Marcus Haley

CL   CL   CL   H
 \\   /   \\   /
   C=C   C=C
 /   \\   /   \\
H   H   H   CL

Cis-dichloroethylene   Trans-dichloroethylene

At first glance both of these structures may appear to be the same, but take a close look and you'll see a slight difference. In the Cis molecule both sets of like atoms are on the same side of the double bond, whereas in the trans molecule the like atoms are on opposite sides. Chemists use the term isomers to describe molecules, which exist in two or more forms. Many fatty acids also exist as Cis and trans isomers. Now here's the kicker. For the most part, the human body evolved to primarily use Cis isomers of food molecules. We have limited ability to digest trans isomers (much the same as the L and D versions of amino acids discussed earlier). Unfortunately the modern food-processing industry, which began in the 1920s, has led to the widespread conversion of Cis isomers into trans isomers. As expected, the human body did not take too kindly to such tinkering and over the past 80 years or so, the incidence of heart disease and stroke has taken a quantum leap upward.

AN OILY SITUATION

Unless you like to live on the edge, or assume that because of your age you're immune to heart disease, we strongly suggest you re-evaluate such misguided thinking. The buildup of arterial fat that causes heart disease usually starts in a person's 20s – earlier for those who are genetically predisposed. By the time you get to your 30s the damage is already advancing. It makes far more sense to prevent heart disease than treat it (and besides, scars from open-heart surgery are hard to cover up with Pro Tan!).

We can't stress enough the importance of reading those labels when you go to the supermarket. Most of the common cooking oils have undergone some degree of processing. As soon as you see the word "hydrogenated" or "partially-hydrogenated", immediately put the bottle back on the shelf. Leave it for those who have less respect for their health than you do. Also, check to see how much saturated and trans fat the product contains. Anything over five grams per serving is considered high.

Hopefully we haven't entirely frightened you away from fats, since there are a number of oils that are both healthy and essential. In the following chapters we'll look at the more popular oils and why small amounts of one or more should be included in your diet on a daily basis.

MEDIUM-CHAIN TRIGLYCERIDES (MCT)

MCT oils are another of those bodybuilding supplements that got their start in the medical field.
Recognizing that many people have trouble absorbing good fats researchers came up with MCTs to help treat people suffering fat-malabsorption diseases. It was also found that MCT oils had the ability to help prevent muscle catabolism in burn patients.

Because of their shorter chains – usually six to 10 carbon atoms – and other unique properties, MCTs bypass the long digestive process that LCTs must go through and are absorbed directly into the bloodstream. Also, unlike LCTs, which go through the intestinal wall and are usually converted to fat and stored, MCTs go directly to the liver where they are rapidly oxidized.

Another difference between the two is that most fatty acids require the amino acid L-carnitine to facilitate their transport into the cell's mitochondria. MCT oils, however, are not dependent on L-carnitine and can go directly into the mitochondria.

BODYBUILDING BENEFITS

Most bodybuilders who use MCT oil say that it increases their endurance and lowers bodyfat. One of the theories for this is that by adding MCTs to the diet the body has a high-density energy source available. This means that glycogen stores are spared for longer more intense workouts. It has also been suggested that MCT oils can increase production of ketones – one of the byproducts of fat metabolism. These in turn can be used as a direct energy source. This helps to suppress appetite and make it easier to stay on a pre-contest diet. It should also be added that the body much prefers to use ketones as an energy source rather than amino acids, particularly branched-chain amino acids. This leaves the amino acids available for muscle repair and growth. It has been shown that MCTs can lower overall cholesterol levels.

SIDE EFFECTS

Side effects from MCT oil are rare but do exist. There have been a few studies that suggest MCTs may reduce the absorption of the fat-soluble vitamins. This is usually of no concern to most bodybuilders given that they take multivitamin supplements. Diabetics may want to avoid MCT supplements because of the ketone relationship. As diabetics already have elevated ketones, MCT supplementing may aggravate the problem producing the condition of acidosis – increased body acidity, which under certain circumstances can be fatal.

People who take MCT oil on an empty stomach or in high dosages (more than one to two tablespoons at a time) may experience diarrhea, stomach cramps, nausea and occasional vomiting. These side effects can easily be avoided by taking the product with meals and only in small dosages. Start out by taking half a tablespoon, and over a period of a few weeks increase it to one to two tablespoons with each meal.

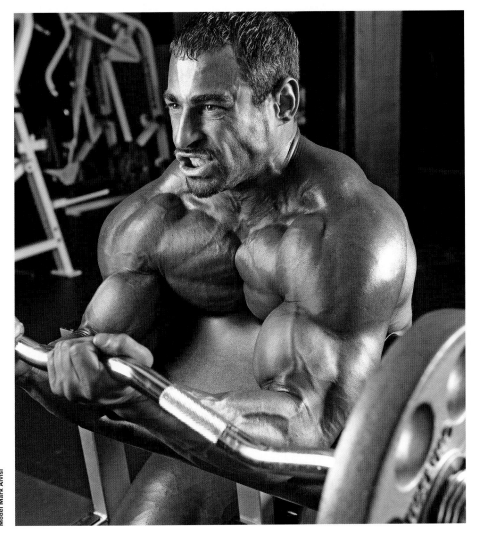

Photo by Ralph DeHaan
Model Mark Alvisi

LEFT: Many bodybuilders choose MCT supplements because the oil is said to improve endurance and help drop bodyfat levels.

317

PRIMROSE OIL

Although at one time shuttled to the fringe of the supplement spectrum, primrose oil has grown in popularity over the last decade. The most well-known member of the primrose family is the Evening Primrose, with the oil being extracted from the seeds (in most species the flowers are yellow and open in the evening hence the name Evening Primrose). The roots have a peppery flavor and can be eaten like a vegetable, while the shoots can be eaten as a salad. Over the centuries, the whole plant has been used to treat various medical conditions. The mature seeds of Evening Primrose contain approximately 7 to 10 percent gamma-linolenic acid (GLA), which is an omega-6 essential fatty acid. This polyunsaturated fat is a "good fat," unlike the saturated fats that contribute to heart disease.

It was originally thought that GLA could be manufactured in all individuals from existing linolenic supplies, but it's now known that many individuals must consume it in their diets. One of the reasons for this is that the body can only make GLA from Cis forms of essential fatty acids, not trans fat. In fact, high levels of trans fats also block GLA production. The following are some of the health and bodybuilding benefits of primrose oil.

FAT BURNING

As with other beta-3 agonists, primrose oil has been linked to fat loss by stimulating brown adipose tissue. It's suggested that high concentrations of GLA stimulate the mitochondria in brown adipose tissue. As we saw earlier, mitochondria are the cell's energy producing organelles and by increasing their activity it causes the body to burn more stored fat as an energy source. This makes primrose oil a valuable addition to your diet – especially during the pre-contest season.

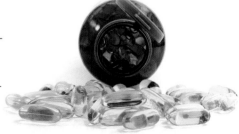

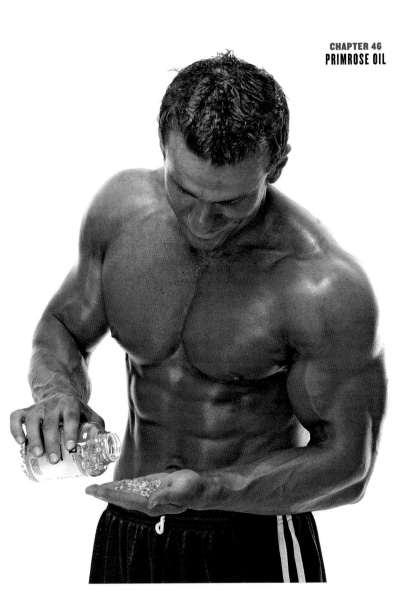

Photo by Alex Ardenti
Model Billy Begovic

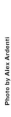

LEFT: Primrose oil supplements have been linked to fat loss and improved heart health.

REDUCING HEART DISEASE

Despite what most people assume, heart disease is a 20th-century invention. Prior to the 1920s, bacteria and viruses killed far more people than heart attacks, but with the addition of trans fat to the diet in the 1920s, cardiovascular-related deaths skyrocketed. Add in the reduced physical activity as people switched from labor to desk jobs, and it's not surprising that heart disease is now the No. 1 killer in western society.

The primary method by which trans fats increase heart disease is by increasing the "stickiness" or clotting ability of blood platelets. While clotting is necessary to prevent bleeding from external cuts, internal clotting can block blood vessels and interfere with the heart's normal pumping activity. Primrose oil, being high in linolenic acid, keeps the blood's clotting mechanisms normal – that is, only coming into play when there is an injury to a blood vessel. In this regard primrose oil would make an excellent substitute for aspirin in those who have a history of heart disease in their families.

"Research has shown that supplementing with good fats such as primrose oil can lower the circulating levels of these 'bad fats' and perhaps help offset some of the potential dangers of steroids. This by no means suggests that supplementing with primrose oil will allow you to stay side-effect free while on long cycles of steroids."

320

PROSTAGLANDIN ACTIVITY

Prostaglandins are hormone-like substances belonging to a family of 20-carbon fatty acids. They are involved in such metabolic functions as raising or lowering blood pressure, regulating digestion, boosting the immune system and regulating blood clotting. There is evidence to suggest that low levels of GLA can interfere with prostaglandin production. Supplementing with primrose oil ensures that the body's synthesis of prostaglandins is always kept at an optimum.

ARTHRITIS

Arthritis is a general term to describe the inflammation and pain found in the tissues and bones at joints. Generally speaking there are two types of arthritis – osteoarthritis and rheumatoid. Osteoarthritis is produced by the daily wear and tear on the connective tissue. Rheumatoid is caused by the inflammation of the membranes surrounding the joints. While primrose oil doesn't seem to help sufferers of osteoarthritis that much, it receives favorable comments from those with rheumatoid arthritis. Although personal preference plays a role, most users find that three to four grams per day helps alleviate the pain. The only catch is that, like glucosamine, it generally takes a couple of months for the pain-killing benefits of primrose oil to kick in.

COMBATING STEROID-INDUCED SIDE EFFECTS

Earlier in this book we looked at the various side effects that users of anabolic steroids may experience. One of the most significant in terms of long-term health was the elevation of fatty acids in the blood. While such effects are transitory and usually disappear after steroid use, those with a history of heart disease in their families or those who stay on steroids for extended periods of time are at risk. Research has shown that supplementing with good fats such as primrose oil can lower the circulating levels of these "bad fats" and perhaps help offset some of the potential dangers of steroids. This by no means suggests that supplementing with primrose oil will allow you to stay side-effect free while on long cycles of steroids. There are still many other factors that come into play, but it may protect you from the negative effects steroids have on your cardiovascular system.

SIDE EFFECTS

It's virtually impossible to overdose on primrose oil. As with most oils, however, users who take the product on an empty stomach or in high dosages all at once may experience nausea, diarrhea, stomach cramps and even vomiting. To reduce if not eliminate the risk of this happening, take the product in small dosages with meals.

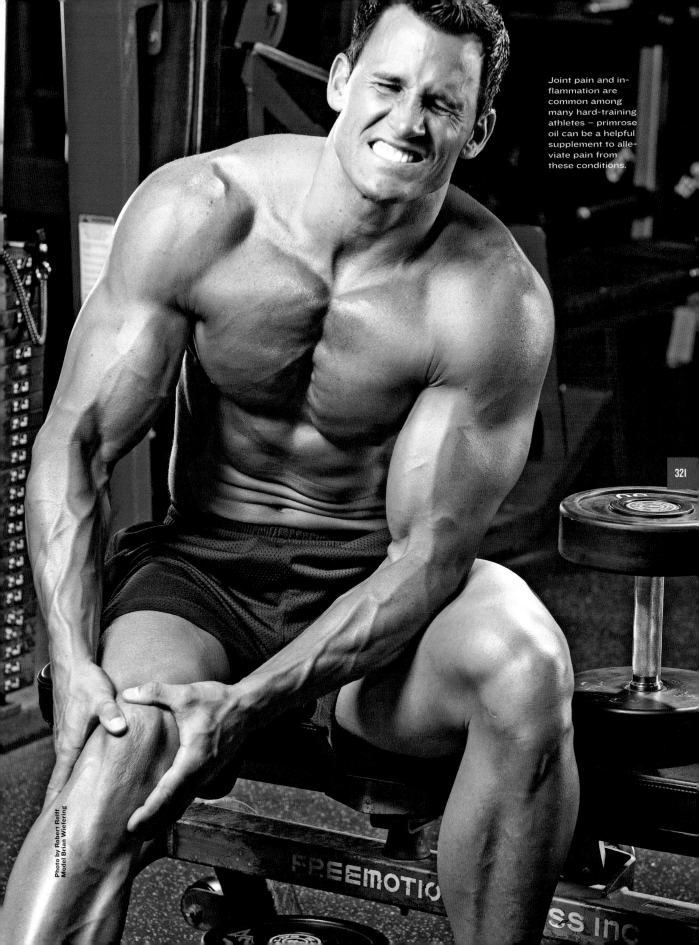

Joint pain and inflammation are common among many hard-training athletes – primrose oil can be a helpful supplement to alleviate pain from these conditions.

321

FLAXSEED OIL

Flaxseed oil is another of those supplements that is held dear to the hearts of many bodybuilders. It's also heavily promoted by nutritionists for its role in improving long-term health. Flaxseed oil is derived from the seeds of the flax plant. Flaxseed oil is a rich source of alpha-linolenic acid (ALA), an essential fatty acid that is known to be beneficial in preventing heart disease, inflammatory bowel disease, arthritis and a variety of other health conditions. Flaxseed also contains a group of chemicals called lignans that may play a role in the prevention of cancer.

ALA, as well as eicosapentaenoic acid (EPA) and docosa-hexaenoic acid (DHA), belong to a group of substances called omega-3 fatty acids. EPA and DHA are found primarily in fish while ALA is found mostly in flaxseed oil and other vegetable oils. Although similar in structure, the benefits of all three may be different.

It is important to maintain an appropriate balance of omega-3 and omega-6 in the diet as these two substances work together to promote good health. For example omega-3 fatty acids help reduce inflammation while most omega-6 fatty acids tend to promote inflammation. It's easy to see how an imbalance of these essential fatty acids could contribute to the development of disease while a proper balance would help maintain or even improve health. Generally speaking a healthy diet should consist of roughly two to four times more omega-6 fatty acids than omega-3 fatty acids. Unfortunately, the typical American diet tends to contain 14 to 25 times more omega-6 fatty acids than omega-3 fatty acids and many researchers believe this imbalance is one of the primary causes of the rising rate of inflammatory diseases in North America.

Omega-3 fatty acids have been shown to reduce inflammation and help prevent such diseases as heart disease and arthritis. Omega-3 fatty acids also appear to be particularly important for cognitive and behavioral function as well as normal growth and development.

Studies suggest that flaxseed oil and other omega-3 fatty acids may be helpful in treating a variety of these conditions. The evidence is strongest for heart disease and problems that contribute to heart

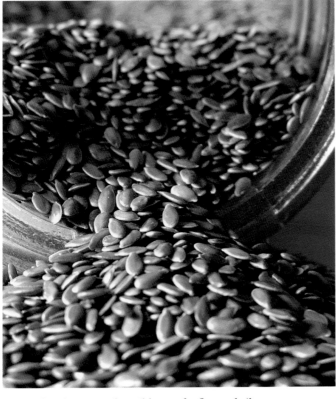

LEFT: Flaxseed is commonly referred to as a super-seed – it positively affects cholesterol and blood pressure, and helps prevent heart disease.

disease, but the range of possible uses for flaxseed oil are numerous and include the following specific areas:

LOWERING CHOLESTEROL

It's known that people who follow a Mediterranean diet tend to have higher HDL ("good") cholesterol levels. The Mediterranean diet consists of a healthy balance between omega-3 and omega-6 fatty acids. It emphasizes eating whole grains, green vegetables, fresh fruit, fish and poultry, olive and canola oils, and ALA, along with avoidance of red meat and high-fat butters and creams.

HIGH BLOOD PRESSURE

Several studies suggest that diets and/or supplements rich in omega-3 fatty acids (including ALA) lower blood pressure significantly in people with hypertension. This is significant for bodybuilders using steroids, as the drugs are known to increase blood pressure.

HEART DISEASE

One of the best ways to help prevent and treat heart disease is to eat a low-fat diet and to replace foods rich in saturated and trans fat with

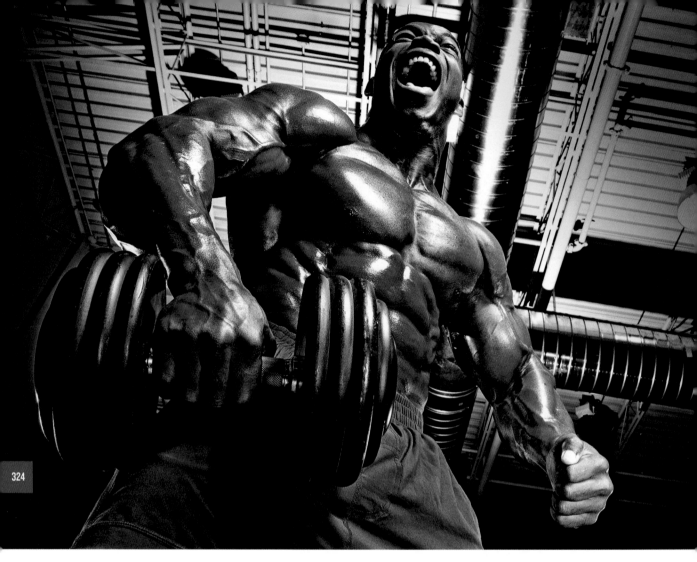

ABOVE: Joint pain and stiffness can often result from hard training; supplementing with omega-3s can reduce these symptoms.

those that are rich in monounsaturated and polyunsaturated fats. Evidence suggests that people who eat an ALA-rich diet including omega-3 fatty acids from flaxseed oil are less likely to suffer fatal heart attacks.

INFLAMMATORY BOWEL DISEASE (IBD)

Studies have shown that many individuals with Crohn's disease have low levels of omega-3 fatty acids in their bodies. Fish oil supplements containing omega-3 fatty acids have been shown to reduce symptoms of Crohn's and ulcerative colitis (another inflammatory bowel disease), particularly if used in addition to medication. Preliminary animal studies have found that ALA (such as from flaxseed oil) may actually be more effective than EPA and DHA found in fish oil supplements, but further studies in humans are needed to confirm these findings.

ARTHRITIS

As with primrose oil, studies suggest that omega-3 fatty acid supplements reduce tenderness in joints, decrease morning stiffness and

Photo by Paul Buceta
Model Chris White

● **ANABOLIC PRIMER** ●

allow for a reduction in the amount of medication needed for people with rheumatoid arthritis.

BREAST CANCER

Women who regularly consume foods rich in omega-3 fatty acids over many years may be less likely to develop breast cancer and to die from the disease than women who do not follow such a diet. Laboratory and animal studies indicate that omega-3 fatty acids can inhibit the growth of human breast cancer cells and may even prevent the spread of cancer to other parts of the body. Several experts speculate that omega-3 fatty acids in combination with other nutrients (namely vitamin C, vitamin E, beta-carotene, selenium and coenzyme Q10) may prove to be of particular value for preventing and treating breast cancer.

DEPRESSION

People who do not get enough omega-3 fatty acids or do not maintain a healthy balance of omega-3 to omega-6 fatty acids in their diets may be at an increased risk for depression. The omega-3 fatty acids are important components of nerve cell membranes. They help nerve cells communicate with each other, which is an essential step in maintaining good mental health.

BURNS

Essential fatty acids have been used to reduce inflammation and promote wound healing in burn victims. Animal research indicates that omega-3 fatty acids help promote a healthy balance of proteins in the body – protein balance is an important factor for recovery and healing after sustaining a burn.

SOURCES

Being a popular supplement, flaxseed oil is available in liquid, powder (as a ground meal) and soft gel capsule forms. As with any oil, flaxseed oil will turn rancid if it is not refrigerated. It also requires special packaging because it is easily destroyed by heat, light and oxygen. The highest quality flaxseed products are manufactured using fresh pressed seeds, bottled in dark or opaque containers, and processed at low temperatures in the absence of light, extreme heat or oxygen.

For those who don't like the taste of the oil or are tired of popping pills, flaxseed meal may be just the thing. For less than $5 you can buy a month's supply of flaxseed meal that can be added to cereal and shakes. Like most meals, flaxseed meal is a powder that is ground down to almost the same consistency of creatine or protein powder. A couple of teaspoons will give you the same benefits of oil or capsules. It's also virtually odorless and tasteless so it won't change the taste of your shake or cereal.

> "For those who don't like the taste of the oil or are tired of popping pills, flaxseed meal may be just the thing. For less than $5 you can buy a month's supply of flaxseed meal that can be added to cereal and shakes."

325

OLIVE OIL

Olive oil has been a staple in the diets of Mediterranean countries for thousands of years. It is used not only in cooking, but also mixed liberally with vinegar as a dressing, and even with cracked black pepper as a dipping sauce for focaccia bread. Decades ago a number of studies were conducted on Greek individuals living on the island of Crete. Researchers were amazed to discover that despite the high fat content in the traditional Greek diet, residents of the island had an exceptionally low occurrence of heart disease. This led researchers to take a closer look at the diets of the Greek people to try to figure out what factors contribute to this low rate of heart disease. Their conclusion? The Greeks do not eat much butter or margarine, but substitute olive oil instead.

By now you should be realizing that by replacing the saturated fats in your diet with monosaturated fat, such as olive oil, you can change your cholesterol profile by decreasing your low-density lipoprotein (LDL) and increasing your high-density lipoprotein (HDL). One of the primary benefits of this is to decrease the amount of dangerous artery-clogging fat circulating in your bloodstream.

Besides the benefits of the monounsaturated fats in olive oil, there are several other compounds that can benefit your health. One in particular can actually stop damage in your arteries before it starts. Polyphenols are powerful antioxidants found in olive oil that disable the free radical oxygen molecules produced naturally by normal metabolism. One of the health benefits of this is to prevent free radicals from increasing the ability of LDLs to attach to arterial walls and block blood flow. The main point here – adding olive oil to your diet helps keep your arteries open.

For female readers there is more good news. Researchers at the Harvard School of Public Health and the Athens School of Public Health studied the effects of olive oil on more than 2,300 women. They discovered that women who consumed olive oil more than once a day had a 25 percent lower risk of breast cancer, and in fact the female population of Greece is much less likely to die from breast cancer than women in the United States. They concluded that the high concentration of both vitamin E (which has been proven to slow or stop cell damage), found in olive oil, as well as polyphenols contribute to this benefit.

SOURCES

To get the most benefit from olive oil, make sure to buy extra virgin olive oil. This oil comes from the very first cold press of the olive and contains the highest and purest amounts of disease-fighting polyphenols. Also, like many other oils, olive oil should be kept cool, either in the refrigerator or other dark cool spot. This will preserve its protective qualities, as well as its great taste.

LEFT: There's no arguing against the health benefits of the Mediterranean diet, and olive oil is a key component.

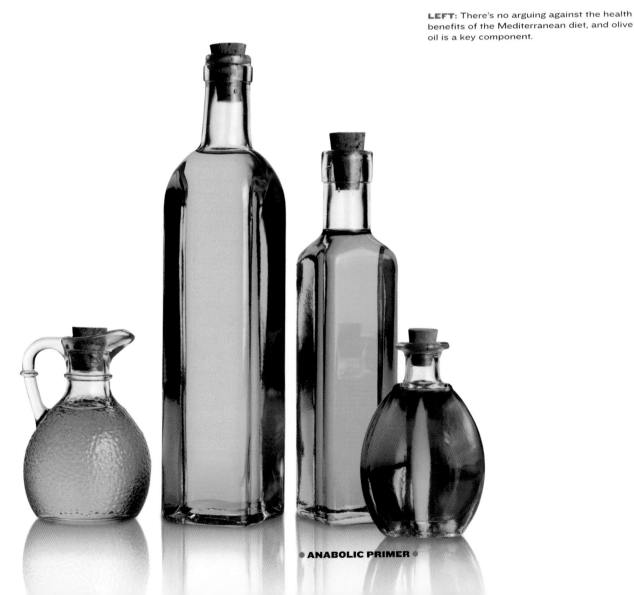

CANOLA OIL

Despite being one of the new "oily" kids on the block, canola oil is gaining fast on the older, more established oils as a healthy alternative.

Canola is a hybridized version of rapeseed developed in 1968 by Baldur Stefansson of the University of Manitoba using the traditional method of selective breeding to create a cultivar that is almost completely free of rapeseed's undesirable substances (erucic acid and glucosinates).

The name canola comes from Canadian Oil Low Acid. The Canadian government smartly coined the term canola due to the negative connotations of the word "rape." Canola is commonly blended with other oils to produce margarine, shortening and vegetable oil. Its mild flavor, light texture and high smoke point make it an ideal choice for stir-frying, deep-frying and sautéing.

Canola has a similar fatty acid profile to olive oil, is high in monounsaturated fats, and contains the lowest amount (seven percent) of saturated fats of all edible vegetable oils. In fact, it's the richest source of essential fatty acids with an omega-6 to omega-3 fatty acids ratio of 2:1. Expeller pressing the seeds of the plant creates the best canola oils, and the oil can be stored for up to a year in a tightly sealed container at room temperature.

COUNTER ATTACK

Just as the major airlines start price cutting as soon as some upstart no-frills airline moves in on their turf, so did the producers of the more established cooking oils launch a negative campaign against canola oil when their sales began to suffer. Banking on the average consumer's lack of knowledge, they began by highlighting canola oil's rapeseed origins. When heated, unprocessed rapeseed oil has been linked to cancer. Natural sources of unmodified rapeseed also contain high concentrations of erucic acid – a compound known to cause heart problems in laboratory animals. They even kept pointing out that rapeseed is a member of the mustard family, the same family that deadly mustard gas is derived from. To the uninformed, such arguments seemed convincing, but what the anti-canola groups conveniently keep forgetting to mention is that in 1974 researchers had developed strains of rapeseed that had levels of erucic all but eliminated and replaced by oleic acid – a healthy monounsaturated fat.

As for the mustard gas association, such other commonly eaten plants as cabbage and horseradish are also members of the same family. Common sense should dictate that there is an enormous amount of chemical modification needed to develop a deadly nerve gas from a plant seed.

Rest assured canola oil is perfectly safe. In fact, it has the lowest saturated fat content of all the common oils and is one of the least expensive. Its mild taste makes it an ideal salad dressing, and its high smoke point makes it one of the best oils for frying foods.

329

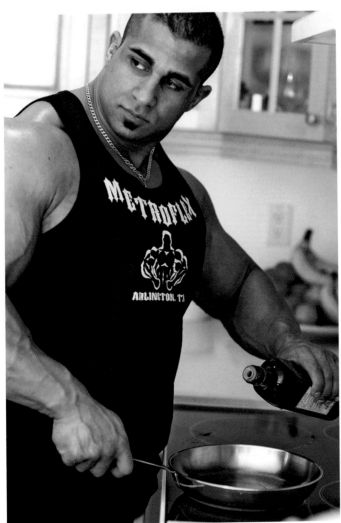

Photo by Paul Buceta
Model Fouad Abiad

LEFT: When your meals require stir-frying or sautéing, a good option is canola oil because of its high smoke point.

TRANS FAT – THE 20th CENTURY'S BLACK DEATH

Throughout this book you'll be seeing us use such phrases as "try to avoid," "limit your intake" or "cut down on" on a regular basis, but if there's one food product that should be avoided at all costs it's trans fat. We touched on trans fat in the earlier chapter on fats and oils, but trans fat is such a killer that it warrants a chapter on its own.

IN THE BEGINNING

Food processors have been tinkering around with trans fats since the early 1900s, and it has been widely available as a food additive since the 1930s. Trans fat includes a number of familiar food additives such as hydrogenated vegetable oil, partially hydrogenated vegetable oil and shortening. You'll notice the word hydrogen in two of the previous examples. This is in reference to the manufacturing technique that produces such silent killers. In simple terms by a series of chemical steps, hydrogen atoms are added to natural fats and oils. This makes them more solid and creamier, and gives them a longer-lasting shelf life – the perfect food additive to increase sales and make more money. Unfortunately such chemical wizardry came with a price – a greatly increased risk of heart disease for the user. It's no coincidence that the increase in heart disease mirrors the food-processing industry. In the case of trans fat, food manufacturers have created a series of compounds that the human body has no ability to handle. It took millions of years for the body's enzyme systems to evolve. Enzymes are used to initiate chemical reactions including breaking down large molecules into smaller sub-units. Enzymes are also specific to certain targets. That is, enzyme A will only break-down target A. Enzymes B, C, and D usually have little or no effect. In the case of fats, they exist in nature as what are called Cis molecules and hence the body's enzymes are designed to only break down Cis fats. But along comes 20th-century food processing and look out – trans fats!

What makes trans fats so deplorable is that the body has no ability to break them down. They are sent to the liver where they are either stored or returned to the blood and deposited in fat cells.

Unlike regular stored fat, trans fat that becomes stored in the body is almost impossible to burn off. Ever wonder why you can't get rid of that last 10 pounds around your waist? Maybe it's all that trans fat you've accumulated over the years.

WAIST NOT – WAIST YES!

It was thought at one time that all fat was stored evenly around the body, but recent research is suggesting that trans fat primarily builds up around the midsection. As bad as this is for the average person, just think what it will mean for your competitive bodybuilding plans. One study found that the bodyfat in subjects who followed a diet high in trans fat was four times higher than those who followed the same diet without the trans fat. Worse, all the fat went straight to the waistline.

Besides the enlarging waistline there's evidence to suggest that trans fat may stimulate the pancreas to produce more insulin, which over time may make the body more resistant to the hormone. Closely related to this is that trans fat may prevent cells from reacting to insulin properly. By now you should be seeing where this could lead. As soon as you start messing around with insulin and insulin sensitivity the end result is diabetes. From there it's only a step or two to insulin needles, your first heart attack or amputation. Not frightened yet? Read on.

If interfering with insulin was not enough, trans fats are also believed to decrease testosterone levels. So a diet high in trans fat will not only cause your waistline to expand, but it will also reduce your muscle-building potential.

331

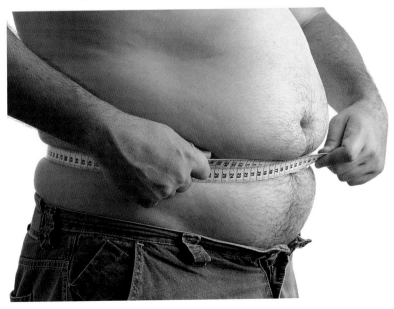

LEFT: The big bellies that have become so common in North America are largely (no pun intended) the result of foods packed with trans fat.

READ THOSE LABELS

At one time you were at the mercy of the food industry when it came to tracking your trans fat intake, but no longer. The FDA has now made it mandatory for food manufacturers to list the amounts of trans fats in their products. Of course there are catches. Most restaurants are still exempt from this law. So if you're in the habit of eating out on a regular basis you can be sure that your trans fat intake is higher than it should be. Also be aware that foods containing less than 0.5 grams of trans fat can still be advertised as "trans fat free" or "contains zero trans fat." The FDA basically went along with the food industry's argument that achieving absolute zero trans fat is virtually impossible.

As you might imagine some of the worst culprits of trans fat loading are the fast- food joints. Those deep-fried wings you love to inhale on wing night just spent a considerable amount of time floating around in trans fat. Granted most establishments are trying to find alternatives, but with few exceptions virtually all the deep-fried food from the other major chains is still drowned in trans fat.

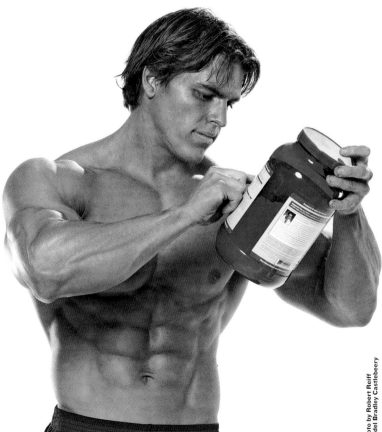

RIGHT: Knowledge is a powerful tool when it comes to nutrition. Always read food labels carefully to ensure what you're eating isn't loaded with unhealthy ingredients.

Photo by Robert Reiff
Model Bradley Castlebeery

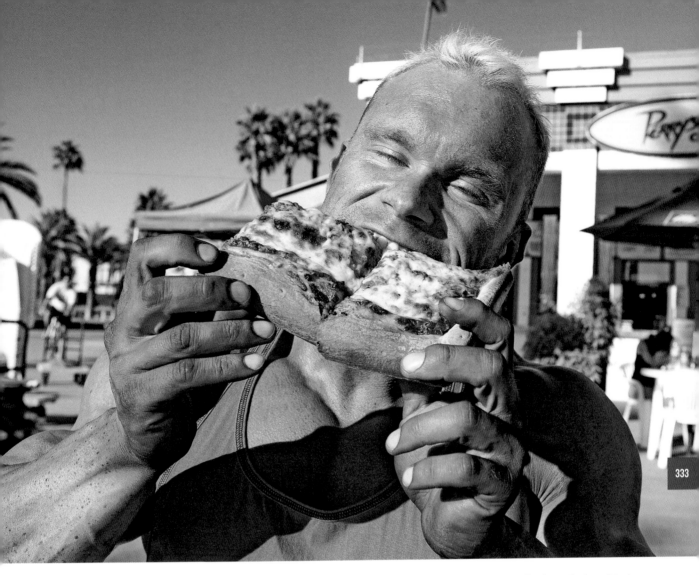

BODYBUILDING IMPLICATIONS

Hopefully by now you are beginning to see the dangers of trans fat consumption. If you're like most bodybuilders you probably allow yourself one greasy junk meal a week. You may even have a cheat day. Unlike simple sugar, however, where the few extra calories won't harm you, no amount of trans fat is safe. In fact, many nutritionists and biochemists recommend that all trans fat be avoided. You may think it's only a small amount, but that small amount builds up over time until your arteries are blocked and your waist is straight from Sumo Wrestling Monthly. Harvard nutritionist Walter Willett has suggested that trans fat consumption is responsible for over 30,000 deaths every year.

If you're concerned about both your appearance and health, then there should be no off-season with regard to trans fat. Avoid all foods that have the terms hydrogenated, partially hydrogenated or trans fat written on their labels. We know it tastes great, but if mom's apple pie crust is made with shortening, forget about it. Shortening is loaded with trans fat. You just have to take a peak at a hunk of shortening to know it definitely can't be good for you!

ABOVE: While fast food may look and taste good, the junk in it will only destroy your bodybuilding efforts.

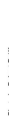
Photo by Robert Reiff
Model Ben Pakulski

VITAMINS AND MINERALS

If protein and creatine are the most popular supplements in the bodybuilding world, then it's safe to say that vitamins and minerals are probably the most popular supplements among the general population. Few houses or apartments can be found without the good old one-a-day vitamin and mineral bottle.

VITAMINS

Much of the early information about vitamins comes from the research on diseases including scurvy and beriberi. Scurvy probably killed more sailors than any enemy gun action. It was a Scottish surgeon by the name of James Lind who discovered that the disease could be prevented by eating citrus fruits, including limes (this is where the popular nickname for British sailors, "limey," came from).

While Lind knew that something in citrus fruit was helping to prevent the condition, it would be over a hundred years before the first vitamins were isolated. The father of vitamin research is considered to be Casimir Funk, a Polish biochemist working in London who was studying the malnutrition disease beriberi. Funk found that he could prevent the disease by administering a powerful compound isolated from rice. Given that the compound was an amine (organic compound containing nitrogen) and vital to life, he coined the term "vitamine" or vitamine. Later, as more similar compounds were discovered that were not amines, the final "e" was dropped and the present term vitamin was adopted.

Vitamins can be defined as inorganic compounds that are necessary for growth, health and normal metabolism. They may act as enzymes (substances that speed up or slow down chemical reactions) or essential components of hormones. Vitamins can be divided into two categories: fat-soluble and water-soluble.

Fat-Soluble Vitamins

Fat-soluble vitamins are named as such because they can be stored in bodyfat. When excess amounts are consumed in the diet and not used right away, they can be stored for later use. Of course this storage can be a double-edged sword. Some of the fat-soluble vitamins can be toxic to the body, particularly the liver, in excessive amounts. Too much vitamin D has even been linked to heart disease and kidney stones.

The primary fat-soluble vitamins are:

VITAMIN	NATURAL SOURCE	USED FOR	AMOUNT PER DAY
Vitamin A	Carrots, green vegetables	Vision	900 mcg
Vitamin D	Fish oil, egg yolk	Growth and repair	5–10 mcg
Vitamin E	Wheat germ, green vegetables	Free-radical fighting	15 mcg
Vitamin K	Cheese, spinach	Blood clotting	120 mcg

Water-Soluble Vitamins

Unlike fat-soluble vitamins, water-soluble vitamins cannot be stored in the body to any great extent and must be consumed in the diet on a daily basis. Under certain circumstances – disease and intense exercise – it may be difficult for individuals to obtain adequate amounts in their diets.

335

The primary water-soluble vitamins are:

VITAMIN	NATURAL SOURCE	USED FOR	AMOUNT PER DAY
Vitamin B-1 (thiamine)	Whole-grain cereals, liver, eggs	Carbohydrate metabolism	1.2 mg
Vitamin B-2 (riboflavin)	Nuts, eggs, whole-wheat cereals	Blood cell formation	1.3 mg
Vitamin B-3 (niacin)	Whole-grain cereals, fish, meats	Lowers cholesterol	16 mg
Vitamin B-5 (pantothenic acid)	Whole-grain cereals, shellfish	Antioxidant	5 mg
Vitamin B-6 (pyridoxine)	Whole-grain cereals, salmon, spinach	Immune-system health	1.5 mg
Vitamin B-9 (folic acid)	Wheat germ, fruits, green vegetables	Energy production	400 mcg
Vitamin B-12 (cyanocobalamin)	Shellfish, cheese, eggs	Carbohydrate metabolism	2.4 mcg
Vitamin C (ascorbic acid)	Citrus fruits, green vegetables	Immune-system booster	90 mg

VITAMIN SUPPLEMENTS

There is considerable misinformation and exaggeration regarding vitamins and exercise. Furthermore, vitamin requirements in athletes generate the same degree of debate as that surrounding protein. Unlike protein, however, there is little to no evidence to suggest that extra vitamins will increase performance or recovery in people who eat properly. Despite what some writers and many supplement manufacturers proclaim, vitamins are not a source of energy. Nor do they hold magical anti-disease fighting properties. Yes they're essential for optimizing health, but they won't elevate your health or performance above what's natural for you. Vitamins will only make a difference if you're deficient in one or more of them.

Generally there are three categories of vitamin supplements. The most popular are the one-a-day multivitamins that contain most of the known vitamins along with the common minerals and trace elements. Prices usually range from $10 to $20 per bottle. To address the child and teen market, there are vitamin products with tablets in the shape of cartoon and other popular characters. While no vitamin tablet can ever take the place of a healthy diet, for a growing child or teen a one-a-day tablet is a good way to ensure they're receiving all the essential vitamins and minerals.

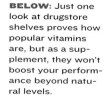

BELOW: Just one look at drugstore shelves proves how popular vitamins are, but as a supplement, they won't boost your performance beyond natural levels.

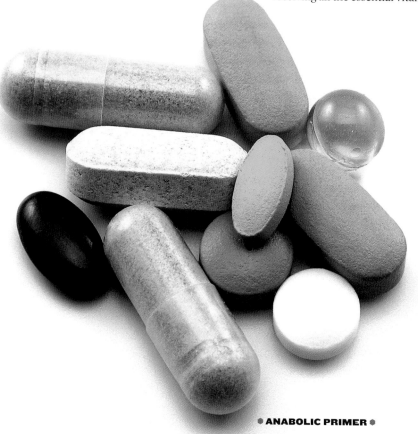

● **ANABOLIC PRIMER** ●

A second category is the products containing two or three vitamins. The most common are the B-complex and B-complex + C products. Unlike the multivitamin products these contain much higher amounts of B-complex and vitamin C. Again prices range from $10 to $20 per bottle.

The third category of vitamin supplements is the single vitamin products. A typical drug store or health-food store looks like a pre-school these days with all the vitamin letters prominently displayed along the shelves. There are advantages and disadvantages to buying vitamins this way. The primary advantage is the dosages available. If you feel (or if your doctor has suggested) that you need a high dosage of one of the vitamins, such single vitamin products are ideal. In most cases a single tablet or capsule supplies more than the daily RDA for that particular vitamin. For those buying vitamin C this way, we suggest buying the 50- or 100-milligram size as the body can only use about 30 to 50 milligrams at any given time. The rest is excreted. Instead of popping one 1,000-milligram tablet, try taking one 50- or 100-milligram tablet a number of times per day. Those 500- or even 1,000-milligram tablets will do nothing but give you the most colorful-looking urine in town!

There are three primary disadvantages to taking high amounts of individual vitamin supplements. For starters, fat-based vitamins are not excreted when taken in excess like water-based vitamins. They could build up to toxic levels. We strongly urge you to only take a fat-based vitamin no more than once a day. In fact, every second day might be a better idea. A second disadvantage is that the body is always trying to find a happy equilibrium. High dosages of one vitamin can interfere with the absorption of other vitamins and minerals. The third disadvantage can be termed "beware of the unknown." No one knows for sure just what the long-term consequences are for taking megadoses of vitamins. Even though vitamin supplements have been around for decades, the megadosing followed by today's bodybuilders is relatively new – say the last 20 years. Who knows what this may lead to 40 or 50 years from now.

ABOVE: Certain vitamins can be purchased in single form; be cautious of these, however, because too much of one may upset your body's vitamin and mineral balance.

337

MINERALS AND TRACE ELEMENTS

The terms mineral and trace element are really just different names for the same substances. Biochemists and nutritionists use the term

Photo by Alex Ardenti

mineral if the body needs more than 100 milligrams of a particular element each day. If less is required, the term trace element is used. Both minerals and trace elements can be defined as inorganic substances that the body needs for growth, maintenance and repair. They are also used for nerve conduction, heart rate regulation and water conservation. Because minerals and trace elements are only required in very small amounts, deficiencies in Western society are very rare. Possible exceptions include athletes who train in hot weather, those suffering from wasting diseases, and women with heavy menstrual periods.

The following are the primary minerals and trace elements:

MINERAL	NATURAL SOURCE	USED FOR
Calcium	Green vegetables, egg yolk	Blood clotting, bone and teeth growth
Chlorine	Meat and fish	Water balance and found in digestive enzymes
Magnesium	Wheat germ, green vegetables	Muscle contraction and nerve conduction
Phosphorous	Fish, poultry, dairy products	Bone and teeth formation
Sodium	Meat and fish	Water conservation and nerve conduction
Sulphur	Eggs, cheese, fish	Hormone production

TRACE ELEMENT	NATURAL SOURCE	USED FOR
Cobalt	Shellfish, meat, liver	Red blood cell production
Copper	Mushrooms, oats, whole-wheat flour	Hemoglobin production
Iodine	Cod-liver oil, seafood	Formation of thyroid hormones
Iron	Shellfish, eggs, whole-grain products	Red blood cell formation
Zinc	Whole grains, fish, meat	Enzyme production
Chromium	Fruit, whole wheat, seafood	Insulin regulation
Magnesium	Bran, coffee, peanuts	Red blood cell production

MINERAL SUPPLEMENTS

Mineral supplements are generally available in three forms. Multivitamin tablets (a misleading name as virtually all multivitamin products contain both vitamins and minerals) are probably the best bang for your dollar, as most contain all the essential vitamins and minerals in sensible amounts (as opposed to mega dosages).

As with vitamins, minerals can be bought as individual products, but unless you've been diagnosed with a specific deficiency, you really shouldn't be consuming individual minerals or trace elements. Pregnant and heavy-menstruating women may need iron, and older individuals often need extra calcium, but for the most part, healthy eating or a multivitamin will provide all the minerals you need.

The third category of mineral supplements is worth billions of dollars a year. These are the mineral drinks usually marketed as electrolyte replenishers. By far the most familiar name in this category is Gatorade. Bodybuilders and other athletes use electrolyte drinks to replenish both their water levels and the minerals lost during exercise in their sweat. While serving as good sources of the major electrolytes (potassium, sodium, calcium, etc.) they are a poor source of the remaining minerals and trace elements.

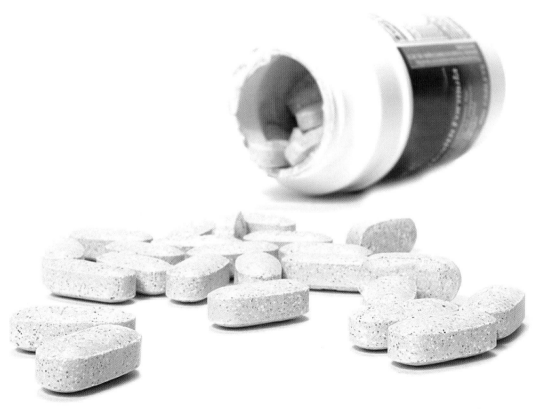

VITAMIN B-6

As most readers are aware, the body uses protein as the major structural component for building and repairing exercised muscle tissue. While it's common knowledge that vitamins and minerals are responsible for many of the chemical reactions that play a role in this, it's not commonly known that vitamin B-6 is the master vitamin for synthesizing protein and processing amino acids. The body utilizes B-6 to both break down and re-assemble amino acids. It also increases their absorption. As an example, B-6 increases the absorption of the amino acid L-methionine, which aids in energy production and muscle development. B-6 is also involved with maximizing the transport and absorption of arginine and ornithine. Both amino acids contribute to growth hormone production and muscle growth. Vitamin B-6 also plays a vital role in the workings of over 100 enzymes that catalyze protein synthesis in the body.

CARB AND SUGAR REGULATION

If protein is the major structural component, then carbohydrate is the body's primary fuel source. Vitamin B-6 plays an important role in the processing of carbs and starches. The process of gluconeogenesis is also heavily dependent on B-6. For those not familiar, gluconeogenesis is the process by which stored glycogen in the liver and muscle cells are broken down into glucose to be used as a fuel source. This fuel source is used as both a back-up energy source as well as helping fatigued muscles recharge after a workout.

READY AND ALERT

Within your nervous system there exists molecules called amines (similar to the amines that combine with acids to form amino acids). These molecules help support the transmission of nerve impulses and messages from one nerve to the next. Two of the best-known amine-derived neurotransmitters are epinephrine and norepinephrine. Among other functions the two help keep you alert and ready to face just about any task including your next workout. Vitamin B-6 plays a major role in the synthesis of both hormones.

BOOSTED BLOOD

Another less-known property of B-6 is its role in hemoglobin production. Hemoglobin is the pigment that red blood cells use to latch on to oxygen and transport it to the various cells in the body. A deficiency in B-6 means less hemoglobin and ultimately a reduced oxygen-carrying capacity of the blood.

THE RIGHT CONNECTIONS

Scientists now know that B-6 is an essential nutrient for the formation and development of connective tissue. Without B-6, the process becomes impeded. B-6 also plays a major role in joint health, including preventing inflammation.

FORMS

Since B-6 is a water-soluble vitamin, the body has neither the means to store nor manufacture it. The vitamin must be obtained through food. Vitamin B-6 exists in six forms, pyridoxal (PL), pyridoxine (PN), pyridoxamine (PM), and the phosphate derivatives pyridoxal 5-phosphate (PLP), pyridoxine 5-phosphate (PNP), and pridoxamine 5-phosphate (PMP). Most of the evidence seems to suggest that PLP is the most biologically active form of the vitamin, so look for this on the label when you buy B-6 in supplement form.

DOSAGES

The recommended dosage for the average adult aged 19 to 50 is 1.3 milligrams. This increases to 1.7 milligrams for men over 50 and 1.5 milligrams for women over 50. But as with most recommended dosages, these numbers are low for athletes engaged in intense exercise and those who follow high-protein diets. Many experts recommend that for every 100 grams of protein, 2 milligrams of B-6 should be consumed. Others go further and suggest 10 to 20 milligrams of B-6 to metabolize the extra protein. If this sounds high, no need to panic as no toxicity for B-6 has been found with an oral intake of up to 200 milligrams.

We're not going to put B-6 in the same category as creatine, branched-chain amino acids and whey protein. Nevertheless, given B-6's crucial role in protein metabolism (not to mention all the other benefits), its relative safety and cheap cost, bodybuilders should definitely add it to their list of "must-use" supplements.

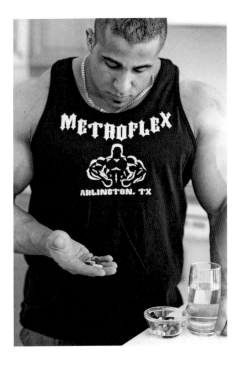

Photo by Paul Buceta
Model Fouad Abiad

LEFT: Regardless of which vitamins and minerals you take, dosing and time are two extremely important considerations.

341

VITAMIN C

Ask anyone off the street to name a vitamin and chances are they'll name vitamin C. Even five-year-olds know that they must drink their orange juice to keep the common cold away. Vitamin C, also known as ascorbic acid, is a water-soluble vitamin. Interestingly enough unlike most mammals, humans do not have the ability to make our own vitamin C. Therefore, it must be obtained through foods in the diet.

FUNCTIONS

Vitamin C is required for the synthesis of collagen, an important structural component of blood vessels, tendons, ligaments and bones. Vitamin C also plays an important role in the synthesis of many neurotransmitters including norepinephrine. Neurotransmitters are critical to brain function and are known to affect mood. In addition, vitamin C is required for the synthesis of carnitine, a small molecule that is vital for the transport of fat molecules to the mitochondria of cells for conversion into energy. Recent studies also suggests that vitamin C is involved in the metabolism of cholesterol to bile acids, which may have implications for blood cholesterol levels and the development of gallstones.

Vitamin C is also one of the body's primary antioxidants and even in small amounts offers protection from free radicals to such important molecules as proteins, lipids, carbohydrates and nucleic acids (DNA and RNA). Free radicals are generated in the body as well as through exposure to toxins and pollutants.

HISTORY

The effects of vitamin C deficiency were among the first to be investigated, and for centuries the fatal disease of scurvy was the scourge of navies. By the late 1700s the British navy was aware that scurvy could be cured by eating oranges or lemons, even though vitamin C would not be isolated until the early 1930s. The symptoms of scurvy include the loss of hair and teeth, bleeding and bruising easily, and joint pain and swelling. Such symptoms appear to be related to the loss of collagen which then weakens blood vessels, connective tissue and bone.

The early symptoms of scurvy such as fatigue are believed to be caused by diminished levels of carnitine, needed to derive energy from fat, or decreased synthesis of the neurotransmitter norepinephrine. Scurvy is rare in Western and developed countries because it can be prevented by as little as 10 milligrams of vitamin C daily (one medium orange contains around 80 milligrams of vitamin C).

In addition to preventing scurvy, vitamin C has been shown in some studies to reduce the frequency and duration of colds and to alleviate their severity. It does not, however, prevent colds. Vitamin C may help prevent lead poisoning, and some scientists believe it holds anti-cancer properties. Again it's not so much a cure as it is preventative medicine.

Vitamin C gets promoted by supplement manufacturers as an athletic aid. This is because of its ability to regenerate collagen. The vitamin's ability to reduce inflammation also makes it popular with bodybuilders and other athletes, even though the scientific evidence to support this is lacking. Given its role in boosting the immune system, many athletes use the vitamin under the belief that it reduces the number of colds and infections that often accompany periods of intense training. In many respects vitamin C is no different than most of the other popular bodybuilding supplements. While the medical research is inconclusive, users swear by it.

EXCESS

As a water-soluble vitamin the body has little ability to store vitamin C so any excess is excreted in the urine (that bright yellow-orange color you notice after chewing one or two 500-milligram vitamin C tablets).

In extreme cases mega-dosing can lead to bladder and kidney stones, and there is some evidence to suggest that mega-dosing can destroy vitamin B-12, reduce the effectiveness of blood thinners, lead to the loss of calcium, and cause diarrhea and nosebleeds.

BEST SOURCES

As you might expect, the best sources of vitamin C are fruits and vegetables. Citrus fruits are most famous for their vitamin C content, but vitamin C can also be found in vegetables such as red peppers and cauliflower. Keep in mind that the actual amount will vary based on climate, growing conditions, time of picking and other factors. The way the food is cooked is also important. To preserve the vitamin C content, refrain from cooking vegetables for too long or at too high a temperature, and retain the water into which the food was cooked. The best option is to eat your vegetables raw whenever possible.

343

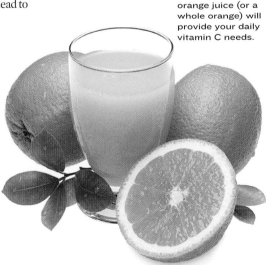

BELOW: Just one cup of 100%-pure orange juice (or a whole orange) will provide your daily vitamin C needs.

VITAMIN E

Given its popularity among the general public (although less so with bodybuilders) it only makes sense to take a more in-depth look at vitamin E.

Vitamin E is made up of seven elements called tocopherols. To differentiate each of the seven elements, biochemists have named them with Greek words: alpha, beta, gamma, delta, epsilon, eta and zeta. For a while it was believed that only alpha had any meaningful biological effects, but recent research has shown that the others also play a major role, including boosting the effectiveness of alpha. There are different vitamin E forms available and while most are fat-based, there are water-based versions. As water-based forms are less than one-fifth as potent as fat-based, you'd need to consume much more to satisfy your requirements. There are also two primary sources of vitamin E available – synthetic and natural. You can tell the difference by reading the label. Synthetic forms will have the prefix dl before the types of tocopherols while natural forms have the prefix d.

BENEFITS

The primary benefit of vitamin E is as an antioxidant. Our bodies are continuously being bombarded with a wide assortment of potentially lethal compounds in the air we breathe, water we drink and food we eat. Some of the most lethal of these compounds are called free radicals – charged ions that go around trying to interact with other charged compounds. The process is called oxidation and is in many respects similar to the rusting process that takes place on cars. Besides causing cell damage, free radicals are also responsible for some forms of disease and cancer. Vitamin E has the ability to neutralize free radicals before they cause cell damage. Of course, in the process of neutralizing free radicals vitamin E is destroyed. Think of it as molecular suicide. This is why you must consume vitamin E on a regular basis.

Vitamin E also guards our health by assisting the liver in detoxifying harmful compounds we encounter every day. Everything from food preservatives and pesticides to exhaust fumes and drugs could potentially cause disease and death, if not for the liver's ability to

"The primary benefit of vitamin E is as an antioxidant. Our bodies are continuously being bombarded with a wide assortment of potentially lethal compounds in the air we breathe, water we drink and food we eat. Vitamin E has the ability to neutralize free radicals before they cause cell damage."

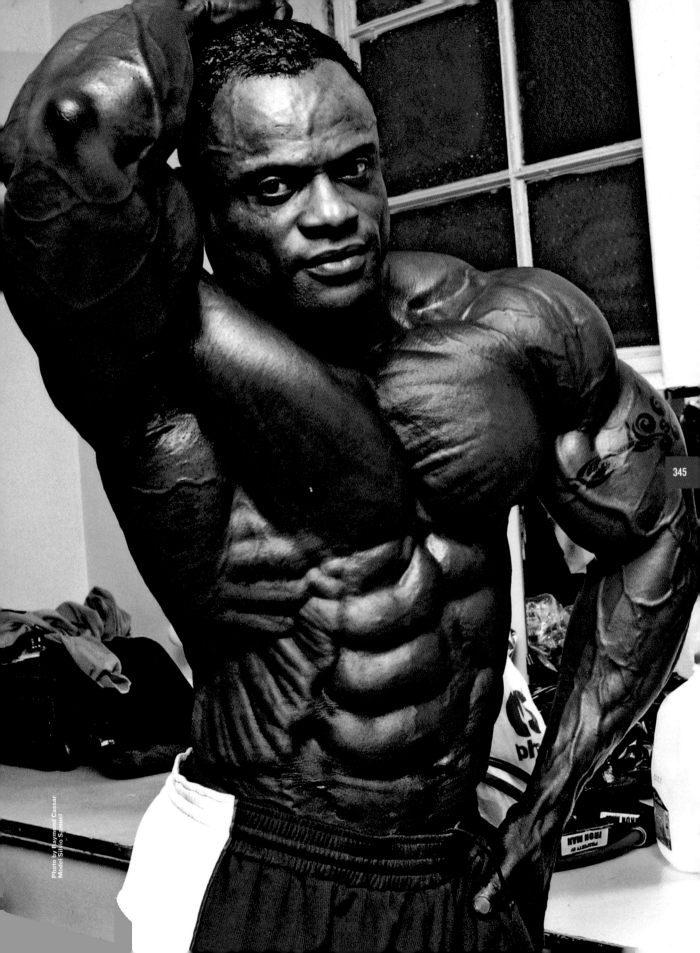

345

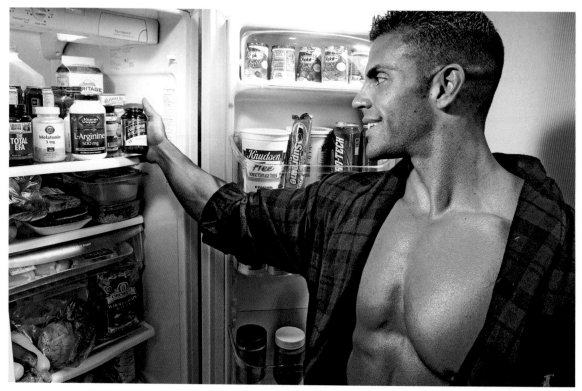

ABOVE: Many people believe that sufficient vitamin E can be consumed in the diet, but because reserves are quickly used during exercise, bodybuilders may benefit from a supplement.

346

break down the compounds . Vitamin E speeds up this process. Another way that vitamin E improves overall health is by boosting the immune system. It does this by increasing production of antibodies such as killer T cells and B cells.

Besides improving overall health, vitamin E may improve exercise performance. When the cells are supplied with a rich source of vitamin E, the muscles are able to perform more efficiently because less demand is placed on the metabolic process. This reduced demand allows the oxygen to be available for other uses such as feeding the muscles and heart during exercise. With adequate vitamin E available the heart doesn't have to work as hard to convey blood to the cells. Research has shown that vitamin E actually strengthens the heart muscle. At the same time vitamin E improves the utilization of oxygen by the heart and prevents the formation of blood clots, which can block the heart's flow.

Another plus to athletes is the fact that vitamin E is a vasodilator. This means that it can expand all the body's blood vessels from arteries and veins to capillaries and arterioles. It doesn't take a nuclear physics degree to see how this would improve exercise performance. Even if the physical activity is not strenuous, vitamin E still has a very positive effect.

Photo by Robert Reiff
Model Chris Jalali

Bodybuilders often dismiss the previous explanation, arguing that a typical bodybuilding workout doesn't place that big a drain on the cardiovascular system, but this logic is flawed. A bodybuilder who is able to move through his workout faster can get more work done in less time than his counterpart who has to take long breaks between sets. A more efficient cardio system also speeds up recovery between workouts.

Still another benefit of vitamin E is its ability to maintain normal cell membrane health. The primary function of the cell membrane is to allow nutrients to pass into the cell and waste products to move out. It also gives the cell some degree of protection and structure. If cell membranes become too hard or worse, impermeable, this selective passage of nutrients and wastes is impeded. Conversely, if the cell becomes too soft or weak, the nutrients may leak out before the cell has a chance to use them.

HOW MUCH?

No doubt many readers may argue that supplementing with vitamin E is not necessary since the vitamin is fat-based, but keep in mind that unlike some of the other fat-based vitamins, vitamin E is stored in small amounts in the pituitary, adrenal and sex glands. These small reserves are quickly used up during exercise, any type of stress including mental and physical, and when you are subjected to toxins and drugs. Reserves are also depleted during illness and when you eat a large amount of fatty food.

You may think that eating vitamin-E-rich foods will give you enough, but unfortunately this is often not the case. Most cereals and bread have up to 98 percent of their vitamin E removed in the refining process. Most of the vitamin E is found in the germ of grains and this part is often discarded to improve the foods longevity. Storing and baking destroy even more. All that remains is a trace amount. For example, most slices of whole-wheat bread contain only four to seven micrograms of vitamin E per gram. Likewise, leafy green vegetables are high in vitamin E, but as soon as you heat them much of the vitamin E is destroyed. So supplementing is a virtual must. Natural versions are best, and one capsule a day is enough.

> "Most bodybuilders have excluded the more mundane vitamins from their nutritional programs partly because they just do not seem very necessary when they're taking more powerful supplements. Another reason people omit vitamins and minerals is simple economics. When a guy lays out $350 for 100 tablets of Winstrol, he doesn't have much left over for ordinary passé vitamins and minerals, even if he does need them."
>
> – Bill Starr, *Musclemag International* contributor

347

FIBER, SALT AND WATER – THE NEGLECTED BIG THREE

FIBER

Fiber is one of those catch-all terms used to describe plant material that can't be digested by the body. Most fiber comes from the tougher parts of plants including stems, roots, seeds and leaves. The primary component of most fibrous compounds is cellulose. Fiber passes through the gastrointestinal tract mostly undigested until it reaches the large intestine where it then helps to form stools and maintain regularity. Dietary fiber has also been shown to play an important role in the prevention of many diseases, including colon cancer. A high-fiber diet has also been proven to help people lose weight. Since the fiber takes longer to move through the digestive system, you feel full longer and therefore do not overeat.

For superior health, it is recommended that people get 25 to 30 grams of fiber each day. The best sources of fiber include whole grains, vegetables, fruit, nuts, seeds and beans. Try to obtain them in natural forms because most processed foods have a lot of the fiber removed.

SALT

Salt is a compound made from two elements, sodium and chlorine. Salt is a mixed bag when it comes to nutrients. On one hand, it's vital for metabolic processes like nerve conduction, muscle contraction and water regulation. On the other hand, excessive amounts can cause heart disease and kidney problems. Most individuals won't need to make a conscious effort to consume salt – they'll get more than they need in their diets. As an example, just two slices of bread supplies the body's daily salt requirements. As salt is in just about every food we eat – especially processed food – your goal is to try and reduce intake.

WATER

In many respects, water is probably the most important single nutrient. You could probably live for weeks if not months without any food, but you'll live only a few days without water. Water is a major component of every cell and makes up about two-thirds of the mass of the human body. It forms most of the volume of human blood, serves as the medi-

"Most individuals won't need to make a conscious effort to consume salt – they'll get more than they need in their diets. As an example, just two slices of bread supplies the body's daily salt requirements. As salt is in just about every food we eat – especially processed food – your goal is to try and reduce intake."

348

um for virtually all chemical reactions, is essential for digestion, helps regulate body heat and plays a major role in waste excretion.

A typical person will lose about two liters of water every day through waste excretion and sweating, more if he or she is involved in intense exercise or working outdoors in hot weather. It's for this reason that water should be consumed on a regular basis. Start with six to eight glasses a day and add more when needed. During a typical workout, you should try to sip and drink at least one to two liters. Try taking a sip of water after every set of an exercise.

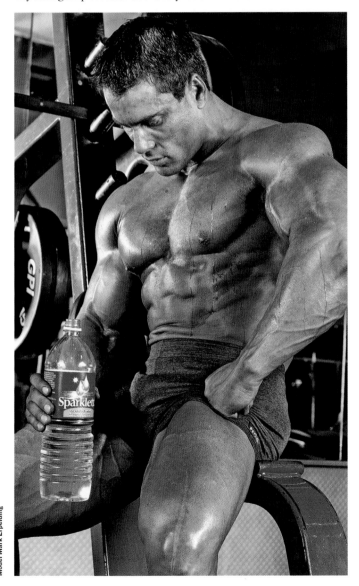

Photo by Irvin Gelb
Model Mark Erpelding

LEFT: The importance of water before, during and after you exercise cannot be underestimated. Six to eight glasses should be your minimum consumption.

SUPERFOODS

In their quest for ultimate muscle size and strength, most bodybuilders worship at the altar of advanced training techniques and state-of-the-art supplements. Anything that can put 20 pounds on their bench press or add 10 pounds of lean mass to their frames is to be treated with the utmost reverence and diligence. Despite all the attention being paid to the bodybuilding side of the equation, overall health should be factored in.

Let's take the element oxygen for example. We all know that we can't live without it. In fact, next to water, oxygen is probably one of the two most vital elements necessary for life (the other being carbon), but despite its importance to respiration and metabolism, oxygen has a downside. Depending on any number of environmental conditions, oxygen may combine with numerous compounds to produce those destructive entities called free radicals.

It's not surprising that something as common as oxygen-produced free radicals would stimulate the body to develop countermeasures. Called antioxidants, such compounds play a major role in combating the damage caused by free radicals. While you can obtain antioxidants in supplement form, there are some foods that are chock-full of these nutrient warriors. This shouldn't surprise you; humans have been eating natural food for about 500,000 years, while supplements have just 50 years or so to their credit. Let's take a close look at a few of the superfoods that should be part of every bodybuilder's nutritional plan.

GRAPE JUICE

Most readers probably know of the relationship between grape juice and creatine absorption. By taking creatine with grape juice, the body increases insulin output to remove the sugar from your bloodstream. At the same time, the hormone speeds up the transport of creatine into the muscles. If you haven't been drinking grape juice (whether for creatine absorption or out of taste) you may want to reconsider. A study published in the *American Journal of Clinical Nutrition* found that test subjects who drank grape juice for just two weeks demonstrated a marked improvement in resistance to damage caused by free radicals.

DARK CHOCOLATE

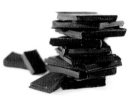

Rare is the individual who hasn't succumbed to the succulent allure of chocolate. Unfortunately most people fall prey to milk chocolate. Milk chocolate can be considered the white bread of the chocolate world. It has been altered with chemicals and other additives, and loaded up with fat and sugar. Dark chocolate, however, with its high polyphenol content is a proven antioxidant. A study published in the *Journal of Cellular Biochemistry* found that dark chocolate contains more of these powerful free radical fighters than green tea and red wine. Then there's the cocoa content that is rich in antioxidant flavonoids called flavanols. Numerous studies have shown that people with high blood levels of flavonoids have a lower risk of heart disease, lung cancer, prostate cancer and Type-2 diabetes. Of course, being a chocolate and containing some sugar, dark chocolate still contains empty calories so don't pig out on it. Just eat enough to satisfy your taste buds.

BRAZIL NUTS

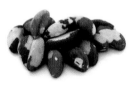

Although typically limited to the Christmas season for many individuals, Brazil nuts have so much going for them that you might consider hoarding them from Santa. Brazil nuts contain protein, fiber, selenium, magnesium, phosphorous, thiamin, niacin, vitamin E, vitamin B-6, calcium, iron, potassium, zinc, copper, and high levels of arginine and flavonoids. Many people avoid Brazil nuts because of the high fat content, but the fat is alpha-linolenic acid, which is converted to omega-3 fatty acid in the body. As with dark chocolate the high calorie content means limiting your intake of Brazil nuts to one or two handfuls per day.

DATES AND FIGS

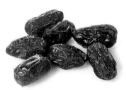

Few foods offer the nutritional charge and taste of dried fruits. Two of the best are dates and figs. Both are dense in phenol antioxidants and other nutrients. They're also loaded with fiber. Dates contain the highest concentration of polyphenols among all the dried fruits and a couple of dried dates or figs each day will provide you with a tremendous amount of antioxidant protection and keep your body in optimal condition.

> "In reasonable quantities, these superfoods can do wonders for your overall health."

351

CREATINE

Since its first mass-production and availability in the early '90s creatine has vaulted to and stayed at the top of the supplement charts. While small numbers of elite athletes were using creatine in the mid-'60s, pro athletes and weekend warriors and everyone in between now use creatine. Unfortunately the combination of creatine's rapid rise and the public's lack of knowledge has lead to numerous myths and misunderstandings about its effectiveness and safety. In this chapter we'll shed some light on the matter.

BACKGROUND

The French scientist Chevreul first identified creatine, a nitrogenous molecule, in 1838. In 1847, another scientist, Lieberg, concluded that the accumulation of creatine in the body is directly involved in supplying muscles with short-term energy. The investigation of creatine supplementation began in the early 1900s using creatine extracted from meats. It wasn't until the early 1960s when synthetic creatine production began, and former East Bloc countries started using it for numerous power sports including weightlifting and track and field. Reports have circulated that several British Olympic athletes were supplementing with creatine before the 1992 Olympic Games in Barcelona. The Olympic Games in Atlanta were jokingly referred to as "The Creatine Games" because a number of athletes supplementing with creatine were awarded gold medals.

To date there have been dozens of highly credible scientific research articles published about creatine in various sports and medical journals, as well as a number of papers presented at various meetings such as the National Strength and Conditioning Association's Creatine Symposium. As of this publication, creatine is one of the most extensively studied nutritional sports supplements available to today's athlete. It's also one of the few supplements that does what the manufacturers claim and in a relatively safe manner.

ATP – THE ENERGY POWERHOUSE

To fully understand creatine, we need to begin with adenosine triphosphate (ATP). ATP is the fuel used by the body for muscle contraction.

> "Creatine loading does for the bodybuilder what carbohydrate loading does for the long-distance runner – it provides more energy-producing materials, which enables more work to be generated."

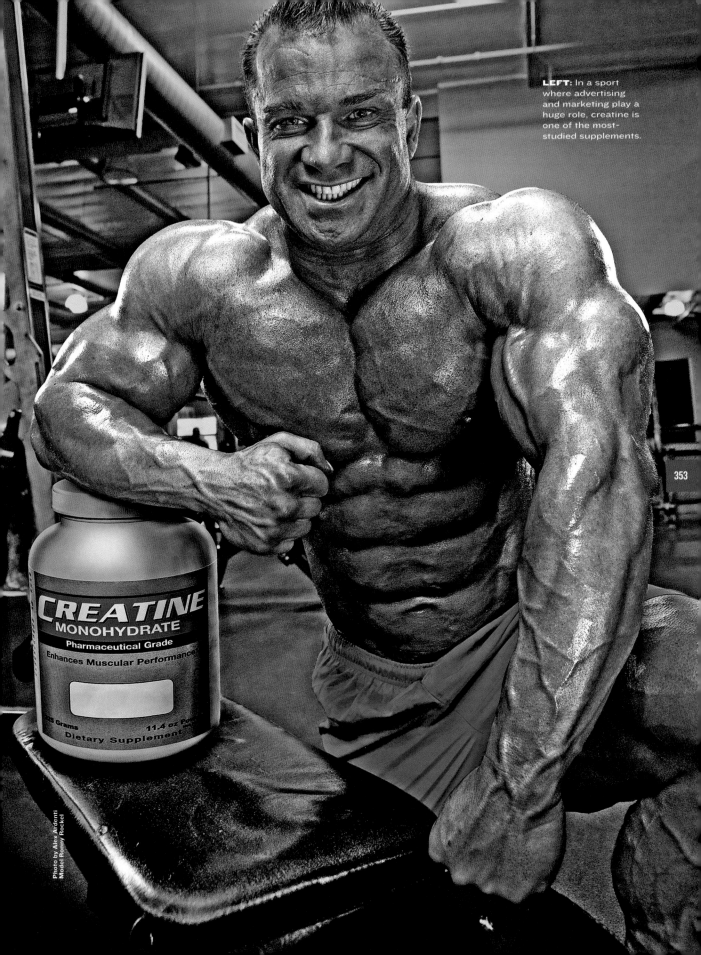

LEFT: In a sport where advertising and marketing play a huge role, creatine is one of the most-studied supplements.

CREATINE
MONOHYDRATE
Pharmaceutical Grade
Enhances Muscular Performance
Grams   11.4 oz
Dietary Supplement

354

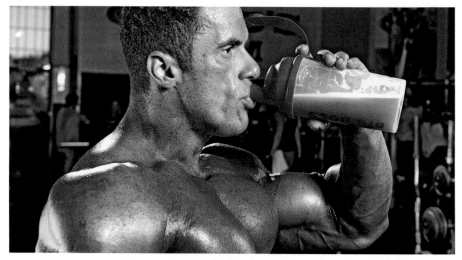

RIGHT: The absorption of creatine is enhanced when it's combined with a substance like dextrose.

From getting out of bed in the morning to those 300-pound bench presses later in the day, ATP is responsible for all of the muscle action we take for granted, but there are limited stores of ATP available in our muscles; therefore, our bodies must continually synthesize it.

THE BIG THREE

The body utilizes three different mechanisms to manufacture ATP: 1) Creatine kinase (anaerobic); 2) Glycolysis (anaerobic); and/or, 3) Oxidative phosphorylation (aerobic). The initial and most effective is accomplished by creatine kinase, which utilizes a non-oxygen dependent process that is responsible for all maximal or near-maximal muscle contractions. Creatine kinase rapidly converts the initial stores of ATP to energy and is responsible for any high-intensity, short-duration activity such as sprinting, jumping and lifting weights. As ATP is used, it loses a phosphate molecule and becomes adenosine diphosphate (ADP), which is useless until it can be converted back into ATP. This is where creatine comes in. Creatine is initially stored in the muscle as creatine phosphate. As creatine phosphate, it can "donate" or give its phosphate group to ADP, thus converting it back into ATP, which is then available as a fuel source. This process is continuously occurring with ADP converting to ATP, and ATP breaking down into ADP + a single phosphate group.

Glycolysis, the second mechanism for producing ATP, is less efficient than the creatine kinase pathway. During glycolysis, a glucose molecule is broken down into two pyruvic acid molecules, yielding two ATP molecules in the process. Glycolysis, however, requires more steps than creatine kinase, which results in a slower yield of ATP. Even though glycolysis provides the energy to perform intense exercise, it has two important consequences. First, it consumes large amounts of

Photo by Robert Reiff
Model Oliver Adzievski

nutrient fuel to yield the ATP molecules. This in turn rapidly depletes the muscle's glycogen stores. Second, the end product of anaerobic glycolysis is lactic acid. Lactic acid is one of the causes of that soreness you feel during and after an intense workout. The lactic acid buildup is also one of the reasons you fatigue after 60 to 90 minutes of exercise.

The third mechanism for ATP production is called oxidative phosphorylation. This is an aerobic process fueled by glucose or fatty acids, depending on the duration and intensity of the activity. Of the three, this is the slowest process for producing ATP because of the high number of steps involved and its dependency on a constant supply of oxygen. Oxidative phosphorylation sometimes works in conjunction with glycolysis. The type and duration of the exercise dictates which of these energy processes will be used.

Now don't let all this biochemistry frighten you. What's important to remember is that in the short term, anaerobic exercise is enhanced with creatine supplementation, which in turn provides the increased supply of creatine phosphate molecules needed to convert ADP back into ATP. Also, by increasing the body's store of creatine phosphate, creatine supplementation prolongs the creatine kinase process. This delays the need for the oxidative phosphorylation and glycolysis pathways, which are slower and less efficient. In the research to date, creatine supplementation has not been shown to enhance aerobic activities.

PREVENTING HEART DISEASE?

While most readers are probably only concerned with the effects of creatine on their skeletal muscles, there is evidence to suggest that creatine can play a role in preserving the health of the most important muscle of all – your heart!

Some research suggests that creatine can reduce the risk of heart disease. How is not fully understood, though. It doesn't appear to be related to reducing cholesterol, but by reducing levels of a compound called homocysteine. Homocysteine is known to irritate blood vessels and lead to blocked arteries.

Some researchers and cardiologists have suggested that homocysteine levels are a better predictor of heart disease than cholesterol levels. One study published in the journal *Neuroscience* found that creatine supplementation could reduce levels of homocysteine.

We should add that men tend to have higher homocysteine levels than women, which is one of the reasons put forward to explain why men traditionally have higher rates of heart disease than women.

CREATINE USAGE

Despite what some supplement manufacturers would have you believe, creatine is naturally synthesized in the liver, pancreas and kidneys from the precursor amino acids, arginine, glycine and methionone. Dietary

"I'm all for progress and new products including new forms of creatine. However, it really burns me when they have to resort to fooling customers. If you make or sell a new form of creatine, great. Use good science and good business practices to promote it, but don't lie about another product to promote your own."

– Will Brink, bodybuilding and nutrition writer

355

> "Some people make their own concoction of creatine and glucose by mixing the creatine in a glass of grape juice. However, grape juice is not all glucose – the juice also contains fructose – and does not contain the other ingredients that some products offer. Some people prefer pre-mixed products because of convenience and the additional ingredients. Experiment and see what works best for you."
>
> – Will Brink, bodybuilding and nutrition writer

creatine is also available in meats and fish, but creatine content is depleted rapidly when foods are cooked. There are approximately two grams of creatine per pound of raw, red meat. Most people, however, store only about 60 to 80 percent of their potential creatine levels. Supplementing with creatine enables individuals to elevate their creatine stores an average of 30 percent. This additional creatine gives the body the necessary ingredients to produce more ATP during the creatine kinase process and to ultimately generate more work. At its simplest, more work equals more muscle stimulation, and more muscle stimulation equals greater muscle size. Creatine does for the bodybuilder what carbohydrate loading does for the long-distance runner – it provides more energy-producing materials, which enables more work to be generated.

The key to proper creatine usage is to find the lowest dosage that supplies the maximum benefit. Currently there is no set dosage determined. However, there is a huge volume of anecdotal evidence. One of the most popular theories is the loading phase, which consists of taking approximately five grams of creatine, three or four times a day for a period of five to seven days. This is followed by a maintenance phase, which consists of 2 to 5 grams per day thereafter. Another theory suggests that the loading phase is unnecessary, wasteful and simply a ploy by manufacturers to get bodybuilders to buy more of their products. An individual who starts supplementing with only the maintenance phase (2–5 grams/day) will have the same muscle saturation in two to three weeks as the individual who loads. In a study published in the *Journal of Applied Physiology*, 31 male subjects were divided into two groups. One group received a loading dose of 20 grams of creatine a day for six days followed by a maintenance dose of two grams a day for 30 days. It was found that muscle creatine stores went up by 20 percent and the participants became stronger and gained lean muscle mass. The other group received a straight three grams per day for 28 days and similar creatine concentrations were seen. The researchers concluded that while the loading phase is a quicker way to get creatine into the muscles, it doesn't produce greater final concentrations of muscle creatine levels or greater increases in strength and size.[1]

Creatine absorption is enhanced when combined with a substance such as dextrose that increases insulin. This increased absorption can be achieved by taking creatine with grape juice or any other beverage high in dextrose. Ingesting creatine with a meal will also provide the same effect because of the increased insulin production. Some studies have also shown that exercised muscles will absorb more creatine than non-exercised muscles. Taking creatine directly after a workout may make some sense although the evidence is not conclusive.

CREATINE AND WHEY TOGETHER?

Every now and then a rumor comes along that leaves you scratching your head. One of biggest that began circulating shortly after the first edition of this book was released concerned taking creatine with whey protein. The gist of the argument was that whey protein could somehow block the absorption and effectiveness of creatine. No one knows who first started this rumor, but it wasn't long before most of the major magazines began suggesting that bodybuilders might want to separate their creatine and whey supplements rather than keep following the standard practice of tossing everything in the same blender.

To address this, researchers at Victoria University's Center for Rehabilitation, Exercise and Sport Science, conducted an experiment involving 33 male bodybuilders. They divided them into four groups: carbohydrate alone, carbohydrate plus creatine, whey isolate alone, or whey isolate and creatine. They then took muscle biopsies and had participants train for 11 weeks.

While all groups gained strength and lean muscle mass after 11 weeks, the group receiving both the whey and creatine experienced the greatest increase in fast-twitch muscle size. Since then, other studies have found similar results. It stands to reason that if whey somehow blocked creatine's absorption, then the whey- or creatine-only groups in the studies would show the greatest strength and size increases. The fact that the whey/creatine combination yielded the best results provided good evidence that the two can, and in fact should, be mixed together.

357

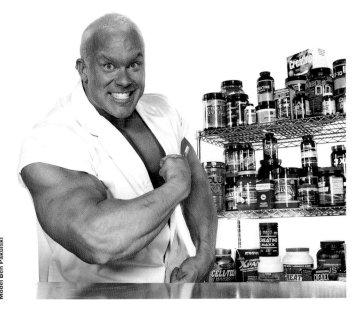

Photo by Jason Breeze
Model Ben Pakulski

LEFT: There's great debate about mixing creatine and whey, but studies seem to show that the two remain just as effective when taken together.

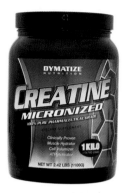

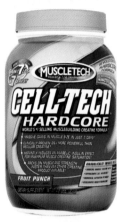

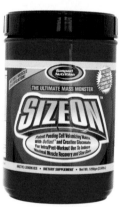

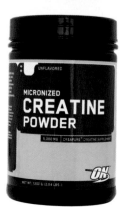

358

CREATINE SUPPLEMENTS

Generally speaking there are three types of creatine supplements available. The most popular, and by most accounts, most effective is creatine monohydrate – a white, odorless, tasteless powder. Creatine powder can be mixed with just about any liquid, but most bodybuilders prefer some sort of fruit drink. Not only does the sugar stimulate insulin release and hence improve creatine absorption, but also it tastes a lot better.

Many bodybuilders also like to add creatine to their protein shakes. Initial reports suggested that taking creatine with protein reduced creatine absorption and storage but as we just outlined, later studies found no such relationship.

Given the link between creatine absorption and insulin, it's not surprising that supplement manufacturers released what are called "pre-loaded" creatine products. Basically they contain a powder of creatine monohydrate mixed with sugar. Although they may be more convenient than creatine monohydrate products, they have a few drawbacks. The first is the amount of sugar. Many manufacturers have dumped 50 or more grams of sugar into their products. They cite studies saying how this is the amount of sugar needed to elicit an insulin response, but this is overkill on their part. As little as five to 10 grams of sugar will cause sufficient insulin release to increase creatine absorption, and at four calories per gram that's an extra 200 calories per serving. If you follow the loading phase and take three or four servings per day, that's 600 to 800 extra calories of simple sugar.

Besides the amount of sugar, pre-loaded creatine products tend to be more expensive. This is surprising given that simple sugar is a lot cheaper to manufacture and add to a product than creatine. In short, you're paying more for less creatine. For less than $5 you can pick up a large bottle of juice or drink-mix powder at the supermarket and pre-load your own creatine.

The third category of creatine supplements is liquid. As the name suggests, liquid products are just that – creatine mixed with a sugar beverage sealed in a plastic or tin container. Again you have to weigh convenience with price. A typical container of creatine liquid is just one serving and costs an average of $2 to $3. At three a day that's $180 to $270 per month! Also keep in mind that creatine is very unstable once dissolved in liquid. The supplement manufacturers claim that they've figured out a way to extend the shelf life, but who knows?

Unless you're really stuck for time (it takes all of one minute to mix creatine powder with a fruit beverage), or like the convenience of the bottle, our advice is to buy creatine monohydrate powder. You'll be getting a lot more of a tried-and-true product.

Photos by Paul Bucera

SIDE EFFECTS

Over the last couple of years, creatine has been getting a lot of bad press. The media maligning of this popular sports supplement has been a surprise to many athletes and coaches, because it is known with relative certainty that creatine can indeed improve muscular strength and size in a variety of different athletes (including football players, bodybuilders, weightlifters, swimmers and cyclists).

The heart of the bad press concerns creatine side effects, which are alleged to include muscle, tendon and ligament strains. In theory, creatine can improve the explosive energy production of muscle cells without actually fortifying the mechanical strength of muscles and their attached tendons, and ligaments holding together the joints across which muscles and tendons act. As a result, the unusually powerful contractions produced in creatine-loaded muscles might literally tear the not-yet strengthened muscle cells, and/or their associated connective tissues.

In the last few years there does seem to have been an increase in the number of injuries experienced by athletes using creatine. However, we must point out that no carefully controlled scientific study has actually linked creatine supplementation with a heightened risk of muscle or connective-tissue damage. In addition, linking two events together – increases in creatine loading with apparent increases in injuries – does not mean that one causes the other. It's also difficult to convict creatine when it's known that most athletes are using any number of other performance-enhancing agents.

The reported deaths of creatine-using wrestlers brought creatine a heap of bad press in the late 1990s. The fact that the wrestlers were taking diuretics and engaging in other weight-loss practices was quietly ignored by the media. Instead, the press focused exclusively on creatine, making it the scapegoat.

Most of the side effects associated with creatine use, such as stomach cramping and diarrhea are dosage related. Most users who experience these side effects are taking 10 grams or more all at once, instead of taking smaller amounts spread throughout the day. There have been no substantiated reports of serious side effects from creatine despite over 12 years of mainstream usage. It is possible that long-term side effects may mainifest themselves down the road, but this is highly unlikely given that creatine is a naturally occurring compound.

Reference

1) Hultman E., *et al*. Muscle creatine loading in men. *Journal of Applied Physiology*. 81: 232–7, 1996.

"Given the link between creatine absorption and insulin, it's not surprising that supplement manufacturers released what are called 'pre-loaded' creatine products. Basically they contain a powder of creatine monohydrate mixed with sugar. Although they may be more convenient than creatine monohydrate products, they have a few drawbacks. The first is the amount of sugar. Many manufacturers have dumped 50 or more grams of sugar into their products."

359

NITRIC OXIDE – NO

Nitric oxide has become extremely popular in body-building circles over the past couple of years. Nitric acid is a free-form gas produced by the body to help cells communicate with each other. At the molecular level, it's composed of the amino acid argi-nine, chemically connected to the compound alpha-ketoglutarate (itself synthesized from the amino acid ornithine and glutamine). Nitric oxide is produced within the flat endothelial cells that line the inside of blood vessels. When endothelial cells are stimulated – for example, during muscle contraction – nitric acid is synthesized and released. Once released, nitric oxide diffuses across the endothelial cell membrane into the adjacent smooth muscle tissue of the blood vessels in the body, caus-ing them to relax and widen (a process called vasodilation).

Bodybuilders have added nitric oxide to their supplement arse-nals for two reasons: to boost recovery and to reduce joint and muscle pain. It is the ability of nitric oxide to increase blood flow that interests bodybuilders. Many bodybuilders believe that the increased blood flow delivers more nutrients to the muscle cells, thus helping them to grow during the adaptation and recovery phase. The anti-inflamma-tion properties of nitric acid are also valued since intense training is hard on the joints and muscles.

In theory NO sounds promising as a supplement, but as with many such supplements there are no legitimate scientific studies showing a relationship between NO supplements and increased strength and muscle size. Most of the NO advocates are taking liber-ties with the available studies to support the use of NO as a muscle builder. For example, they believe that NO could help muscle gains because of the increased blood flow to the muscles. Other studies show an increase in NO production after resistance exercise.[1] This has led some to suggest that NO may then be involved in increasing pro-tein synthesis post-workout.

NITRIC OXIDE SUPPLEMENTS

It may surprise you to learn that most nitric acid supplements don't contain nitric acid. Instead, they contain the precursor, arginine. The

"Bodybuilders have added ni-tric oxide to their supplement arsenals for two reasons: to boost recovery and to reduce joint and muscle pain."

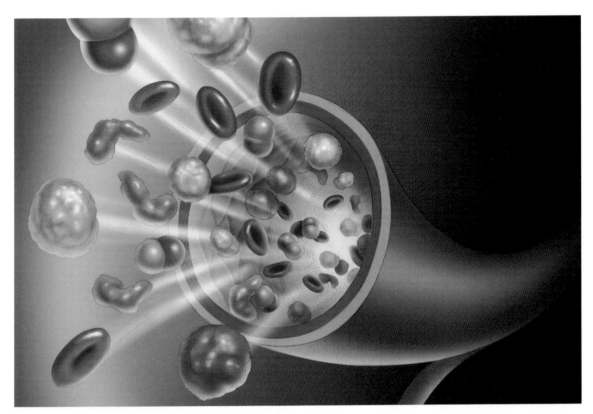

problem with these supplements is that arginine doesn't seem to convert to nitric oxide at the recommended dosages. If you examine most of the studies involving high doses of arginine, you will see no increase in vasodilatation (increased blood flow). It leads to vasodilatation only at high doses which can be achieved only by injection. The reason users can't get to those levels orally is that such dosages would invariably lead to stomach upset.

ABOVE: NO is produced in the endothelial cells lining the blood vessel walls. Muscle contractions cause NO release, which opens blood vessels.

SIDE EFFECTS

Given that most nitric oxide supplements are really nothing more than high dosages of arginine, the side effects experienced would be the same as taking high dosages of this amino acid. Since the body evolved to use amino acids in proportion and balance, the long-term risks associated with high dosages of individual amino acids are unknown. In the short-term, it has been reported that many users experience nausea and diarrhea when supplementing with more than 5 to 10 grams of arginine per day.

Reference

1) *Am J Hypertens*. 2007. Aug;20(8):825–30.

Illustration by Molly Borman

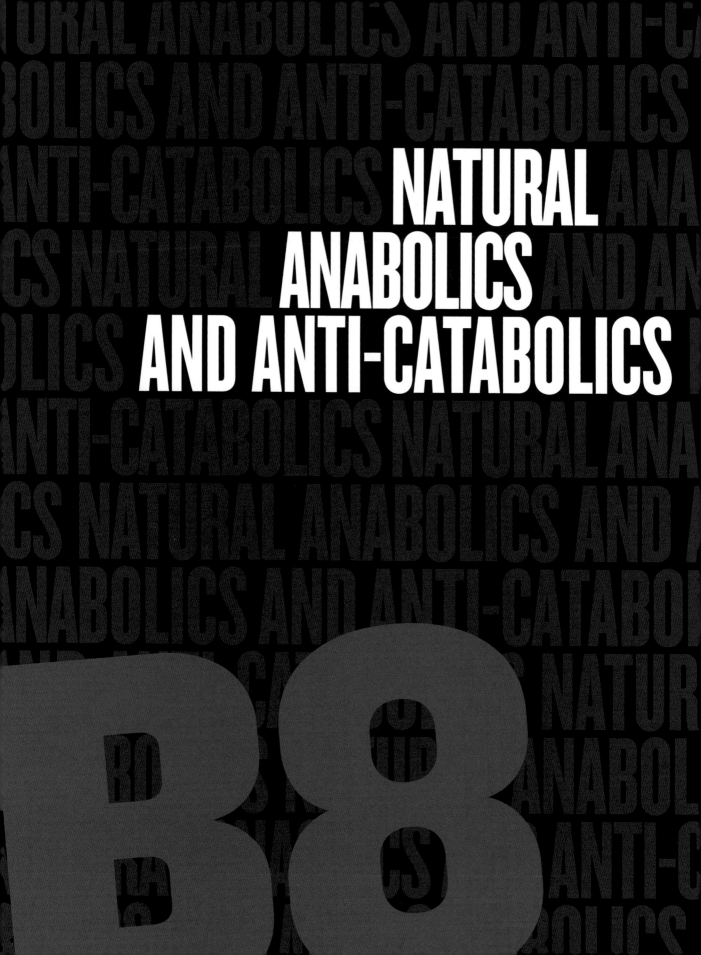

NATURAL ANABOLICS AND ANTI-CATABOLICS

B8

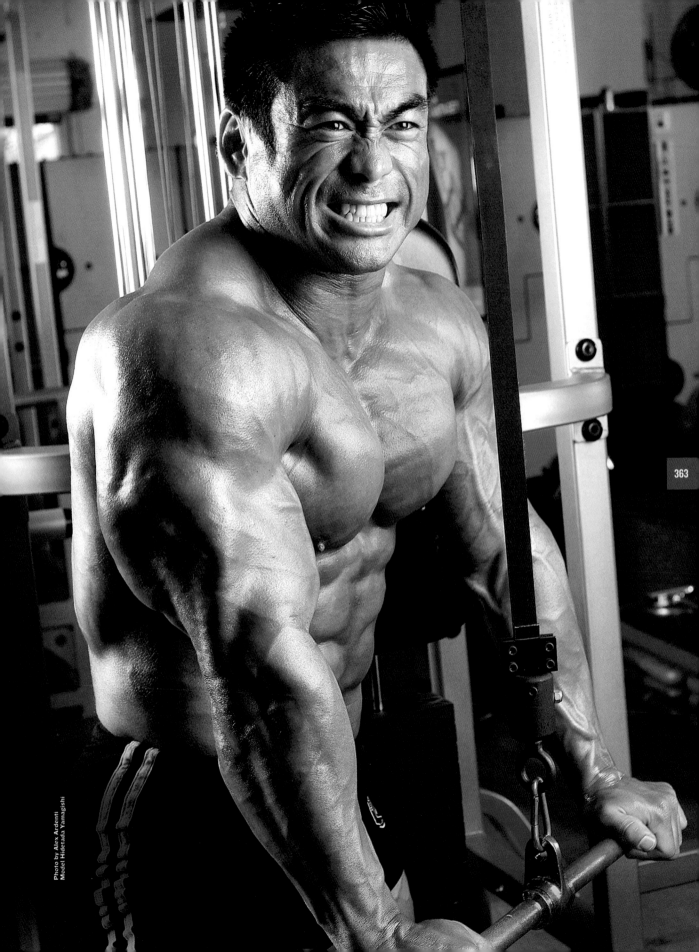

363

INTRODUCTION

The crackdown on steroids in the early 1990s meant that supplement manufacturers had to begin looking for new substances to promote as legal alternatives to anabolic steroids. Often marketed as "steroid replacers" or "testosterone boosters," most products are nothing but vitamin and mineral combinations and other common food nutrients. Certain substances such as prohormones seemed to show promise but were quickly classified as illegal under the Anabolic Control Act. Another popular form of replacement is herbal supplements produced from herbs that have been around for thousands of years in traditional and Chinese medicine. Despite the professional look and creativity of the advertising, and the fact that many have their advocates who swear by the effects, the vast majority of these compounds have no firm science behind them.

The following chapters will discuss some of the more popular substances marketed as "natural" alternatives to steroids and other illegal performance-enhancing drugs.

RIGHT: Herbal supplements have become extremely popular, but the use of herbs for health reasons dates back to ancient Chinese medicine.

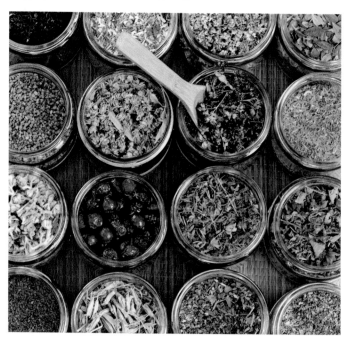

Because of the strict drug laws, many athletes now seek out natural supplements to improve their physiques.

365

Photo by Rich Baker
Model David Henry

PROHORMONES AND RELATED COMPOUNDS

Tribulus terrestris **is an herb with a long history in traditional medicine as an aphrodisiac. Its primary** method of action is believed to be stimulating the pituitary to release more luteinizing hormone (LH). LH is the main hormone responsible for signaling the testes to increase testosterone production. Tribulus received its big break when reports began leaking out of East Europe that Bulgarian weightlifters were using the plant with great success. The documented effects of this herb are split, though: Some studies have found increased sperm production and motility, and elevated testosterone levels after administration; other research has yielded no testosterone or sperm changes. We should also add that despite the anecdotal reports by bodybuilders, few studies have conclusively shown Tribulus products to positively impact muscle strength and size.

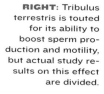

366

RIGHT: Tribulus terrestris is touted for its ability to boost sperm production and motility, but actual study results on this effect are divided.

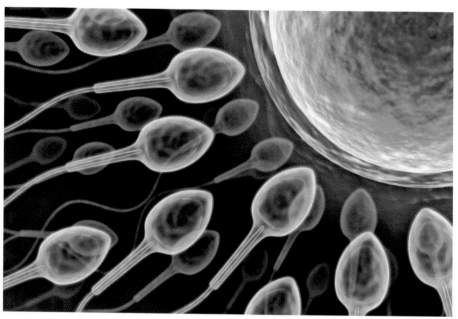

FALSE EVIDENCE?

Arguments for the efficacy of Tribulus are based largely on a few unsubstantiated studies and accounts of traditional use in Chinese medicine. The ancient Greeks also supposedly used it as a diuretic, mild laxative and general tonic. Similarly, homeopaths have long valued the herb for its diuretic and aphrodisiac qualities, often including it in rejuvenative formulas for remedying sexual problems. In China, Tribulus is still frequently used to treat a variety of diseases affecting the liver, kidneys, urinary tract (including urolithiasis, or urinary stones) and cardiovascular system.

Citing the results of a clinical trial from India, some supplement companies claim that Tribulus can decrease fatigue. Researchers in that study gave a preparation of the herb to 50 men and women who were suffering from general fatigue and lacked interest in daily activities. Subjects reported that their symptoms improved by 45 percent after taking the herb.[1]

What initially prompted researchers at the Chemical Pharmaceutical Research Institute in Sofia, Bulgaria, in the mid-1970s was the search for a safe, non-hormonal treatment for infertility and other reproductive disorders. The promising results led Eastern European drug companies to start releasing standardized Tribulus preparations in 1981. This particular investigation is now out of print, but is still often quoted by supplement makers, as it demonstrated that Tribulus boosted blood levels of luteinizing hormone. No part of the study, however, looked at the effects of the herb on muscle strength or size. But because it's now out of print and poor records were kept, verifying important details such as by how much luteinizing hormone levels were increased and whether the herb increased testosterone is impossible.

Another study, first published in the Russian journal *Farmatsiya* and mentioned in a 1996 *Muscle and Fitness* article by James Wright, M.D., reported that 750 to 1,500 milligrams of Tribulus administered daily for 30 to 60 days increased testosterone levels of men suffering from impotence and infertility.[2] But as with the Bulgarian study, the Russian researchers did not examine changes in muscle size and strength.

So what's the bottom line? The anecdotal reports don't provide solid evidence to confirm the theory that Tribulus enhances muscle growth and/or strength. Even if it does increase LH levels, there is nothing in the scientific literature to suggest that such increases lead to meaningful boosts in testosterone and ultimately muscle size and strength. Tribulus is more of a fad herb (albeit a highly profitable one for supplement manufacturers). Until further research is conducted on healthy individuals with no libido or hormonal problems, there's no guarantee this product will bring about any improvements to your physique.

> "Whether you decide to take 4-androstenedione, or any other substance for that matter, remember that the only constant in bodybuilding is regular, serious training. No amount of hype can substitute for sweat."
>
> – Will Brink, bodybuilding and nutrition writer

367

ANDROSTENEDIONE

"Andro" is another supplement that got its first promotion through research carried out in former East Germany. Because success in athletics was a substantial part of the Communist statement, those in the sports community were always on the lookout for substances that could boost performance but go undetected in a drug test. According to declassified reports from the East German doping program, many of the athletes were using an andro nasal spray that would elevate testosterone levels for a few hours – the amount was enough to increase performance but not fail a drug test. This development marked the beginning of the science of testosterone precursors.

If the East Germans are credited with introducing andro to the athletic world, then baseball player Mark McGwire holds the honor of bringing andro to the masses. Although banned by most sports federations, andro is perfectly legal in professional baseball. All it took was a snooping reporter who spotted it in McGwire's locker, and the media frenzy ensued. So-called "experts" came out of the woodwork to denounce McGwire for using anabolic steroids. The fact that andro is not a classified anabolic steroid, however, conveniently seemed to be ignored. At that point, the genie had already been let out of the bottle and supplement companies made a fortune – ironic because andro was at the time on its way out of bodybuilding circles. The supplement had seen one or two good years, but the results had been less than expected, and it was slowly beginning to disappear. But along came McGwire and andro jumped to the top of the charts, all thanks to the power of the media!

At a biochemical level androstenedione is an intermediate precursor to testosterone – the two differ by a single enzyme and one step. While theoretically this may sound great, a host of variables must occur in order for andro to be converted into the desired hormone. Even when it is, the outcome isn't all it's cracked up to be. Most andro marketers say the product "increases testosterone levels" and leave it at that. What they don't tell you, however, is that only a small amount (five to 10 percent is the range most commonly quoted) makes the journey from andro to testosterone. Another deterring point to consider is that andro stays active in the body for only a short period of time – roughly a few hours. From a biochemical perspective, andro thus has a short half-life (the time needed for half of the substance to degrade or be converted into another substance). We also must point out that there's little research to suggest slightly elevated testosterone levels can make much of an impact on athletic performance. Unless you were to consume andro every couple of hours on an ongoing basis, a few capsules a day probably isn't going to lead to any meaningful muscle growth.

> "If the East Germans are credited with introducing andro to the athletic world, then baseball player Mark McGwire holds the honor of bringing andro to the masses. Although banned by most sports federations, andro is perfectly legal in professional baseball. All it took was a snooping reporter who spotted it in McGwire's locker, and the media frenzy ensued."

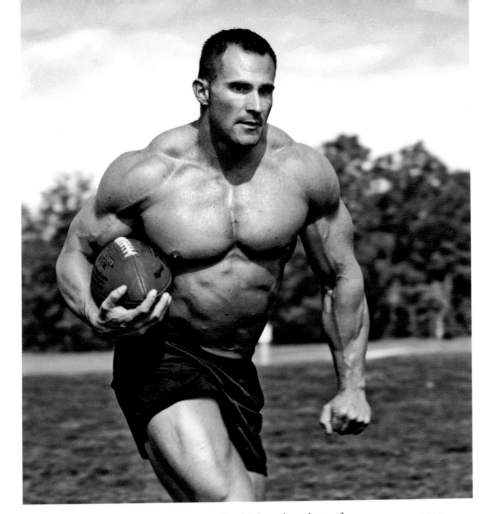

Photo by Jason Breeze
Model Mark Richmond

In addition, testosterone is only one of multiple end products of andro metabolism. Andro can also be converted into estrogen. Now, even though there's limited evidence showing that estrogen can stimulate testosterone levels, greater evidence supports higher estrogen levels as a factor for increased fat storage (one of the primary reasons women on average have higher bodyfat percentages than men).

With respect to side effects, andro is not in the same category as some of the harsher anabolic steroids (e.g., Anadrol-50), but there are still risks. Many users of this hormone experience increased facial and torso acne. Remember, testosterone and its derivatives also have androgenic effects (i.e., development of secondary sex characteristics such as hair growth, etc.). This is why acne is common during the teenage years and especially in males – higher levels of testosterone. If you had severe or even moderate acne as a teenager, then you're more prone to developing the condition when taking andro.

One particular side effect may offer an athletic edge for those who use this supplement: elevated aggression levels. The link between high testosterone levels and aggression has been hypothesized and examined in the scientific community for quite some time. Numerous studies with prisoners have confirmed that a relationship does exist between the two (of course, there are many more variables that lead to incarceration). For athletes in a sport requiring a certain combative mentality (i.e., football, rugby, judo, etc.), andro might offer a slight advantage.

ABOVE: While andro was marketed as a performance booster, athletes weren't told that only a small percentage actually converts to testosterone.

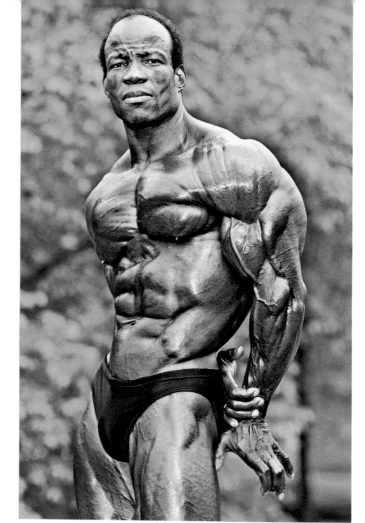

RIGHT: Albert Beckles achieved and maintained a physique that carried him through over 100 bodybuilding contests – now *that's* performance at its best!

> "One particular side effect may offer an athletic edge for those who use this supplement: elevated aggression levels. For athletes in a sport requiring a certain combative mentality (i.e., football, rugby, judo, etc.), andro might offer a slight advantage."

A less common but potentially more severe side effect concerns the prostate gland. This small organ in the lower groin of males is very sensitive to high androgen levels. Many men (20 to 25 percent by some accounts) are genetically predisposed to develop prostate problems later in life. Taking any substance that's biochemically similar to (or converted to) testosterone increases the risk of prostate issues, including cancer.

Finally, assuming andro actually does get converted to testosterone, you are still faced with the problem of feedback interference. Most of the body's hormones, including testosterone, are regulated by a biofeedback mechanism – in effect the body increases or decreases levels depending on how much of the hormone is circulating. As soon as you introduce an outside source, the body's natural hormonal axis becomes disrupted.

The "accepted" dosage for androstenedione is 100 to 200 milligrams per day – preferably split evenly over three or four dosages. This is probably enough to slightly elevate testosterone levels (though it's difficult to confirm this) without producing the unwanted side effects. The bottom line, however, is that the efficacy of this hormone depends on the individual. If you have a history of hair loss, prostate problems or acne in your family, we strongly advise against using andro products.

Model Albert Beckles

19-NOR-4-ANDROSTENEDIONE (19-NOR)

Like androstenedione, 19-Nor is another example of a group of substances called prohormones. They work in one of two primary ways: They either convert to testosterone or they convert to another anabolic hormone. 19-Nor does the latter – the liver modifies it into nandrolone. Now this name may not ring any gym bells for many readers, but perhaps nandrolone decanoate will. Nandrolone is the active ingredient in the very effective anabolic steroid Deca-Durabolin (also called "Deca" for short). Deca has a cult-like following of bodybuilders because the substance is highly anabolic, but low in androgenic properties. This steroid also has a reputation of being one of the safest anabolic steroids ever manufactured.

Taking 19-Nor gives users the option of naturally creating nandrolone in the body without having to worry about any legal ramifications. Now by no means are we saying that 19-Nor is as powerful as Deca. But for a natural trainer who has never used steroids, 19-Nor will make a significant difference.

BELOW: John Hansen competed as a natural bodybuilder, and his two biggest victories came at the 1998 Natural Olympia and 1996 Natural Mr. Universe.

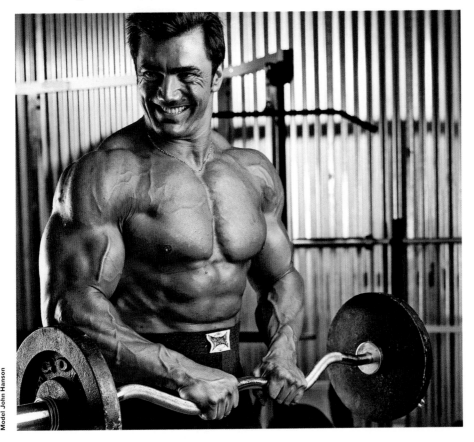

Photo by Rick Schaff
Model John Hansen

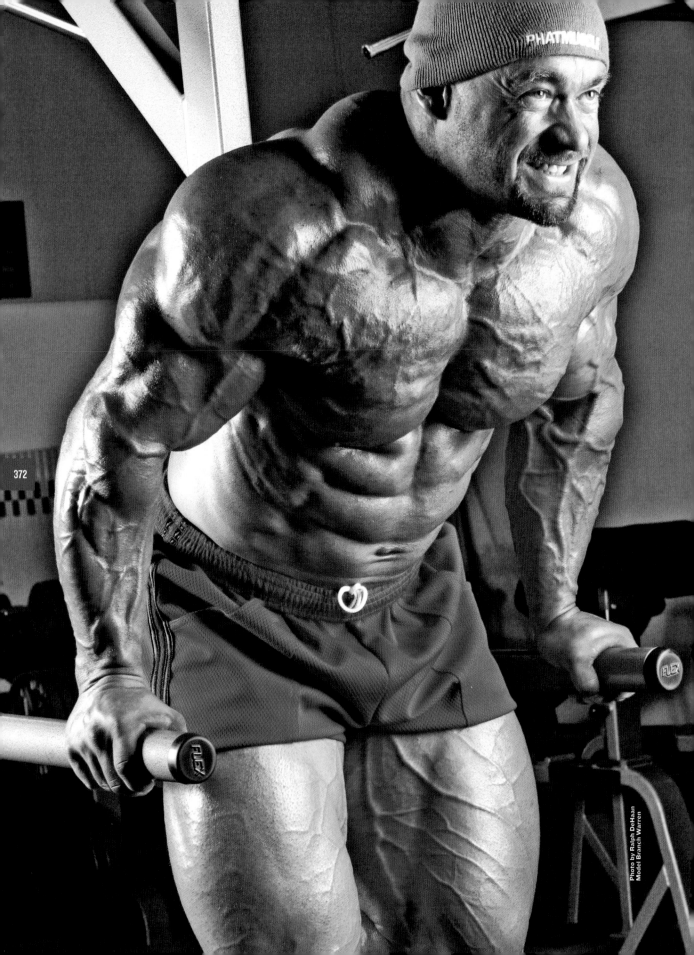

372

A final point to note about 19-Nor and other nandrolone derivatives is that they are among the easiest to detect in a drug test. The 1999 Pan American Games in Winnipeg, Canada, is a prime example when numerous athletes tested positive for nandrolone. Most of the athletes claimed they never used injectable nandrolone products, but many admitted to taking over-the-counter 19-Nor. For those who were in fact telling the truth, those failed drug tests help to confirm what many considered merely the hype generated by supplement manufacturers – that 19-Nor could biochemically change and become nandrolone. And not only that, it could convert at a rate high enough to be detected in a drug test. And for those of you who have recently stopped taking nandrolone and its relative compounds, you are not out of the woodwork just yet. Nandrolone can be detected in the body for as long as 18 months after its last ingestion. That's right. It may take your body over a year and a half to clear the product from your system. Please keep this in mind if you plan on competing in a sport that has a reputable drug-testing policy.

7-KETO-DIHYDROEPIANDROSTENDIONE

Dihydroepiandrostenedione is a derivative of the popular supplement DHEA. Produced naturally by the adrenal glands, DHEA is one of the most dominant hormones in the body. It functions as somewhat of a "mother" hormone, giving birth to a host of other hormones depending on what the body needs. One exciting feature shown from studies is that supplementing with DHEA can increase circulating testosterone levels. Other investigations have demonstrated that users of this hormone gain more muscle mass and lose more bodyfat than non-users. Once again, DHEA is not a replacement for anabolic steroids, but depending on the individual, may increase levels of testosterone in the bloodstream.

It's important to note, however, that most studies on DHEA and its efficacy have focused primarily on the elderly or those deficient in the hormone. Long-term trials involving bodybuilders or other healthy athletic subjects are few and far between in medical literature. While there is a mountain of positive anecdotal evidence to suggest that DHEA may help promote muscle size and fat loss, the scientific backing is limited, at best.

5-ANDROSTENEDIOL (DIOL-5)

Diol-5 is a close cousin of 19-Nor and is also reported to be converted to nandrolone in the liver. It is sold in many countries as methandriol. According to the substance's manufacturers, Diol-5 produces three main effects in the body. First, it's supposedly anti-catabolic, which means it suppresses cortisol and other stress hormones released by

> "The 1999 Pan American Games in Winnipeg, Canada, is a prime example when numerous athletes tested positive for nandrolone. Most of the athletes claimed they never used injectable nandrolone products, but many admitted to taking over-the-counter 19-Nor. For those who were in fact telling the truth, those failed drug tests help to confirm what many considered merely the hype generated by supplement manufacturers – that 19-Nor could biochemically change and become nandrolone."

373

intense training. Cortisol causes protein to be leeched from muscle tissue, leading to muscle wasting. The higher cortisol levels are, the harder it is for the body to recover from exercise.

Another noted property of Diol-5 is its ability to bind to estrogen receptors. The more estrogen receptors that are "blocked," the fewer effects this feminizing hormone can have. And closely related to this, Diol-5 also has the ability to prevent the conversion of testosterone to estrogen (called aromatization).

A final benefit of Diol-5 is that like glutamine, it can strengthen the immune system by increasing the activation of lymphocytes. As many bodybuilders will admit, a couple of months of intense training often leaves them in a drained state and open to every flu or bug that goes around. Diol-5 may act to boost the immune system, helping to ward off such stress-induced ailments.

As with most prohormones, precise dosages have never been calculated for Diol-5. Most anecdotal reports suggest taking 50 to 100 milligrams of Diol-5 per day.

4-ANDROSTENEDIOL

4-AD is the brainchild of chemist Patrick Arnold and his company LPJ. This supplement is promoted as the best among the current generation of precursors because it converts to testosterone three times faster than other precursors like androstenedione. In one study presented at a major conference in Finland, 100 milligrams of 4-AD was found to raise testosterone 42.5 percent as compared to only 10.9 percent for an equal amount of androstenedione.

4-AD is found in several tissues of the body including the adrenal cortex, hypothalamus and testes. Besides raising testosterone levels higher than other precursors, 4-AD may have another advantage – it doesn't seem to aromatize to estrogen like many other similar substances. Without insulting the biochemists out there, suffice it to say 4-AD is missing a side group (in this case a ketone) that most of the others have. Of course, the extra testosterone produced by 4-AD can and will aromatize to a certain degree, but such is the price you pay when you play chemist with your hormone levels.

FINAL COMMENTS

There are two primary questions to ask when discussing the topic of prohormones: 1) Are they effective? 2) What are the long-term dangers? To answer the first question, while they're not in the same category as anabolic steroids, prohormones will give most natural bodybuilders an increase in size and strength beyond what they'd gain without the substances. Of course, this calls into question the actual meaning of "natural." Is taking a substance that converts to an anabolic steroid molecule in a different category than injecting the com-

"Prohormones have only become a major player in athletics over the last 10 years or so (excluding the East German use of androstenedione back in the '70s and '80s). As such, there simply aren't any long-term studies to use as a point of reference. Therefore, no one knows what will happen to current users 10 or 20 years from now."

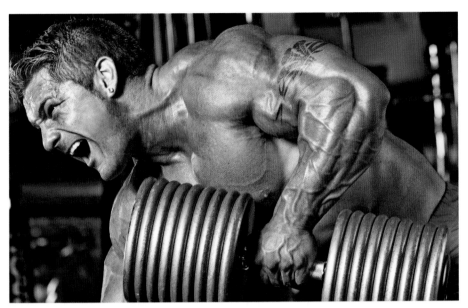

pound directly? As we explained earlier, there is a large gray area in the realm of modern supplements, and prohormones are among the leaders for debate.

The second question is much more difficult, if not impossible, to answer. Prohormones have only become a major player in athletics over the last 10 years or so (excluding the East German use of androstenedione back in the '70s and '80s). As such, there simply aren't any long-term studies to use as a point of reference. Therefore, no one knows what will happen to current users 10 or 20 years from now. The fact that most prohormones are found naturally in the body would suggest that no side effects should occur. But then you have to consider that these compounds are not usually found in the dosages routinely taken by bodybuilders. The common analogy of alcohol use rings true here: small amounts are not dangerous and in some cases can actually be beneficial, but heavy alcohol consumption leads to a whole host of problems. The same logic could be true for prohormones, but only time will tell.

Since the first edition of this book was published, prohormones have been reclassified as controlled substances and now fall under the same legislation as anabolic steroids. So even if they are as effective as manufacturers claim, you'll still face jail time if you get caught in possession of any of these hormones.

ABOVE: Many prohormones are claimed to convert to testosterone, hence why some bodybuilders choose to take them as a "natural" means to boost their muscle gains.

References

1) Jayaram S., *et al. Indian Drugs.* 1993. 30(10):498–500.
2) Milanov., *et al. Farmatsiya* 1987. 37(6):142.

GAMMA ORYZANOL, YOHIMBINE, SMILAX, BORON

376

> "The theory behind yohimbine as a performance enhancer is somewhat flawed, but the supplement is still heavily promoted in the industry. Many manufacturers claim (and get athletes to believe) that if yohimbine has aphrodisiac properties, then it must likewise elevate hormone levels – including testosterone – by some means. And more testosterone in the body translates into greater muscle-building potential."

Though the popularity of this substance seemed to peak in the 1980s (thanks to heavy promotion in Joe Weider's *Muscle and Fitness* magazine), gamma oryzanol still has its fans. Gamma oryzanol is a mixture of plant hormones (called sterols) and ferulic acid esters derived from the bran in barley, corn and rice. The majority of this substance used for nutritional supplements is harvested in Japan.

What made gamma oryzanol so attractive to bodybuilders (and supplement producers) were early reports that the compound could increase levels of testosterone, growth hormone and other anabolic (muscle-building) hormones. As with many such supplements, however, these initial studies were conducted on animals and primarily involved poor research methods. There is still no hard evidence confirming that gamma oryzanol either boosts these hormones or enhances performance. In fact, the few thorough studies that have been conducted show just the opposite – the product has no effect on any anabolic hormones in the human body. For example, one double-blind study found that consumption of gamma oryzanol for nine weeks at a dose of 500 milligrams daily affected neither anabolic hormone nor performance levels.[1]

The standard dosage used by bodybuilders is 5 to 30 milligrams, two to three times per day; when you take into account the aforementioned study, it comes as no surprise that most users don't experience any performance-boosting effects from gamma oryzanol.

YOHIMBINE

This alkaloid compound is derived from the inner bark of the yohimbe evergreen tree that grows in West Africa. Yohimbine has been used for thousands of years as an aphrodisiac, and is now primarily used in veterinary medicine and in general medicine for the treatment of erectile dysfunction. In general, bodybuilders use yohimbine to boost their hormones levels and increase fat loss.

While yohimbine has not been researched as thoroughly as many other fat-loss aids, the existing data on this substance is promising.

One example is a three-week study conducted in 1991 on 20 obese females. Participants were placed on daily diets of 1,000 calories; one group was given 20 milligrams of yohimbine per day and the other group received a placebo. The study results showed that subjects taking the supplement experienced increased weight loss of three pounds more than the placebo group.[2] Other research has demonstrated that yohimbine increases the amount of non-esterfied fatty acids (NEFAs), which is a product of lipolysis (breakdown of fat), in the bloodstream in both lean and obese individuals.[3,4] This effect was shown to persist for at least 14 days, a finding indicative that rapid tolerance to this supplement does not develop.

Although the exact mechanism of action has not been singled out, it is believed that yohimbine works by blocking alpha-2 adregenic receptors. There are a number of feedback mechanisms that prevent the release of norepinephrine (NE), one of the body's primary lipolytic hormones. When NE is released, such as in periods of stress or after

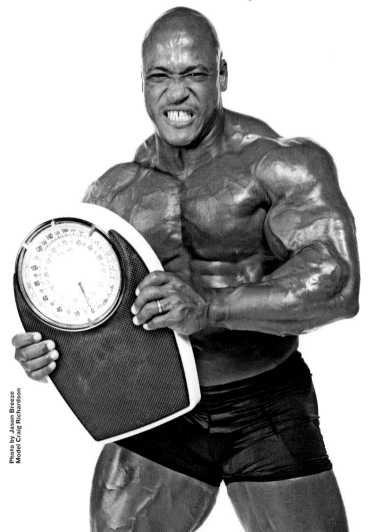

Photo by Jason Breeze
Model Craig Richardson

LEFT: In the battle against the scale, some athletes opt for yohimbine as a tool to aid fat loss.

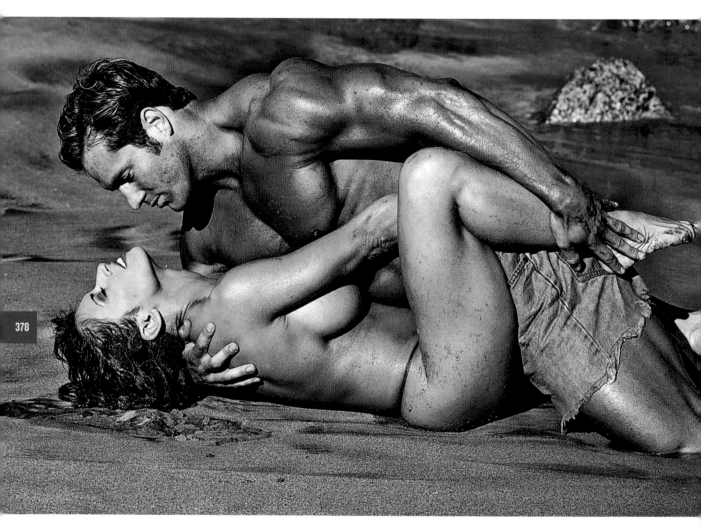

378

ABOVE: Many yohimbine users take this supplement not just for fat loss, but also because of its claimed aphrodisiac qualities.

taking a sympathomimetic (such as ephedrine), it stimulates both the alpha and beta adrenoreceptors. Stimulation of the beta adrenoreceptors specifically causes the breakdown of fat while stimulating the alpha-2 receptors has the opposite effect, preventing the release of NE and lipolysis. Yohimbine prevents this negative feedback mechanism, thus increasing NE release and lipolysis.

In addition to its positive role in fat loss, yohimbine is well-known as a sexual stimulant. Though most published studies are those on animals, findings indicate that this natural amine increases copulatory behavior and reduces sexual exhaustion in male rats.[5,6] A review of the literature also seems to indicate that when yohimbine is combined with drugs that increase the action of nitric oxide, results show great promise in the treatment of male erectile dysfunction.[7]

Photo by Jim Amentler
Models Jeff Dwelle and Devon Michaels

As an alpha-2 receptor antagonist, yohimbine blocks receptors in the brain, leading to physiological responses such as increased heart rate and blood pressure, improved motor function and vasodilation. And it's the last function that plays a central role in treating impotence. The blood vessels leading to all the extremities become dilated and blood flow increases. More blood reaches the penis and therefore the male should be able to achieve an erection (assuming the problem is related to blood flow).

The theory behind yohimbine as a performance enhancer is somewhat flawed, but the supplement is still heavily promoted in the industry. Many manufacturers claim (and get athletes to believe) that if yohimbine has aphrodisiac properties, then it must likewise elevate hormone levels – including testosterone – by some means. And more testosterone in the body translates into greater muscle-building potential.

While this perhaps looks great on paper, there are practical considerations that detract from claims made by manufacturers about this compound. For starters, there is no scientific evidence to demonstrate that yohimbine can in fact elevate testosterone levels. Most aphrodisiacs owe much of their success to the placebo effect. Like other touted sex promoters such as Tiger Penis and Spanish Fly, most of these substances are psychological in nature. And despite yohimbine's ability to increase blood flow to the genitalia, this alkaloid simply has not been proven to increase sexual prowess by elevating hormone levels.

Another reason yohimbine is questionable as a hormone booster is that it's derived from a plant. Although some plant hormones do have bioactivity in humans, most do not – the majority of drugs that come from plants need to be chemically modified in order to have any effect in humans. What supplement manufacturers have done is banked on the fact that many consumers aren't familiar with the scientific terminology. Companies capitalized by using the word sterol, confusing buyers through advertising by making it sound similar to steroid. But the fact remains that no plant sterol is going to act the same as an anabolic steroid in the human body.

Also adding to the puzzlement around this supplement is that yohimbe bark sometimes contains small amounts of methyltestosterone. The debate still rages as to whether or not methyltestosterone from plants is bioactive in humans. And even if it is, the amounts present are nowhere near enough to cause any anabolic effect.

USING YOHIMBINE

If you decide to use yohimbine, the recommended dosage is 15 to 20 milligrams per day. Take note, however, that these amounts are for treating impotence; no doubt many bodybuilders are taking many times the suggested dosage.

379

"Another reason yohimbine is questionable as a hormone booster is that it's derived from a plant. Although some plant hormones do have bioactivity in humans, most do not – the majority of drugs that come from plants need to be chemically modified in order to have any effect in humans."

> "One fact remains constant: to formulate a true high-quality supplement, manufacturers must invest significant amounts of money, which then gets passed on to you, the consumer, in the price. And while we'll readily admit that expensive ineffective supplements are out there, the odds of finding a cheap effective product is extremely unlikely."

Finally, while yohimbine may hold some merit as an aphrodisiac (and some bodybuilders swear that it gives them greater pumps before a workout) because of its vasodilating effects, science has found little relevance for this substance as an anabolic agent.

SMILAX

Smilax is yet another supplement that has seen its glory days come and go. Smilax (or Smilax officinalis) is derived from the herb Sarsaparilla; you can obtain the compound naturally from the herb, but supplement manufacturers have produced more concentrated forms (in the same manner that ephedrine is available from the herb Ma Huang). To give the supplement greater credibility, manufacturers often strategically market the product in drug-like bottles. We can only guess how many bodybuilders fell for such false misleading advertising during the 1980s – the heydays of Smilax.

In very similar fashion as the marketing of yohimbine, Smilax was (and still is to a lesser degree) labeled as a natural testosterone booster. Supplement companies frequently cited studies to back their claims – unfortunately the studies were mainly out of Bulgaria, giving way to much skepticism because of the degree of steroid use in former East Bloc countries. North American researchers have never confirmed any testosterone-boosting capabilities of Smilax.

As we noted earlier, plant compounds generally have little or no effect on human hormone biochemistry, so it seems logical that Smilax lacks the ability to increase testosterone. As soon as plant sterols are consumed, they immediately get broken down in the digestive system into their component nutrients – vitamins, minerals, protein and carbohydrates.

We must also take into account the potential legalities of such claims by advertisers. If Smilax could boost testosterone production to the degree that manufacturers claim, the FDA would reclassify the compound as a drug. Soft drink companies would also have to remove it from the ingredient list in some of their products (Smilax is often used as a flavoring ingredient in root beer).

It's also amusing to hear supplement manufacturers attempt to claim that Smilax will produce great increases in testosterone without the side effects produced by steroids. Even the most dedicated of steroid users, however, will admit that all anabolic steroids generate side effects (just usually not to the same extent that anti-steroid groups argue). You have to ask yourself, "How can Smilax be 'side-effect free' while steroids are 'dangerous and to be avoided at all costs'?" This question alone should be enough to raise big warning flags.

With regards to pricing, Smilax is one of the cheapest supplements available – usually ranging from $10 to $20 for a month's sup-

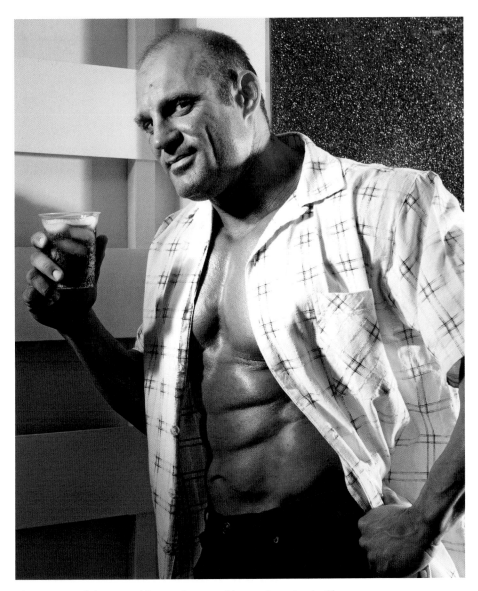

LEFT: Smilax is often used as an ingredient to flavor root beer. If it was as potent as manufacturers claim, soft drink companies would have to remove it from products.

381

Photo by Robert Reiff
Model David Bourlet

ply. As most of the reputable supplements (the products backed by credible scientific research) are much more expensive, you can bet that Smilax doesn't cost much to produce. This is not to say, however, that price is the only factor for rating a supplement. But one fact remains constant: to formulate a true high-quality supplement, manufacturers must invest significant amounts of money, which then gets passed on to you, the consumer, in the price. And while we'll readily admit that expensive ineffective supplements are out there, the odds of finding a cheap effective product is extremely unlikely.

BORON

Boron is perhaps the most blatant example of how some shady supplement manufacturers selectively used research studies to make false claims about their product.

Boron is a trace mineral that functions in the metabolism of other minerals like magnesium, phosphorus and calcium. There is also evidence indicating that it can reduce the adverse effects of arthritis and osteoporosis.

Boron became one of the most popular supplements in bodybuilding during the 1980s when researchers discovered that test subjects experienced testosterone increases of 200 to 300 percent from using boron. Taken at face value, such results seemed to suggest that boron's efficacy was comparable to that of anabolic steroids. What the supplement manufacturers conveniently failed to mention was that the "test subjects" were post-menopausal women! How anyone could compare this group to hard-training male bodybuilders is incomprehensible. Nevertheless, millions of dollars were made from this scam, and it was only after a few well-respected writers exposed the truth in bodybuilding magazines that boron slipped out of popularity. A 20-year-old male bodybuilder would be wasting his time taking boron with the hopes of boosting his testosterone levels.

References

1) Fry A.C., Bonner E., Lewis D.L., *et al*. The effects of gamma-oryzanol supplementation during resistance exercise training. *Int J Sport Nutr*. (1997) 7:318–329.

2) Kucio C., Jonderko K., Piskorska D. Does yohimbine act as a slimming drug? *Isr J Med Sci*. (1991) Oct;27(10):550–6.

3) Berlan M., Galitzky J., Riviere D., Foureau M., Tran M.A., Flores R., Louvet J.P., Houin G., Lafontan M. Plasma catecholamine levels and lipid mobilization induced by yohimbine in obese and non-obese women. *Int J Obes*. (1991) May;15(5):305–15.

4) Galitzky J., Taouis M., Berlan M., Riviere D., Garrigues M., Lafontan M. Alpha 2-antagonist compounds and lipid mobilization: evidence for a lipid mobilizing effect of oral yohimbine in healthy male volunteers. *Eur J Clin Invest*. (1988) Dec;18(6):587–94.

5) Carro-Juareza M., Rodriguez-Manzo G. Yohimbine reverses the exhaustion of the coital reflex in spinal male rats. *Behav Brain Res*. (2003) Apr 17;141(1):43–50.

6) Rodriguez-Manzo G., Fernandez-Guasti A. Participation of the central noradrenergic system in the reestablishment of copulatory behavior of sexually exhausted rats by yohimbine, naloxone, and 8-OH-DPAT. *Brain Res Bull*. (1995) 38(4):399–404.

7) Tam S.W., Worcel M., Wyllie M. Yohimbine: a clinical review. *Pharmacol Ther*. (2001) Sep;91(3):215–43.

382

"Boron became one of the most popular supplements in bodybuilding during the 1980s when researchers discovered that test subjects experienced testosterone increases of 200 to 300 percent from using boron. Taken at face value, such results seemed to suggest that boron's efficacy was comparable to that of anabolic steroids. What the supplement manufacturers conveniently failed to mention was that the 'test subjects' were post-menopausal women!"

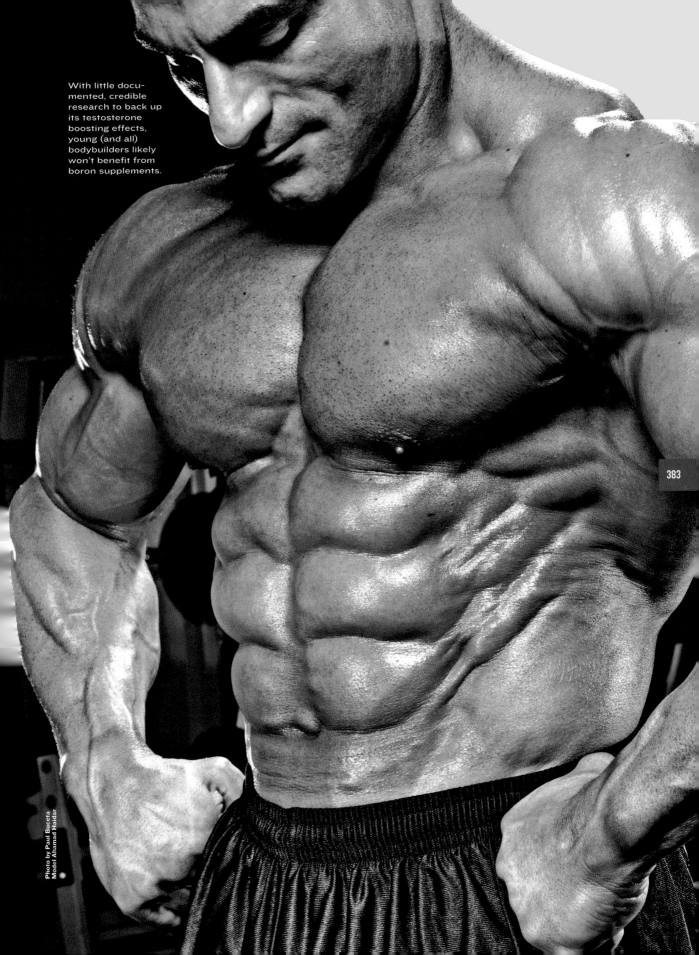

With little documented, credible research to back up its testosterone boosting effects, young (and all) bodybuilders likely won't benefit from boron supplements.

383

CHROMIUM

When most people hear the word chromium, they think of the shiny chrome metal plating that adorns many expensive sports cars. Few individuals are aware that this trace element is actually a vital tool for maintaining health. The importance of chromium in the body went unnoticed until the 1950s when animal experiments discovered that a deficiency in this chemical element could lead to serious health issues. Prior to such research, most assumed chromium's uses were limited to steel manufacturing, dyes and paints, and leather tanning processes.

Much of what we now know about chromium in human bio-chemistry comes from the works of Dr. Walter Mertz. In the 1950s, Dr. Mertz first isolated the biologically active form of chromium called GTF – glucose tolerance factor. Later research determined that GTF is an organic chromium complex, which helps bind insulin to cell

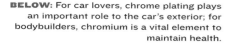

384

BELOW: For car lovers, chrome plating plays an important role to the car's exterior; for bodybuilders, chromium is a vital element to maintain health.

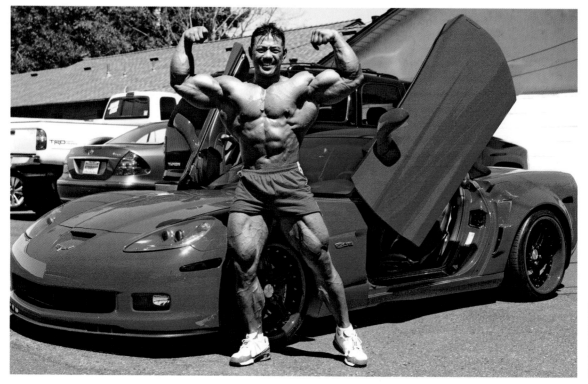

Photo by Ralph DeHaan
Model Ray Arde

membrane receptors. If this structure is not present, insulin's ability to metabolize and transport glucose becomes hindered. Dr. Mertz also discovered that not all forms of chromium are biologically active and capable of affecting insulin. Only those bonded to nicotinic acid and the amino acids glycine, cysteine, glutamic acid and aspartic acid are believed to be effective.

ACTIONS IN THE BODY

From Dr. Mertz's works and more recent studies, it is believed that chromium has three primary effects in the human body. We've already touched on the first, which is glucose modulation. The element carries out this function by increasing the efficiency of insulin, especially as it relates to improving binding power to cell receptors.

The second action of chromium is to reduce blood cholesterol levels. When researchers combined data from five double-blind, placebo-controlled studies, involving more than 300 patients, they discovered a significant change in total blood cholesterol levels. On average, subjects who were taking chromium experienced their levels drop more than 20 points, going from upward of 220 milligrams per deciliter to less than 200 milligrams per deciliter. Study participants were not on any lipid-lowering medications. Supplementation with 1,000 micrograms had the greatest effect, although doses as low as 200 micrograms also substantially lowered blood cholesterol.[1] Chromium's positive impact on cholesterol is further supported by another study that was presented at a meeting of the American College of Nutrition. Researchers found that the element may also be important for blood cholesterol reduction and lessening the risk of diabetes and heart disease; on average, people receiving a chromium picolinate supplement had a total blood cholesterol decrease of more than 20 points.[2]

Chromium's third role is what's made it such a popular bodybuilding supplement. A number of studies have demonstrated that chromium may hold promise as a fat-burning product. One such investigation involved test subjects who took a daily dose of either 400 micrograms of chromium or a placebo. Changes in bodyfat, fat-free mass and weight were then measured over a 90-day period. The study was a double-blind format with 122 moderately overweight people and lasted for three months. The results indicated that the chromium group experienced an average loss of 6.2 pounds of bodyfat, as opposed to 3.4 pounds in the placebo group. This data demonstrated a statistically significant reduction in bodyfat (and fat mass) in those individuals who took chromium, without the sacrifice of any valuable lean body mass. The outcomes of this study (among others) suggest that chromium can help you lose fat without compromising muscle.[3,4,5]

"The person who needs to be careful about chromium intake is the diabetic. You need to take into account the blood sugar levels that have already been adjusted by medicine intake. If you are a diabetic, you should not take chromium supplements unless you and your physician are monitoring your blood sugar, so you can make the appropriate changes to your medication."

– Dwayne Hines II, *MuscleMag International* contributor

385

THE EVOLUTION OF CHROMIUM SUPPLEMENTS

Chromium supplements are not without an interesting history. "Older" readers may remember the original chromium supplement, brewer's yeast tablets, made popular by the Muscle Beach bodybuilders back in the 1950s and 1960s. Despite the favor they received at that time, brewer's yeast is actually a poor source of chromium with less than 2 micrograms per gram (less than half of what's in the biologically active GTF form) – not to mention the flatulence-producing side effects the tablets were known for!

The second generation of these supplements consisted of the chromium salts chloride, acetate and oxide. Again, however, the problem of bioavailability rears its ugly head as less than one percent of chromium salts is absorbed and utilized by the body.

The next wave of this compound appeared in the early 1970s and consisted of chromium bound to amino acids. Despite the improved absorption, these supplements didn't seem to influence insulin to any degree.

The first step in the right direction occurred in the 1980s when chemists began to synthesize biologically active GTF complexes. This was achieved by adding chromium to yeast cultures. The one main drawback, however, was that only about 20 to 40 percent of the added chromium was converted into the biologically active GTF structure.

It would take until the late 1980s and even into the early 1990s before chromium supplements became refined enough to affect insulin and fat levels. And much like the Beta and VHS wars of the early 1980s, or the more current DVD and Blu-Ray competition, two forms of chromium supplements were put head to head to battle for control of the market.

CHROMIUM PICOLINATE

Chromium picolinate is a form of chromium combined with picolinic acid, which is one of the metabolites (breakdown products) of the amino acid tryptophan. Structurally, it is very similar to the B-complex vitamin, niacin. Chromium picolinate received its biggest promotional boost from a study carried out by Dr. Gary Evans at Bemidji State University in Minnesota. From his research, Dr. Evans claimed that test subjects supplementing with chromium picolinate reduced bodyfat, increased muscle mass and decreased cholesterol levels. At face value such results seem promising. The problem, however, was that few other researchers could manage to replicate Dr. Evan's findings. Another troubling factor was that the test subjects in Dr. Evan's study were college football players who were not tested for anabolic steroids or other performance-enhancing drugs. Without confirming that these athletes weren't taking other substances, it's dif-

> "It would take until the late 1980s and even into the early 1990s before chromium supplements became refined enough to affect insulin and fat levels. And much like the Beta and VHS wars of the early 1980s, or the more current DVD and Blu-Ray competition, two forms of chromium supplements were put head to head to battle for control of the market."

LEFT: Certain research results on the effects of chromium picolinate may have been skewed by the sample group – college football players – guys who train hard and already eat large amounts of protein.

ficult to conclude if the results were from the chromium or another "supplement." Another consideration is the fact that college-aged football players generally don't make good test subjects for such research. Steroids or not, athletes in this age group are going to be in a naturally high anabolic state to begin with. They train hard, eat large amounts of high-protein foods and their bodies are probably in one of the biggest muscle-building stages of their lives.

Finally, Dr. Mertz, the father of chromium research, himself pointed out that chromium picolinate complexes are likely too tightly bound to be biologically active and capable of influencing the action of insulin. He conceded that chromium picolinate would probably be excreted almost as fast as it's absorbed.

CHROMIUM POLYNICOTINATE

Supplement manufacturers jumped on the knowledge that the biologically active form of chromium is a complex with niacin and designed a supplement with that exact molecular arrangement. Of course, just because a chromium supplement contains niacin doesn't necessarily mean it's bioactive. As molecular chemists are quick to point out, there are numerous ways that chromium can be bonded to niacin.

WHICH IS BEST?

The wide availability of two forms of chromium has left many consumers scratching their heads about which is the better product. From a marketing and popularity point of view, chromium picolinate seems to be winning the sales war. But science seems to indicate the opposite.

Photo by Irvin Gelb
Model Vander Van Assche

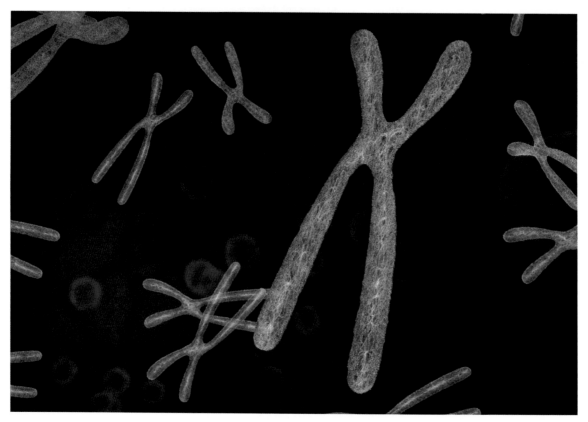

ABOVE: The side effects of chromium picolinate may be much more severe than polynicotinate. Animal studies have indicated that the picolinate form can damage chromosomes.

Chromium polynicotinate is the more bioavailable form of chromium. An animal research study conducted at the University of California found that chromium polynicotinate is absorbed and retained up to 311% more effectively than chromium picolinate (and 672% better than such salts as chromium chloride).

As we noted, chromium polynicotinate is created in complex with niacin, a B-vitamin, whereas chromium picolinate is compounded with picolinic acid. The long-term health effects of picolinic acid on the body remain largely unknown. While chromium picolinate does provide chromium to the body, little evidence supports this form as a naturally occurring substance or one that can influence glucose and cholesterol metabolism. It's even quite possible that long-term supplementation with high doses picolinate complexes may prove to be harmful. Biochemically, picolinic acid competes with niacin, leaches iron from cells and has been shown to alter glandular functioning in laboratory animals. We're fairly certain that none of these effects are what you're looking for in a nutritional supplement.

Chromium picolinate became popular as a result of smart marketing. Virtually all of the claims about the benefits of this supplement originated from the few studies carried out by the product's inventor (who as you might guess had a vested financial interest in the sale of the product). This conflict of interest has raised serious questions as to the validity of the research used to promote this form of chromium. The statement that chromium picolinate is "Patented by the U.S. Department of Agriculture" is also somewhat misleading. The USDA only received this patent because the inventor worked there at the time he developed the product. It's important to note that the USDA currently does not endorse chromium picolinate for use in human nutrition.

Conversely, the nutritional use of chromium polynicotinate is backed by numerous studies performed at independent universities and government labs. For example, research conducted at Auburn University has shown that chromium in polynicotinate form lowers cholesterol in humans by 14 percent. And tests at New Zealand's Massey University have demonstrated that this type is many times more potent than other forms of chromium.

SIDE EFFECTS

We touched on a few of the side effects earlier in this chapter, but a few additional points are necessary here. While polynicotinate supplements have never been linked to serious health issues, the same cannot be said for picolinate. Animal studies have revealed that picolinate supplements can cause chromosome damage. And while most of the studies involved dosages far beyond what humans would take, there is still cause for concern given the mega doses some bodybuilders ingest.

Finally, those with diabetes or insulin-related conditions need to consult their physicians before using any chromium-based supplement. While the effectiveness of such complexes may not be as powerful as the advertisers claim, you should nevertheless consider all your options before attempting to modify your insulin levels.

References

1) Kaats G.R., Blum K., Pullin D., *et al.* A randomized, double-masked, placebo-controlled study of the effects of chromium picolinate supplementation on body composition: a replication and extension of a previous study. *Current Therapeutic Research*. June 1998. 59:379–388.

2) Hoeger W.W.K., Harris C., Long E.M., *et al.* Four-week supplementation with a natural dietary compound produces favorable changes in body composition. *Adv Ther*. 1998. 15:305–314.

3) Grant K.E., Chandler R.M., Castle A.L., *et al.* Chromium and exercise training: effect on obese women. *Med Sci Sports Exerc*. 1997. 29:992–998.

4) *Journal of the American College of Nutrition*. Nov. 2000. 19:687.

5) *Whole Foods Magazine*, Jan. 2001. Newslinks, 22.

"Chromium polynicotinate is the more bioavailable form of chromium. An animal research study conducted at the University of California found that chromium polynicotinate is absorbed and retained up to 311% more effectively than chromium picolinate (and 672% better than such salts as chromium chloride)."

DIBENCOZIDE

Dibencozide is yet another substance that gained heavy promotion during the '80s as a natural alternative to anabolic steroids. Like arginine and Smilax, Dibencozide's effects were heavily exaggerated by supplement manufacturers. In fact, "exaggerated" is probably an understatement given the actual lack of scientific evidence showing any performance benefits in healthy individuals.

Like many unproven natural anabolic compounds, Dibencozide got its main boost from reports out of the Soviet Union and Bulgaria where weightlifters were using the supplement in their training. And because these athletes seemed to dominate the sport during the 1970s and 1980s, anything they took was assumed to be quite effective. The logic, however, isn't that simple. Further investigation into the "strategies" these athletes used revealed that they were ingesting many more "supplements" to gain a competitive edge.

WHAT IT IS

Dibencozide is the biologically active form of vitamin B-12, also known as coenzyme B-12. As many readers know, the B-complex vitamins, including B-12, are essential to the maintenance of proper health. The vitamins in this group can be found in both animal and plant sources (except B-12, which cannot be derived from plant foods), and once in the stomach are bonded to other factors to form a complex that is immune to further breakdown. Absorption only takes place at specialized receptor sites in the lower part of the small intestine, called the ileum. Once the ileum has been exposed to high concentrations of B-12, it blocks further absorption of the complex for four to five hours. During this time period the B-12 structure breaks down and the vitamin gets transported in the bloodstream by a specialized carrier called transcobalamin II. From here, B-12 is taken to the liver where it's then either stored or converted to coenzyme B-12, as the need arises. Coenzyme B-12 can then be released back into the bloodstream and absorbed by the body's various tissues.

MECHANISM OF ACTION

Describing the array of metabolic roles of B-12 could fill an entire book; our discussion will instead focus on the major functions of B-12 in the body.

> "The claim that Dibencozide won't be detected in a drug test is proof of just how far some supplement companies will go to sell a product. Of course this substance won't be detected in a drug test – remember, it's a vitamin. And for the most part, sports federations don't focus their efforts on looking for performance-enhancing vitamins."

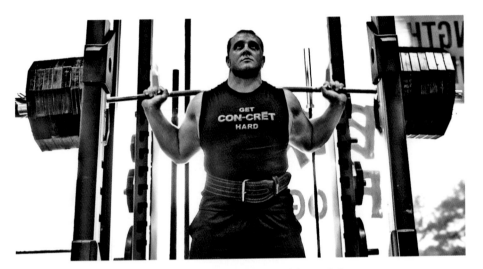

At the molecular level B-12 is involved in synthesis of the nucleic acids DNA and RNA, and protein. This vitamin's primary mechanism of action is to assist in methylation, which is the process of attaching methyl groups (CH_3) to protein and nucleic acids. Because of this important role, it should be easy to understand why a deficiency in B-12 could lead to impairments in protein synthesis, cell maintenance and ultimately overall body growth.

Another vital function of B-12 is to help with the oxidation of fats, which is carried out by processing fats with odd-numbered carbon chains. This allows the maximum amount of energy to be utilized from fat sources.

A final metabolic action of B-12 is to help regulate the nervous system. Of particular importance is the role it plays in maintaining the myelin sheath. The sheath acts like the plastic barrier to insulate the nerves from one another and from surrounding tissues, ensuring no loss of signal and therefore rapid nerve conduction. A deficiency in B-12 can disrupt this intricate process, resulting in poor muscular contraction and muscle weakness.

ABOVE: During the '70s and '80s many Soviet and Bulgarian weightlifters were using Dibencozide ... and winning. This helped the supplement catch on in North America.

EFFECTIVENESS DEBATE

There are conflicting opinions when it comes to the effectiveness of Dibencozide – the medical community holds one perspective while supplement manufacturers argue the opposite, and many users add a third opinion. As with most of the other "steroid replacers" that are on the market, Dibencozide has its merits, but some of its touted benefits may in fact be misleading. If coenzyme B-12 products generated the degree of strength and size gains that manufacturers claim, the supplement would need to be classified as a drug and be available by prescription only.

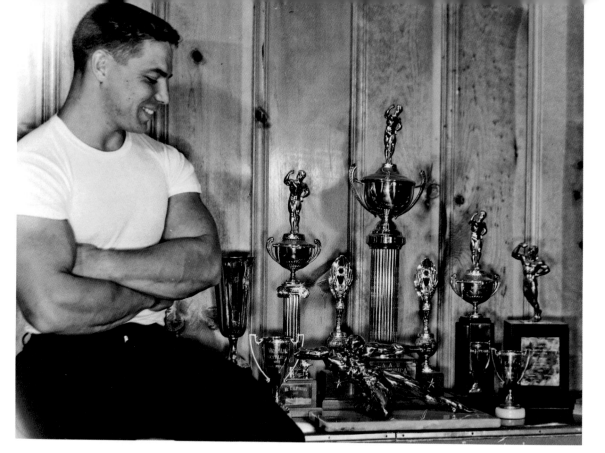

ABOVE: Bill Pearl (shown here) was a vegetarian – one group who may benefit nutritionally from Dibencozide because they can often lack B-12 from not eating enough animal products.

For those who have bought into assertions about Dibencozide, such as that it's "safer than steroids," or "more powerful than steroids," or "guaranteed to pass a drug test," it's necessary to take a closer look at such statements.

For starters, Dibencozide should be safer than steroids – after all, it's a vitamin and not a drug. And because it's a water-based vitamin, the occurrence of side effects is fairly limited. Second, the claims about this substance being "more powerful than steroids" came in large part from a few European studies in which researchers administered sick children and teenagers either Dibencozide or steroids. The Dibencozide group gained more muscular bodyweight, which at base level seems to be solid evidence for the supplement's growth-producing abilities. What the manufacturers failed to share is that the steroid dosage in the study was far less than what's generally used by athletes. In addition, sick children and teens who are put on healthy diets under the care of physicians almost always gain healthy bodyweight – it's called normal growth! Therefore, the Dibencozide more than likely had little to do with the results that were reported.

The claim that Dibencozide won't be detected in a drug test is proof of just how far some supplement companies will go to sell a product. Of course this substance won't be detected in a drug test – remember, it's a vitamin. And for the most part, sports federations don't focus their efforts on looking for performance-enhancing vitamins. Granted, the name itself may influence some less-informed individuals to assume that Dibencozide is a drug. But rest assured, you're not doing anything illegal or breaking any sporting rules by taking this supplement.

Model Bill Pearl

When you break it down, these claims are used by supplement manufacturers as a strategy to entice consumers to buy their products. And while aggressive marketing using legitimate medical studies is a perfectly acceptable business practice, exaggerating and misrepresenting studies solely for financial gain is not. While science will no doubt continue to provide bodybuilders with compounds that are anabolic in nature, the fact remains that no OTC supplement currently available comes close to duplicating the effects of steroids. Dibencozide may have its place in general nutrition – especially for vegetarians who may lack B-12 from not consuming animal sources of food – but don't be misled into thinking this coenzyme is some powerful anabolic agent.

DIBENCOZIDE SUPPLEMENTS

For those who decide to use Dibencozide, the first issue is choosing the right form. Most supplement manufacturers only sell straight B-12, which is a quality vitamin but not in the same category as its coenzyme B-12 derivative. You should only buy the bioactive form labeled as Dibencozide or coenzyme B-12. Also, capsule forms are recommended over the liquid versions, which tend to be less stable and deteriorate quickly.

While most biochemists suggest taking it about a half-hour before working out, most bodybuilding experts advise that best results are experienced when the capsules are consumed in the morning and evening. The average dosage is 5,000 to 10,000 micrograms per day. For those not familiar with micrograms, all you have to do is simply divide these numbers by 1,000 to get the measurement in grams (in this case 5 to 10 grams per day). The reason we've listed micrograms is because most supplement manufacturers market their Dibencozide products in these units (likely because 5,000 micrograms sounds much more impressive than 5 grams!).

SIDE EFFECTS

As a derivative of a water-based vitamin, side effects associated with taking Dibencozide are not very prevalent whatsoever. Some users may experience nausea or diarrhea, but supplementing with B-12 or B-12 derivatives for the most part is safe.

We must note, however, that some B-12 preparations become toxic when they are left for long periods of time or are exposed to light. This occurs because the element cobalt, which is part of the B-12 molecule, is highly toxic when it becomes split from other atoms. While being an extreme case, nevertheless, it's not a good practice to use old B-12 products or those that have been exposed to light.

> "While science will no doubt continue to provide bodybuilders with compounds that are anabolic in nature, the fact remains that no OTC supplement currently available comes close to duplicating the effects of steroids. Dibencozide may have its place in general nutrition, but don't be misled into thinking this coenzyme is some powerful anabolic agent."

393

VANADYL SULFATE, VANADATE

"In theory, any substance that mimics insulin should have anabolic properties. Insulin causes glucose and amino acids to be forced into muscle tissue at a faster rate and in larger quantities than would normally be absorbed."

In similar fashion to the promotion of chromium, vanadyl sulfate (VOSO4) got its first big break via diabetes research. And like chromium, there's limited science to back vanadyl sulfate, but many bodybuilders swear by it for performance enhancement.

Vanadyl sulfate and its cousin compound vanadate are derivatives of vanadium. A trace element, vanadium is used by the body for numerous metabolic actions including glucose and fat regulation. In its natural state vanadium is toxic, but when combined with other compounds such as sulfate, it becomes quite safe.

MECHANISM OF ACTION

Animal studies seem to indicate that vanadate functions very well to regulate glucose in animals with diabetes, obesity and insulin resistance. Researchers believe the compound has the ability to mimic insulin in both the liver and peripheral tissues. Other investigations have also demonstrated that vanadate stimulates lipogenesis in animals with reduced insulin levels.

One of the interesting outcomes from these studies was that vanadate simulated insulin's effects on glucose but didn't seem to have any of insulin's anabolic effects. In fact, test subjects often lost bodyweight (which could be explained by a decrease in appetite). This point has become significant in bodybuilding as many supplement manufacturers promote vanadate as an "anabolic" compound. Furthermore, there are bodybuilders who swear by the supplement's role in promoting muscular weight gain.

In theory, any substance that mimics insulin should have anabolic properties. Insulin causes glucose and amino acids to be forced into muscle tissue at a faster rate and in larger quantities than would normally be absorbed. Insulin also helps increase glycogen storage in muscles and improve protein synthesis. This not only causes the muscle to become rock hard and pumped, but it also creates the perfect anabolic environment in muscles that have just been exercised.

DOSAGE

Because this substance has a poor scientific pedigree, personal preference is an influential factor when determining the best dosage for vanadate. Most bodybuilders take 40 to 50 milligrams per day, but as you might expect, some individuals pump in 200-plus milligrams every day. If you do decide to mega dose – which is a practice we advise against – treat the supplement as a drug and cycle it, going four to six weeks on, and then two to four weeks off. Doing so will not only reduce your chances of developing side effects, but theoretically should also increase it's efficacy since there's less chance you'll build up a tolerance.

SIDE EFFECTS

The risk of developing side effects is low, but certain research indicates that high dosages of vanadyl sulfate may throw off liver enzymes. And because of the compound's impact on glucose levels, those with diabetes or diabetes-like conditions may want to avoid vanadate or any vanadyl-related substances.

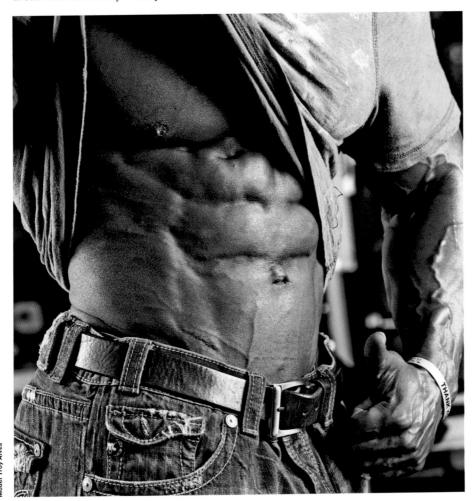

LEFT: Claims have been made that vanadate mimics insulin. Therefore, by boosting glycogen storage and protein synthesis, advertisers say vanadate supplements will cause muscles to become rock hard and pumped in an anabolic environment.

Photo by Ralph DeHaan
Model Troy Alves

ALPHA-LIPOIC ACID (ALA)

ALA is yet another supplement that owes its origins to diabetes research. Although the compound is largely touted for increasing muscle mass and boosting energy, the two areas where ALA seems to hold credible scientific results are as an antioxidant and a facilitator for glucose. It's the latter that has captured the attention of both diabetes researchers and supplement manufacturers. Numerous studies have shown promise in ALA's ability to reduce insulin resistance, which is common among individuals with Type-2 diabetes. While many individuals with this particular condition produce sufficient amounts of the hormone, their body's receptors have

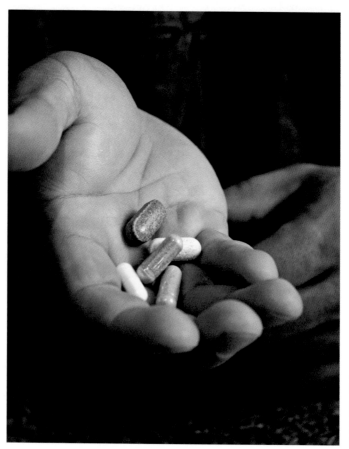

RIGHT: ALA has been widely researched as it relates to diabetes. But the supplement lacks study in healthy, non-diabetic individuals.

Photo by Michael Butler

trouble recognizing or bonding with the hormone. The end result is a decreased capability of glucose to be absorbed by cells.

The cells in the human body use glucose for numerous vital functions, including growth and repair as well as energy production. In situations when blood glucose levels are elevated (called hyperglycemia) the amount of oxidative stress on body cells becomes increased. This interaction between oxygen and bodily cells produces unstable molecules called free radicals. And free radicals cause damage to cell membranes, genes and proteins – a form of stress that has been linked to various diseases including certain forms of cancer. One class of free radicals, called reactive oxygen species (ROS), is especially destructive on the human system. Research has shown that a relationship exists between ROS and increased insulin resistance and beta-cell dysfunction. The second condition is significant since one group of beta cells located in the pancreas synthesizes and secretes insulin.

Studies have also demonstrated that ALA accelerates the removal of glucose from the bloodstream and decreases insulin resistance. This compound also reverses beta-cell dysfunction. Medical researchers use such findings to promote ALA as a non-drug form of diabetes therapy. And supplement manufacturers jump on this research to market ALA as a fat-loss supplement (by way of better glucose utilization) and a creatine absorption booster.

A point that needs to be stressed, however, is that the research concerning ALA supplementation in healthy individuals and non-diabetics is very limited. One study in particular involved subjects who consumed creatine, sucrose and ALA. The first group received 20 grams of creatine per day. The second group was given 20 grams of creatine and 100 grams of sucrose. The third group received 20 grams of creatine, 100 grams of sucrose and 1,000 milligrams of ALA. All participants were asked not to exercise for seven days and were given the same diet to follow. While all three groups had significant increases in total muscle creatine, it was the ALA group that showed the greatest measurable improvement.[1]

> "Although the compound is largely touted for increasing muscle mass and boosting energy, the two areas where ALA seems to hold credible scientific results are as an antioxidant and a facilitator for glucose. It's the latter that has captured the attention of both diabetes researchers and supplement manufacturers."

USE AND DOSAGES

So, should you use ALA supplements to increase your creatine absorption? When you consider the cost, relative safety and positive research (albeit limited), you have nothing to lose by trying alpha-lipoic acid. The recommended dosage is 600 to 1,000 milligrams combined with about 50 grams of carbs and 10 grams of creatine. You could even add 10 grams of glutamine to really jazz up your post-workout cocktail.

Reference
1) Evans J.L., *et al*, Oxidative stress and stress-signaling pathways: a unifying hypothesis of Type-2 diabetes. *Endocr Rev.* 23:599–622.

GLANDULARS

> "The theory behind the effectiveness is that whatever gland the supplement was derived from, the corresponding gland in your body would become stimulated. We need only look at historical records to see that such beliefs are not the invention of 20th-century supplement advertisers – the ancient Greeks believed that by slaying a mighty warrior and then eating his heart, those who consumed it would add that person's strength to their own. Philosophers of the time also maintained that eating the brains of dead colleagues would improve intelligence and create future geniuses."

Glandulars went through a phase of popularity back in the '70s and '80s but have since been replaced by more credible supplements. Nevertheless, these perceived natural hormones are still sold in health-food stores and some bodybuilders still waste their money on these ineffective products.

The name glandular refers to substances derived from the tissues or extracts of animal glands and organs. The theory behind the effectiveness is that whatever gland the supplement was derived from, the corresponding gland in your body would become stimulated. We need only look at historical records to see that such beliefs are not the invention of 20th-century supplement advertisers – the ancient Greeks believed that by slaying a mighty warrior and then eating his heart, those who consumed it would add that person's strength to their own. Philosophers of the time also maintained that eating the brains of dead colleagues would improve intelligence and create future geniuses. Even as recently as the last century, African tribesmen were known to eat the hearts of lions to improve their courage.

Once preparation techniques improved, supplement manufacturers expanded on these "traditional" notions and processed and bottled just about every gland or organ for human use. Some of the more popular choices are pituitary extracts to increase that gland's output of growth hormone; adrenal glandulars to stimulate the release of adrenalin, thus generating more workout energy; and, heart glandular supplements to increase blood flow. Even animal testes have been processed into supplemental form to boost testosterone and bedroom prowess! While all this may sound great in theory, there are a number of reasons that glandulars fall way short of the manufacturer's claims.

TOO GOOD TO BE TRUE

One of the biggest pieces of evidence for dismissing the efficacy of glandulars lies in the fact that they're perfectly legal. If these substances modified and influenced the body's endocrine system to the degree that manufacturers attest to, the FDA and other drug-regulatory agencies would more than likely classify the products as drugs requiring a prescription. Anything that can alter a person's endocrine system is a drug – the fact alone that glandular supplements are easily obtainable at health-food stores should cause you to stop and rethink the advertiser's promotional interests.

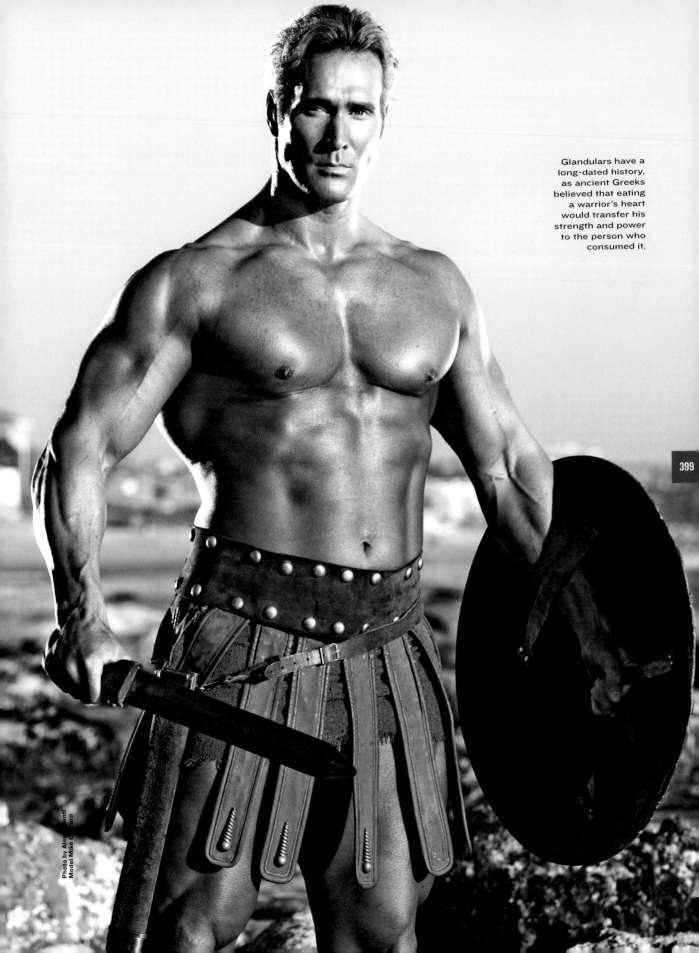

Glandulars have a long-dated history, as ancient Greeks believed that eating a warrior's heart would transfer his strength and power to the person who consumed it.

399

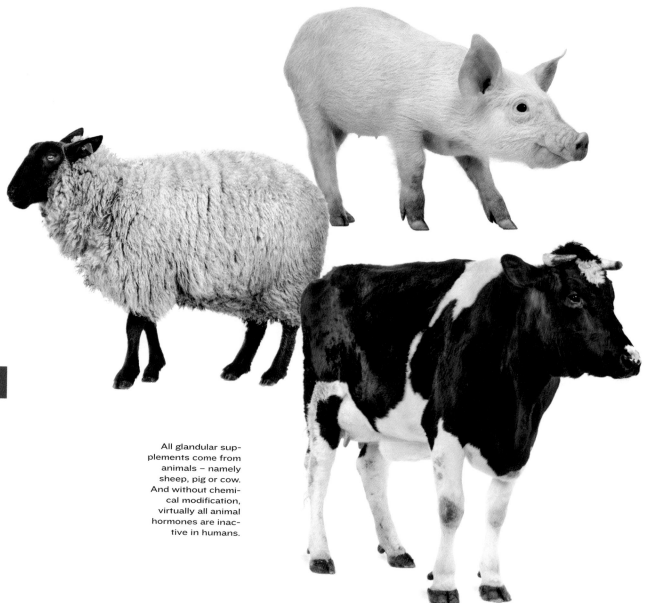

400

All glandular sup-
plements come from
animals – namely
sheep, pig or cow.
And without chemi-
cal modification,
virtually all animal
hormones are inac-
tive in humans.

A second factor that denounces glandulars as a viable supplement is their origins. All products of this type are made from the dried and ground-up remains of animal sources. For example, if you buy a pituitary glandular, odds are that it came from a sheep, pig or cow. Despite what manufacturers may assert, virtually all animal hormones without chemical alteration are inactive in humans. There are numerous reasons to account for this, one of which is the differing pH levels between animals and humans.

One of the simplest reasons to leave glandulars on the store shelf is the price. Such products are among the cheapest available, averaging $10 to $15 for a month's supply. But for every ounce of biologically active hormone that is produced in the lab, hundreds and in some cases thousands of pounds of animal glands and/or organs must be processed using techniques that require both time and money. This is one of the reasons prescription drugs are so expensive. Common sense should tell you that a product costing $10 per bottle of 100 didn't go through the complex and costly manufacturing procedures. If it did, such costs would be reflected in the price of the supplement.

A final point that raises the question as to the value of glandulars is their oral route of administration. While there is minimal evidence that injected gland tissue may actually make its way to the targeted glands, all glandular supplements are taken orally. As soon as these products enter your mouth, they begin to be digested, first by the salivary glands and then by the acids in your stomach. This is why oral anabolic steroids are chemically modified, to allow them to survive digestive processes (and hence why oral steroids are so much harsher on the liver than injectable drugs). So even if by some remote chance glandulars did contain some bioactive material, it would quickly get broken down into its protein, carbohydrate and other nutrient constituents via digestion.

ARE THERE ANY BENEFITS?

About the only positive statement we can make about glandulars is that they'll be recognized by the body as another source of protein, fat, vitamins and minerals, etc. And while animal organs qualify as a decent source of protein (albeit often with a high fat content), for the same amount of money you could buy 10 to 20 times as much whey protein. Our advice: use your money wisely.

ASSOCIATED RISKS

Though we've just discussed that glandulars are virtually useless because of their lack of activity in the body, taking them still involves a certain level of risk. The primary reason humans cook meat is to kill any pathogens. Eating raw meat puts individuals in danger of picking up a tapeworm or developing salmonella poisoning. Most glandular products are well processed (the intense heat acts as a sterilizing agent), but the same cannot be said of "basement-created" products. Just as there are bogus forms of steroids on the blackmarket, so too are there fake glandulars. Who knows what might be contained in pills or capsules produced by a non-reputable manufacturer? And if someone offers to inject you with animal hormone – don't even consider it. Animal hormone preparations contain some of the deadliest diseases known to man. As we noted earlier in the book, the AIDS virus is believed to have originated from rhesus monkeys. Do you really want to inject some mystery concoction into your quads that may kill you in six months?

> "One of the simplest reasons to leave glandulars on the store shelf is the price. Such products are among the cheapest available, averaging $10 to $15 for a month's supply. But for every ounce of biologically active hormone that is produced in the lab, hundreds and in some cases thousands of pounds of animal glands and/or organs must be processed using techniques that require both time and money. This is one of the reasons prescription drugs are so expensive. Common sense should tell you that a product costing $10 per bottle of 100 didn't go through the complex and costly manufacturing procedures."

401

HMB – BETA-HYDROXY BETA-METHYLBUTYRATE

HMB is a metabolite of the amino acid leucine. It received its biggest boost in the supplement industry from Bill Phillips back in the mid to late 1990s. HMB is a mixed bag when it comes to how the substance functions as a bodybuilding supplement. Many bodybuilders swear by its anti-catabolic effects while others find it worthless. Similarly, there are some quality scientific studies to back up the manufacturer's claims; most of these often-quoted studies that yielded positive results, however, have been funded by the very same supplement companies. Cash-strapped researchers will very quickly bias their results when millions of dollars of funding is on the line.

THE RESEARCH

While numerous findings have been published, the main study that laid the groundwork for HMB's promotion as a bodybuilding supplement was conducted at the University of Iowa in 1997. Two groups of untrained subjects were given a daily dose of either 3 grams or a placebo. The participants were put on a weight-training program for three weeks and then analyzed. It was discovered that the HMB group had increased their strength levels by 18 percent while the placebo group had improved their strength by 9 percent.

Another study performed in Queensland, Australia, in 2000 involved 22 experienced athletes. They were given 3 grams of HMB for a period of six weeks. Contrary to the findings from the University of Iowa, at the end of this study it was found that subjects had no significant increases in strength or muscle size.

Also of interest is that HMB has even been tested by NASA as a dietary approach for astronauts to prevent muscle wasting associated with the weightlessness of prolonged spaceflight. Daily supplementation with 1.5 to 3 grams of HMB, in combination with a weight-training program, for three weeks increased muscle mass and strength and decreased exercise-induced muscle damage.[1]

Back here on Earth, researchers in a separate study investigated the effects of HMB supplements on muscle breakdown, strength and

> "HMB has even been tested by NASA as a dietary approach for astronauts to prevent muscle wasting associated with the weightlessness of prolonged spaceflight. Daily supplementation with 1.5 to 3 grams of HMB, in combination with a weight-training program, for three weeks increased muscle mass and strength and decreased exercise-induced muscle damage."

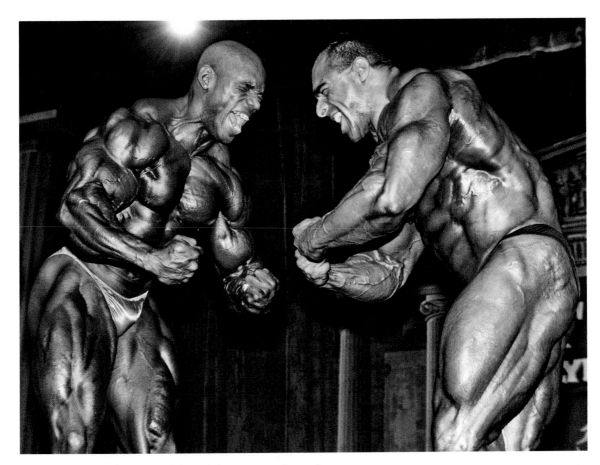

body composition during a weight-training program (seven hours per week for a time frame of four weeks). The study sample was 40 experienced weightlifters who received either 3 or 6 grams of calcium HMB or a placebo. Results showed that HMB supplementation resulted in a significant increase in blood levels of HMB but no marked difference in muscle anabolic/catabolic status, lean body or fat mass, or overall muscle strength.[2]

Further findings come from a study that looked at the impact of HMB supplements in 39 men and 36 women (aged 20 to 40 years of age). Subjects received 3 grams of HMB per day while training three times per week for four weeks. Among the HMB group, blood levels of creatine phosphokinase (an indicator of muscle damage) were reduced compared to the placebo group, and both upper-body strength and fat-free mass were increased. Overall, the study showed that a short-term period of HMB supplementation can increase upper-body strength and minimize muscle damage when combined with an exercise program in both men and women.[3]

ABOVE: Just as bodybuilders face off head-to-head in posedowns onstage, they also have conflicting opinions on HMB – some swear by it; others consider it useless.

Models Flex Wheeler and Nassar El Sonbaty

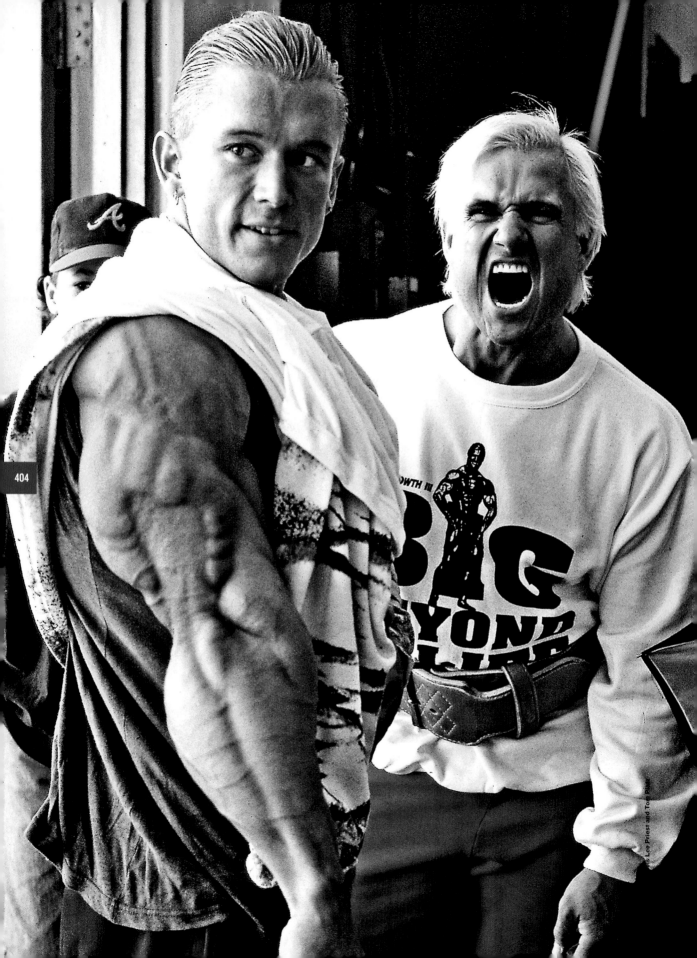

MECHANISM OF ACTION

Both the researchers and manufacturers of HMB are the first to admit that the exact system of action for HMB, as it applies to increasing muscle size and strength, is unknown. One theory is that HMB is a powerful anti-catabolic compound that prevents the normal muscle breakdown brought on by intense weight training. Another theory suggests that it can modify the signals between hormones and target cells. Finally, as a metabolite of leucine, HMB may play a role in increasing muscle-protein turnover.

DOSAGE

Both the scientific and anecdotal reports seem to suggest that 3 to 5 grams per day is the optimum dosage for HMB. The late Dan Duchaine suggested that given its short half-life (a couple of hours), the efficacy might improve if individuals took six smaller dosages of 500 milligrams spread over the day, rather than one or two large amounts. For those who think it might be cheaper to take more leucine and let the body convert it into HMB, only about five percent of leucine actually becomes HMB. You'd need to ingest 60 grams of the amino acid to obtain the 3 grams of HMB – an approach that would be very expensive and more important – downright dangerous.

References

1) Kreider R.B. Dietary supplements and the promotion of muscle growth with resistance exercise. *Sports Med.* 1999 Feb;27(2):97–110.
2) Mero A. Leucine supplementation and intensive training. *Sports Med.* 1999 Jun;27(6):347–58.
3) Clarkson P.M, Rawson, E.S. Nutritional supplements to increase muscle mass. *Crit Rev Food Sci Nutr.* 1999 Jul;39(4):317–28.

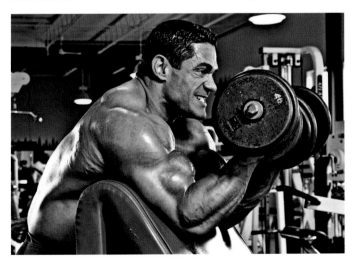

Photo by Jason Breeze
Model Gustavo Badell

LEFT: Regular intense weight workouts cause muscle breakdown – HMB is thought to prevent this from occuring as an anti-catabolic substance.

405

GLUCOSAMINE

Glucosamine is another product kidnapped by the bodybuilding industry from another area of legitimate medical research – in this case, arthritis. Glucosamine functions as a natural building block of bone cartilage, formed by the combination of glucose and an amino acid. This amino sugar is part of a larger molecule known as glycoprotein, which is a structural component for the building and repairing of cartilage.

Glucosamine helps to lubricate the joints by stimulating the production of the synovial fluid that acts as a cushion. In addition, glucosamine contains numerous anti-inflammatory properties that make it very useful for treating osteoarthritis, a condition that occurs when the cartilage between the joints wears away. Glucosamine also helps prevent further deterioration of the cartilage around the joints.

Though our bodies produce glucosamine naturally, the ability to produce sufficient quantities is decreased with age. Adequate levels of this amino sugar are essential for producing the nutrients needed to create synovial fluid and for repairing the associated joint structures.

When you have a glucosamine deficiency, the cartilage hardens and bone spurs may develop, which over time could lead to deformities in the joints. This in turn reduces your mobility and could eventually lead to osteoarthritis. It's for this reason that glucosamine supplements are extremely popular among athletes and bodybuilders – they use it to ease pain and repair damage to cartilage around overused and injured joints.

As soon as the scientific relationship between glucosamine and joint health was established, the major supplement companies began marketing the substance as an athletic product. These days, virtually all of the large manufacturers market a version of glucosamine.

SUPPLEMENTAL FORMS

Glucosamine is available in several forms, the most popular of which are glucosamine sulfate and glucosamine hydrochloride. Most studies are conducted using the sulfate type, since it appears to be the version that is most easily absorbed. Molecules of glucosamine sulfate are relatively small, so they can actually penetrate cartilage tissue and then act as building blocks that may repair and/or prevent damage. There are other less expensive forms of glucosamine on the market, but the alternatives are not considered nearly as effective.

> "As soon as the scientific relationship between glucosamine and joint health was established, the major supplement companies began marketing the substance as an athletic product. These days, virtually all of the large manufacturers market a version of glucosamine."

Most glucosamine sulfate supplements are usually derived from the cartilage of shellfish. And many of these products are often found in combination form with chondroitin (another building block of glycoprotein), because when used together glucosamine and chondroitin appear to produce a synergistic effect.

DOSAGES

In most studies, the dosage of glucosamine sulfate found useful for treating mild to moderate osteoarthritis is 1,500 milligrams per day. This supplement should be taken for 10 to 12 weeks to determine its efficacy for alleviating joint pain or preventing further damage.

SIDE EFFECTS

Glucosamine is one of the safest supplemental products available. It has been extensively studied since the early '80s, meaning that people have been taking it with certainty for over 25 years. Still there are a few concerns you need to be aware of when taking glucosamine.

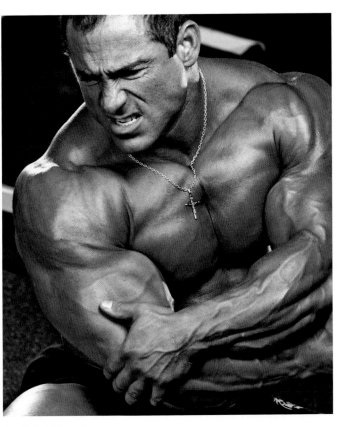

407

ABOVE: For hard trainers, joint pain is an all-too-common complaint. Glucosamine helps to lubricate the joints and also offers anti-inflammatory benefits with long-term use.

Most glucosamine products are derived from shellfish (although a few manufacturers produce it from corn), so you should consult your doctor prior to using glucosamine if you have specific allergies. Odds are that you'll be fine even if you are allergic to shellfish because generally, the allergic reaction occurs from the proteins and not the chitin (the carbohydrate glucosamine is derived from). As a precautionary measure though, you'll still want to consult your physician.

Those with diabetes or diabetic-like health issues may also want to check with a medical professional before using this supplement. Glucosamine is technically a carbohydrate (a sugar), though the body is not able to convert it into pure glucose. Hence, glucosamine should not affect your blood sugar levels, but we suggest talking to your doctor first.

The most common side effects reported from glucosamine use are those related to mega-dosing. Taking more than the recommended dosage can cause gastric upset such as cramps, diarrhea or nausea. Some people may even be prone to these effects from consuming small dosages. If that's the case, ingesting the glucosamine with meals should alleviate such problems.

Photo by Alex Ardenti
Model Mike Ergas

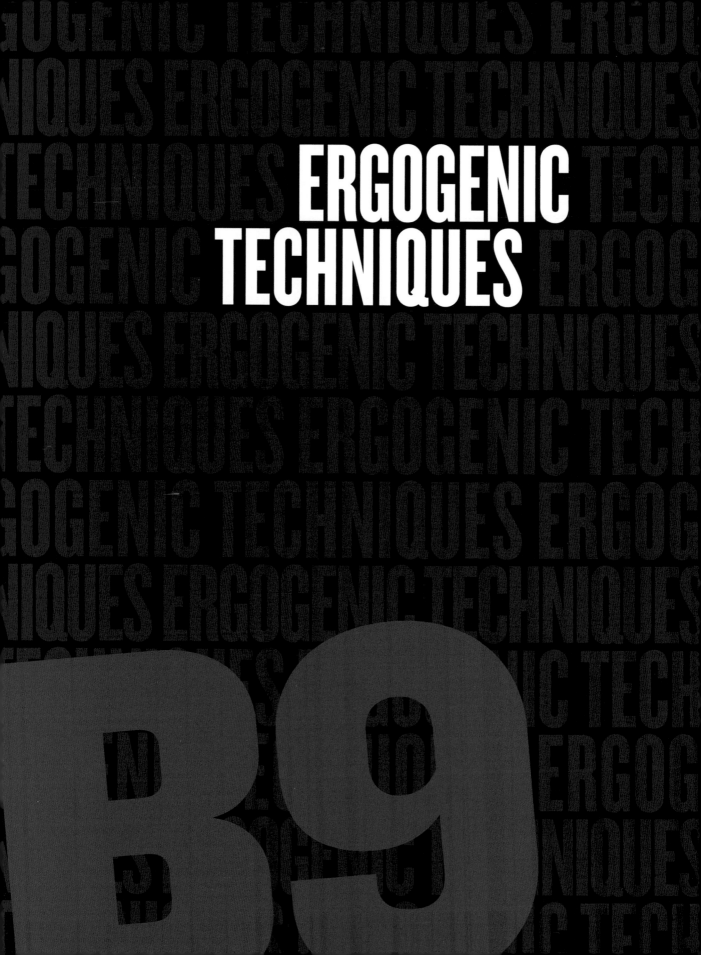

ERGOGENIC TECHNIQUES

B9

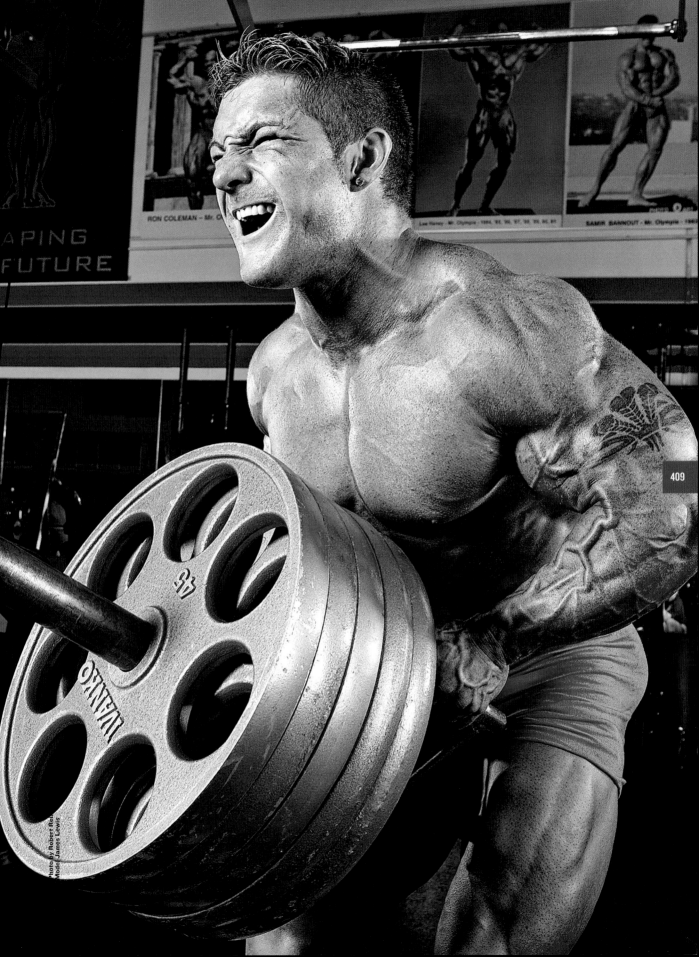

RON COLEMAN – Mr. O

Lee Haney – Mr. Olympia – 1984, '85, '86, '87, '88, '89, '90, '91

SAMIR BANNOUT – Mr. Olympia – 198

409

APING

FUTURE

45

IVANKO

Photo by Robert Reiff
Model James Lewis

INTRODUCTION

When the original *Anabolic Primer* was released, many readers wrote in suggesting that if we ever did a follow-up book, we should include chapters on the numerous techniques athletes use to boost performance, or in the case of body-building, to improve a physique's appearance. A lot has been learned over the past 10 years about employing exercise as a means to naturally boost hormone levels. Likewise, the emergence of Synthol has left many bodybuilders looking for answers. The following chapters attempt to address some of these concerns.

BELOW: In front of the scrupulous eyes of the judges, every competitor wants to display the best-looking physique from all angles.

410

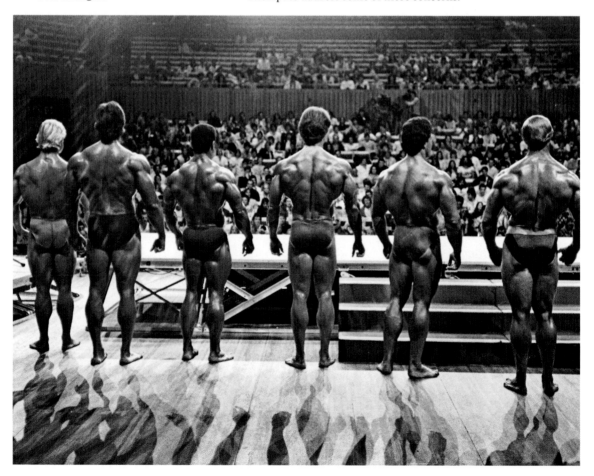

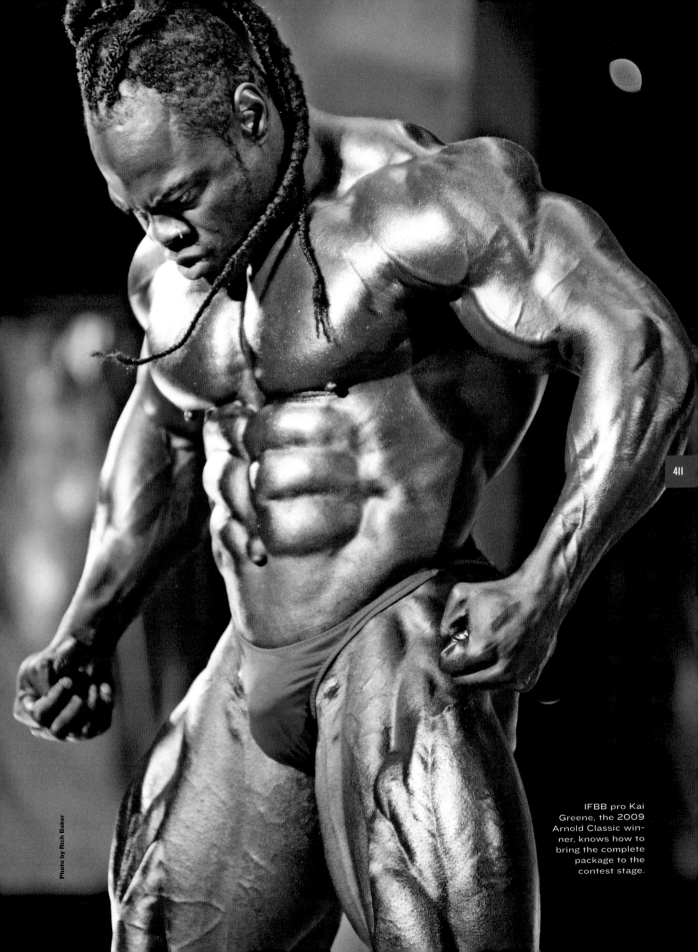

411

IFBB pro Kai Greene, the 2009 Arnold Classic winner, knows how to bring the complete package to the contest stage.

SYNTHOL

412

> "The effect is quite obvious as the Synthol-enhanced muscles take on shapes never found on any natural human being. You can go to any contest or large fitness expo and see several men who have injected enough oil into their bi's and tri's to satisfy their most extreme desires. Gains of two inches or more in the arms alone are quite commonplace."
>
> – Ron Harris, *MuscleMag International* contributor

> "All it takes is one little glob of this crap to plug one of your ventricles or the blood supply to your brain and that's it – you're dead."
>
> – Ron Harris, *MuscleMag International* contributor

The genesis of Synthol was an Italian steroid called Esiclene that was quite popular in the 1980s. For those unfamiliar with the drug, Esiclene was used immediately before a contest as a quick-fix for visually weak bodyparts.

Acting primarily as a muscle inflammatory agent, competitors injected it directly into their calves, arms or shoulders for a bit of extra size and fullness in lagging muscles. The effect was fleeting, but the drug served its short-term purpose. In the early '90s, a German man named Chris Clark began to toy with the idea of an injectable substance that would yield more permanent gains in size. He came up with a formulation initially named Synthol but soon learned that was already a registered and trademarked pharmaceutical name. So Clark renamed his product Pump 'N Pose, though the original name stuck. Now the word Synthol is as much a part of hardcore bodybuilding vocabulary as Dianabol or Deca. Clark hit upon a gold mine, as there were thousands of steroid-using bodybuilders who were dissatisfied with the size of their arms, delts and calves. Let's face it – few have the genetics to build an upper arm of 20-plus inches in lean condition, even with a boatload of anabolics and the most brutal training regimens imaginable. In fact, one of the drug's first users was a German strongman who billed himself as having "the world's largest arms" at 27 inches.

The downside to Synthol is that the effect is quite obvious – the enhanced muscles take on shapes never seen on any natural human being. You can go to any contest or large fitness expo and see several men who have injected enough oil into their bi's and tri's to satisfy their most extreme desires. Gains such as two inches or more in the arms are quite commonplace. Synthol is also often injected into the side delts and calves, as was Esiclene. Ironically, this liquid substance is available legally, since the $400-bottles are strategically labeled as posing oil. Despite the high price tag, however, makers still find it difficult to keep up with the worldwide demand from bodybuilders.

WHAT IS SYNTHOL?

Synthol is composed of 85 percent medium-chain triglycerides (a fatty acid), 7.5 percent Lidocaine (painkiller) and 7.5 percent Benzyl alcohol. The preparation is directly injected deep into the muscle where it becomes encapsulated between the fascicles (bundles of muscle fibers). With repeated injections, a larger volume of oil builds up inside the muscle, expanding its size much like a balloon is filled with air. About 30 percent of the injected substance gets metabolized by the body. The other 70 percent remains lodged in the muscle, where it breaks down very slowly over the course of three to five years. There seems to be some debate among bodybuilders as to whether or not Synthol actually lasts in their systems this long, though some believe the time frame is even longer. Inventor Chris Clark is convinced that the oil somehow leads to permanent muscle growth in the effected areas, though his claim is not supported by data on the specific mechanisms that would make this possible. Synthol users report amazing pumps while training, but this could simply be a result of the extra pressure from the accumulated oil.

RISKS OF SYNTHOL USE

Although Mr. Clark has claimed Synthol is completely safe, he's also made sure to reinforce that he is not legally responsible for bodybuilders who use the injection for anything other than what it's sold as, a posing oil. Of course, injecting any amount of fatty-acid material intramuscularly can be perilous, which is only complicated by the fact that few bodybuilders have any medical training when it comes to needles. Without knowing the exact location of major nerves, it's easy to hit one by accident and cause permanent paralysis of muscle fibers in that area. Another possible complication of injections of any type is abscess infections at the injection site; these buildups of infected tissue are often extremely painful and can sometimes even require surgery to remove, not unlike a tumor. You haven't heard the worst yet. Even more serious risks are involved should you inject into a vein or artery by mistake (generally avoided by drawing back on the syringe to make sure there is no blood, a simple precaution many individuals are too squeamish to utilize). If this happens, the fatty acids could be transported to your lungs, causing a pulmonary embolism; to your heart, causing a heart attack; or, perhaps even into your brain, leading to a cardioembolic stroke. These cases are all potentially fatal. It's been alleged that IFBB pro Milos Sarcev had a close call when, supposedly, some of the Synthol in his arms traveled to his heart. Sounds like an enormous amount of risk simply for the benefit of inflated arms and calves, doesn't it? Stereotype or not though, some bodybuilders have been known to try just about any substance or method in their quest for an extra inch or two on a lagging bodypart. To some, the risk of death is outweighed by the prospect of finally achieving 21-inch arms just like the big genetic freaks they idolize. While there aren't currently any known deaths related to Synthol or any of the several knock-offs, this is a fairly new product and use has skyrocketed over the past five to 10 years. Ultimately, Synthol users are adults responsible for their own health and safety and are free to make their own choices.

Model Greg Valentino

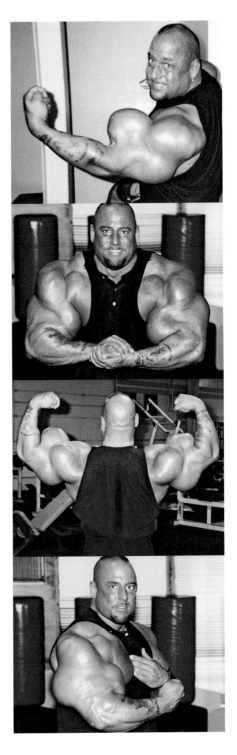

BLOOD MODIFICATION

Many substances and compounds discussed in this book have some impact on the blood. The bloodstream after all is the body's primary transport route and is vital for carrying the various nutrients, supplements and drugs to the tissues. While numerous substances affect the blood secondarily, certain drugs and techniques are used by bodybuilders and other athletes to directly modify their circulatory systems. Some of these forms are perfectly legal, while others have been banned.

BLOOD DOPING

Because the body's transport medium is blood, some athletes have sought ways to improve their performance abilities by improving circulatory function or "boosting their blood." Numerous techniques exist, all of which fall under the umbrella phrase blood doping when used by athletes to gain a competitive edge.

The simplest method to increase the oxygen-carrying capacity of the blood is to inject more of it. While some athletes roll the dice by using another person's blood, the safest method is to recycle their own. In preparation for an upcoming competition, some athletes will draw out a liter or so of their own blood and freeze it for a couple of weeks. Then, a few days before the given event they'll re-inject it. The

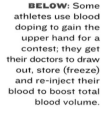
BELOW: Some athletes use blood doping to gain the upper hand for a contest; they get their doctors to draw out, store (freeze) and re-inject their blood to boost total blood volume.

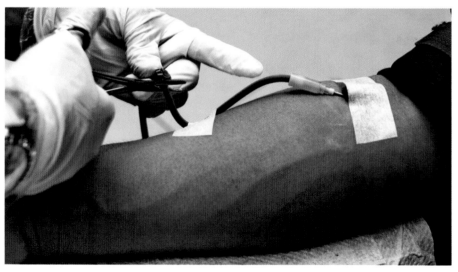

414

theory behind such an approach is that the body will replenish the lost blood over the course of those weeks, thus making the athlete a "liter ahead" when the drawn blood is injected back in. The boost in volume means more oxygen-carrying red blood cells (RBCs) are present and the speed at which waste products are cleared from the muscles is faster. Now, while this may sound fairly straightforward, there are risks involved. For starters, you can't simply take a liter of blood and store it in your freezer – proper safeguards must be in place. Without using the correct storage procedures, you run the risk of infusing pathogen-laden blood into your body. You also need to be aware that once your body replaces the initial blood withdrawn, the re-injection of that liter will greatly increase your blood pressure. This brings with it the possibility of heart attack and stroke. It's for these reasons that most top athletes in the world who use this technique have physicians to handle the drawing, storing and re-injecting processes.

The second popular method of blood doping involves using EPO (erythropoietin), which is the primary hormone responsible for increasing the rate at which RBCs are manufactured. When the body detects low RBC levels, EPO amounts go up and stimulate the RBC generating centers (i.e., the spleen) to increase production of RBCs.

While this hormone is not overly popular among bodybuilders, it is probably the drug of choice for marathon runners, distance nordic skiers and cyclists. Few Tour de France races get from start to finish without one or more athletes being caught with high levels of EPO in their bodies.

Much like growth hormone, there are now genetically-engineered versions of EPO available. The most popular is called Epoetin and while it is used medically to treat such diseases as anemia, AIDS and cancer, this form has also become popular among athletes.

FAMILIAR SOURCES

Athletes who want to get their hands on EPO or Epoetin for the most part have no trouble obtaining it. Many simply approach team doctors who can legally prescribe the drugs. If that avenue falls through, some individuals opt for the black market. High-performance athletes prefer the former, however, as they get medical supervision. This monitoring is not just for safety reasons, but more so because most sports organizations have legal limits for RBC levels on the event or race day. For example, the Tour de France officials allow a 50-percent level; any higher than that amount is considered a failed drug test – whether blood boosters are found or not. With that in mind, athletes rely on the doctors for appropriate dosages and timing. Obtaining the substances on the black market, however, means self-injections, potential medical problems and the chance of buying fake or even contaminated drugs.

"While this hormone is not overly popular among bodybuilders, it is probably the drug of choice for marathon runners, distance nordic skiers and cyclists. Few Tour de France races get from start to finish without one or more athletes being caught with high levels of EPO in their bodies."

415

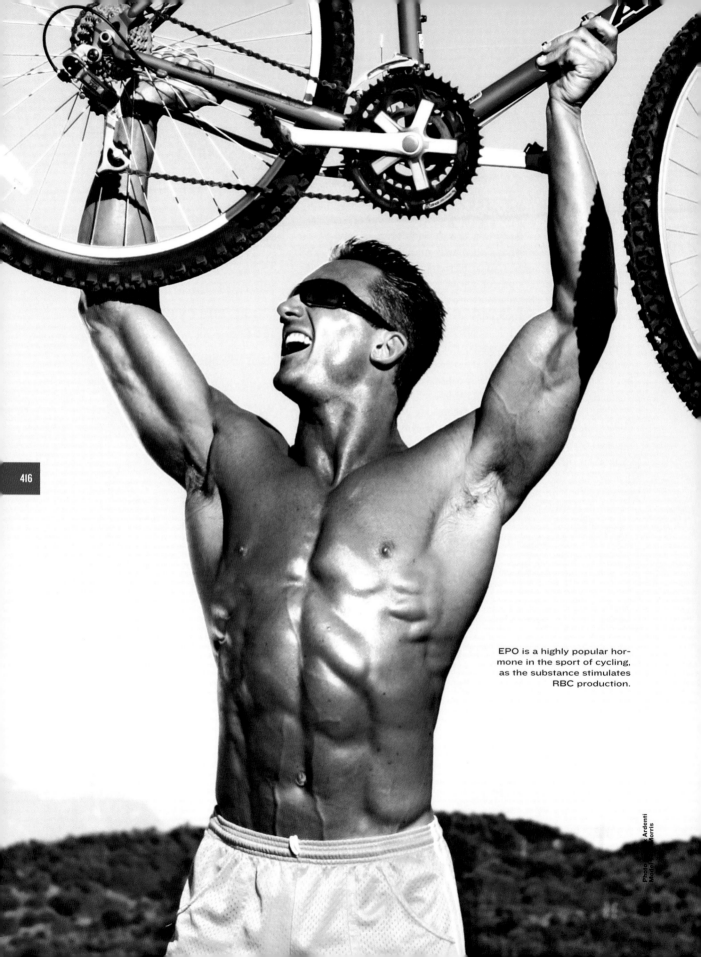

416

EPO is a highly popular hormone in the sport of cycling, as the substance stimulates RBC production.

SIDE EFFECTS

Despite the perceived safety of having medical supervision, there still aren't any guarantees when using blood boosters. The most serious complication has to do with dehydration. When athletes increase their RBC counts without maintaining proper hydration, they put themselves at increased risk for heart attacks, strokes and clotting. This is because all of the extra RBCs require additional fluids to be transported. When fluid levels drop, the blood becomes thick and syrupy. This bodily state puts more stress on the heart and ultimately increases blood pressure.

Of course athletes tend to turn a blind eye to this potential side effect, instead focusing on the literature showing that EPO conveys a five- to 15-percent performance advantage. Translated into minutes, a five-percent boost would have meant the difference between first and 140th in a number of cycling tour events. And while studies about the permanent health effects from EPO use are inconclusive, it's been shown that the sludge-like blood can linger in your system for up to 120 days. Since the 1980s, there have been dozens of deaths among competitive cyclists attributed to EPO usage. In most European countries the deaths were documented as heart attacks because no autopsies were conducted. North American heart specialists argue, however, that such a high number of deaths in young, perfectly healthy athletes is abnormal, statistically speaking.

417

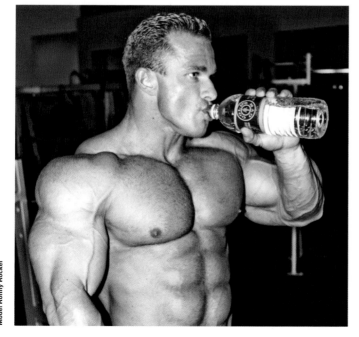

LEFT: Blood-boosting products are known to cause dehydration because the extra RBCs need additional fluid for transport.

Photo by Raymond Cassar
Model Ronny Rockel

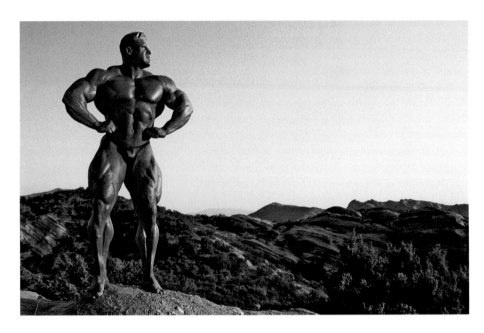

RIGHT: Athletes who live at higher land elevations gain training and competitive advantages because their oxygen-carrying capacity is boosted.

THE NATURAL ROUTE

Just as it's possible to increase testosterone and growth hormone by natural means, so too can athletes take advantage of Mother Nature to boost their RBC counts. It's well-studied and documented that individuals who live in high-altitude locations have proportionally higher RBC levels in their blood. This is nature's way of compensating for the lower oxygen content at high elevations. From an athlete's perspective, the added bonus is that the modification doesn't take years. Within a few days, the body acclimatizes and begins increasing RBC levels; after a few months, visitors to these regions have RBC counts nearly as high as local inhabitants.

The U.S. Olympic team has been using this phenomenon to their advantage for decades. Prior to the Games, many athletes take up residence in places farther above sea level for a couple of months. They still train at lower elevations but live in higher areas to adapt to the decreased oxygen content. By doing so, their oxygen-carrying capacity improves thus giving them a training advantage, allowing for longer, more intense workouts. It also facilitates a competitive advantage – their raised RBC levels will stay elevated for a few weeks after returning to lower elevations.

BLOOD BUFFERING

As most readers are aware, muscular strength and endurance decline with time. Depending on the exercise involved, the downturn can occur within seconds or may take a few hours. Although decreases in

Photo by David Paul
Model Jay Cutler

energy account for some of the performance drops, the most prevalent theory for muscle weakening is changes in the blood's pH from basic to acidic. This in turn interferes with the muscle's contractive abilities. Before going any further with the discussion, however, we need to take a brief look at acid-base chemistry.

BIOCHEMISTRY 101

Although the terms can mean many different things in normal day-to-day vernacular, in chemistry, acids and bases have precise definitions. Within most solutions there exists negatively charged hydroxide ions (OH-) and positively charged hydrogen ions (H+). To compare the ratios of both in solutions, chemists came up with a rating system called the pH scale. The scale ranges from one to 14, and seven represents neutral. Solutions with more H+ ions are placed below seven and are called acids. Those with more OH- ions are ranked above seven and are called basic solutions. The most potent acids score close to one and the strongest bases are at the opposite end of the spectrum, ranking close to 14.

HUMAN APPLICATIONS

Over the years of human evolution, the body's systems have adapted to work most efficiently at the slightly basic level between 7.4 and 7.7 on the pH scale. And though it may not sound like much, a change of even one small percentage point can have major effects on human biochemistry. During exercise, lactic acid buildup from fatiguing muscles can tip the body's pH from basic toward acidic. This biochemical change is believed to increase muscular fatigue.

BUFFERS

One of the ways chemists keep solutions fairly stable is by using buffers, which are substances that soak up and neutralize excess ions to help keep the pH constant. One of the ongoing areas of athletic research is the investigation for compounds that will combat the negative effects of lactic acid. The most popular substance at the moment is sodium bicarbonate (baking soda). Classified as a base, it works by neutralizing excess H+ ions right as they get produced during muscular contractions. Although little research has been conducted in which the participants were bodybuilders, numerous studies involving runners and cyclists suggest that ingesting 0.3 to 0.5 grams of sodium bicarbonate per kilogram of bodyweight before exercise may be beneficial. Now, before some readers decide to mega-dose on baking soda, be aware that certain adverse reactions are quite common. Many users experience nausea, vomiting and diarrhea when they ingest amounts above 0.5 grams per kilogram of bodyweight.

"Over the years of human evolution, the body's systems have adapted to work most efficiently at the slightly basic level between 7.4 and 7.7 on the pH scale. And though it may not sound like much, a change of even one small percentage point can have major effects on human biochemistry."

419

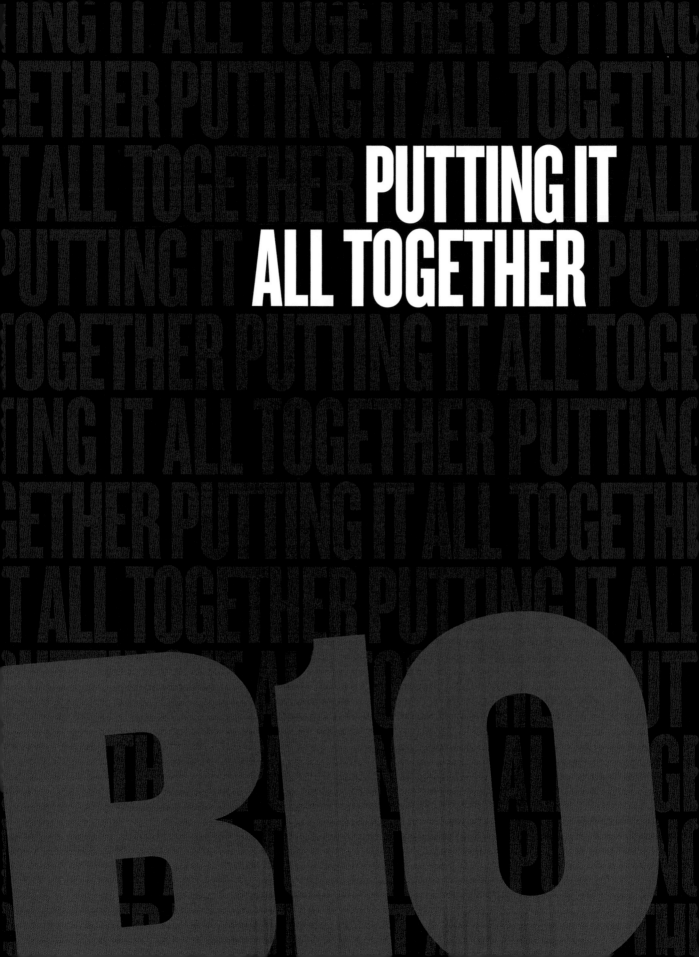

PUTTING IT ALL TOGETHER

BIO

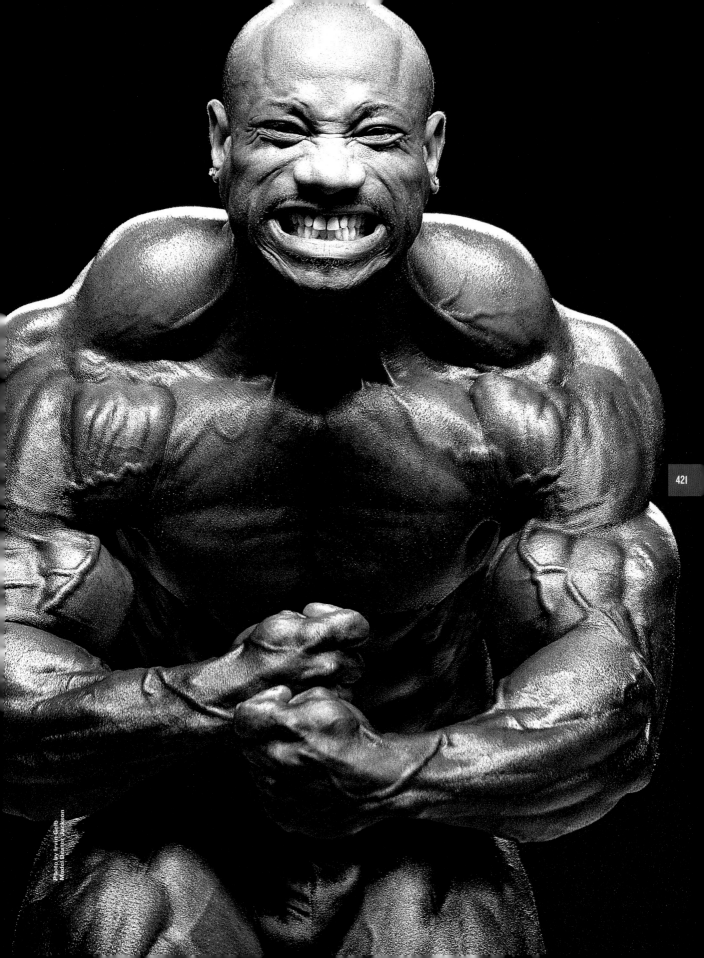

421

ACNE

Although we could have easily included this topic in the earlier chapter on physiological side effects of steroids, the widespread scope of acne is large enough that it warrants a separate chapter. We also took into account that acne can be caused by more than just steroids. Almost every drug that changes your hormonal systems or increases the activity of the skin's sebaceous glands can lead to the condition. And the act of exercising is itself known to promote the development of acne in some individuals.

Acne, however, is probably one of the few side effects that virtually all steroid users will experience. The degree of the skin problems can range from a few facial abrasions (commonly called whiteheads) to widespread blood-filled cysts spanning the entire body, particularly the back. Whiteheads are fairly uncomplicated and usually disappear after steroid use is stopped, but the cystic forms are more serious and often leave scarring since they penetrate into deeper skin layers. While the process is not fully understood, it is believed that steroids and testosterone increase activity in the skin's oil-producing sebaceous glands. The extra oil then traps dirt and other toxins – a perfect breeding ground for acne-causing bacteria.

Studies have shown that there seems to be a relationship between the degree of acne experienced during a steroid cycle and prior acne development. Those who had mild to severe acne in their teens and early 20s tend to develop the worst forms of acne while on a steroid cycle.

Another common cause of acne is the heavy use of cosmetics – which is typically seen in girls during their late teens and early 20s. The condition is not caused by a lack of cleanliness but rather a blockage of the pores from various oils in the cosmetics.

Contrary to popular belief, there is limited evidence of any connection between diet and acne. Chocolate and soda pop do not increase an individual's risk of developing acne. The reason these food (and drink) culprits tend to get tarnished is that some of the biggest consumers of chocolate and soft drinks are teens – and teens just so happen to develop the most severe acne because of their active hor-

"Acne, however, is probably one of the few side effects that virtually all steroid users will experience. The degree of the skin problems can range from a few facial abrasions (commonly called whiteheads) to widespread blood-filled cysts spanning the entire body, particularly the back."

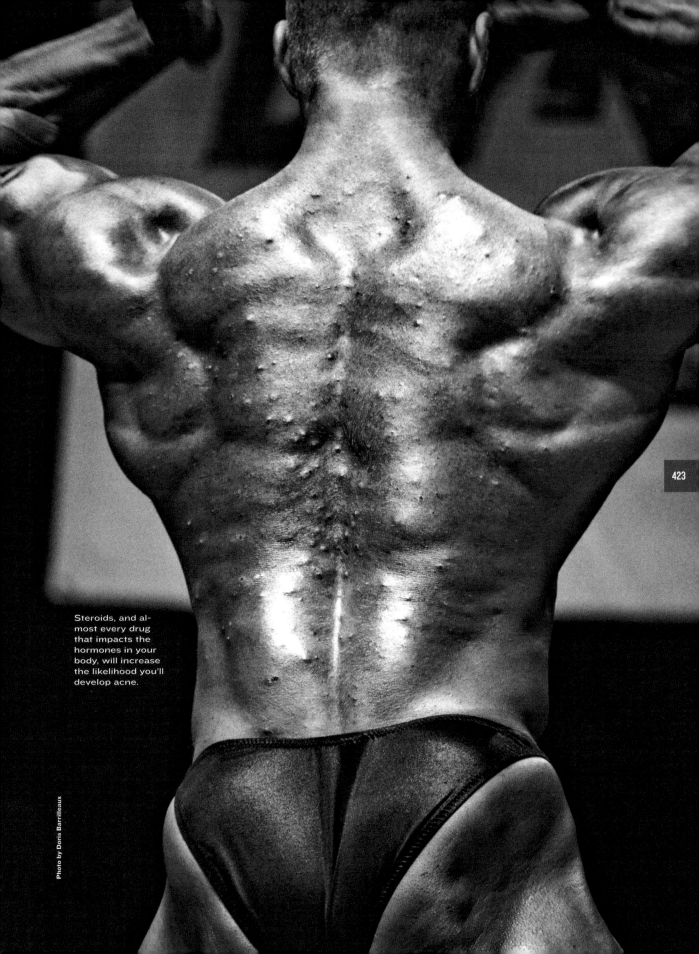

Steroids, and almost every drug that impacts the hormones in your body, will increase the likelihood you'll develop acne.

423

monal systems. This so-called relationship, as research has demonstrated, is nothing more than a coincidence.

While the unpleasant cosmetic effects of acne are not life threatening, individuals with low self-esteem – especially teenagers – often have difficulty coping with the condition. But for those who choose to take steroids, knowing all the risks involved, it all comes down to priorities. Most bodybuilders will gladly trade unsightly skin for an extra 20 or 30 pounds of muscle. A track star trying to shave a half-second off his 100-meter sprint likely couldn't care less about his skin's appearance. For those who take pride in healthy-looking skin, however, or bodybuilders who intend to compete, a severe case of acne will need to be treated.

TREATMENT OPTIONS

Numerous treatment options are available for acne sufferers. One of the most common, however, could also be one of the most dangerous. Because of the link between acne and oily skin, many individuals take the "dry-out" route and try tanning. Exposure to sun or artificial light may indeed yield decent results, but people who do this have essentially fixed one problem at the expense of another – the UV rays from tanning make you more prone to developing skin cancer, which can potentially become deadly.

A safer option is to experiment with some of the OTC anti-acne products. We say "experiment" because there are so many creams and gels out there, some of which yield little or no results. Most contain alcohol or peroxide solutions and while moderately effective for facial pimples, these products probably won't have any remedying effect on severe cystic acne. For cases of complicated acne, you'll likely need to look into using certain drugs.

The first step in addressing severe cystic acne (aside from coming off the juice, which is probably what caused the problem in the first place) is to go see your physician. Most types of acne are caused by bacteria, so your doctor can prescribe an appropriate antibiotic. These medications are very effective at treating cystic acne and clear up the condition in the vast majority of patients. If you're one of the few who doesn't respond to antibiotics, the next step might be Accutane. Be aware, however, that while probably the most effective anti-acne drug, Accutane also has numerous side effects. Many users report experiencing dry skin, itching, muscle soreness, joint pain, headaches, fatigue and nausea. In some cases, users may even develop bone spurs. Pregnant women are advised not to use Accutane because of the risk of birth defects associated with the drug.

For cases of extreme acne, a doctor may recommend cryotherapy, which is a method that involves using liquid nitrogen to freeze the cyst. Once this has been done, the cyst will then either fall off on its

"Most bodybuilders will gladly trade unsightly skin for an extra 20 or 30 pounds of muscle. A track star trying to shave a half-second off his 100-meter sprint likely couldn't care less about his skin's appearance. For those who take pride in healthy-looking skin, however, or bodybuilders who intend to compete, a severe case of acne will need to be treated."

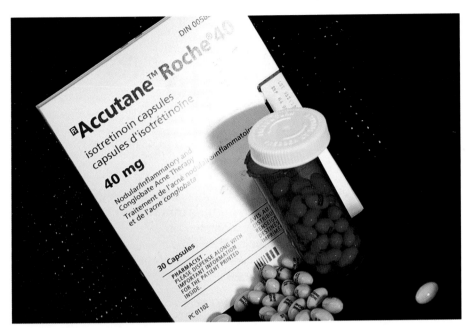

425

own or be surgically removed. For someone with a back covered in blood-filled cysts, the procedure is long and expensive, but may be the only option.

Besides drugs there are other treatment options that offer some degree of success. Believe it or not, one of the simplest is increasing your water intake. If you're a regular reader of *MuscleMag International* you're probably doing this already. But if not, you should start. Water helps keep the skin stay hydrated and flushes away acne-causing bacteria and wastes. Another alternative is to give the sauna a try. Some researchers suggest that by having regular sweat sessions in a sauna, your pores will be kept open, creating less chance for bacteria and dirt to accumulate. Of course, there's a flipside to that coin. Other researchers claim saunas might be the worst option, as clogged pores may not clear but will instead produce bigger pimples. Our advice? Experiment and see what happens.

Those with acne can also try having a regular facial. Don't laugh – some of Hollywood's most macho actors have routine facial treatments! Although expensive, this spa procedure will keep your skin clean and free of dirt and acne-causing bacteria.

Whatever method you decide to use, be sure to check with your doctor first. Acne is a very prevalent health issue, so there's a great deal of research on the topic. Every year seems to bring a new generation of products and treatments, and you and your doctor can discuss what the best option is for you.

ABOVE: Accutane is one of the anti-acne drugs prescribed to those who don't respond well to antibiotic treatment.

PRE- AND POST-WORKOUT NUTRITION

While it's safe to say that each and every one of your meals and snacks is important to your bodybuilding success, probably the two most crucial are the ones immediately before and after your workouts. Appropriately called pre- and post-workout nutrition, both meals are vital to enhancing the recovery and muscle-building process.

PRE-WORKOUT

We know that certain foods and supplements are beneficial before a workout, and the latest research suggests that this time period is just as critical as if not more important than post-workout nutrition. One particular study involved test subjects who were given an amino acid/carbohydrate solution prior to and following exercise. It was found that while delivery of the amino acids was increased in both groups, the transport was greater in the participants who consumed the mixture before their workout compared to the post-exercise group.

Another study, though it used rats and not humans, shed additional light on the subject. Three groups of rats were exercised for two hours daily over a five-week period. Each group ingested one of the following substances beforehand: glucose, whole milk or whey protein. The results were quite telling. The glucose group showed increased glucose oxidation and decreased fat oxidation during and after exercise – they burned sugar instead of bodyfat for energy. The whole-milk and whey groups preserved fat oxidation and increased protein oxidation, – they kept fat burning stable and used protein as a fuel source. Not surprisingly, the whey group showed the most protein oxidation, probably because whey was the fastest-absorbed protein.

Another finding from this study was the source of the weight increases. For the group getting glucose or whole-milk protein, the gains were from bodyfat; for the whey group, however, it was muscle mass that increased and bodyfat that decreased. The researchers theorized that the outcome was primarily due to whey's ability to rapidly deliver amino acids during exercise.[1]

So what does this mean for you? Before you hit the iron in each

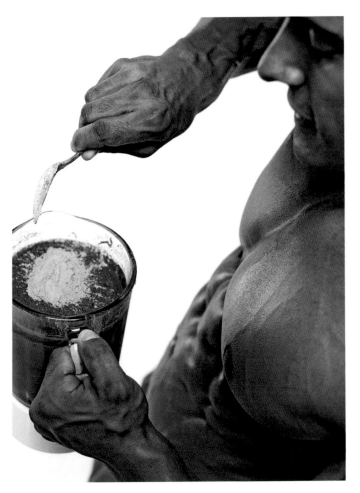

"No doubt most readers have heard the old saying, 'You don't grow in the gym but outside of it.' The reason is that after an intense training session, your muscle glycogen levels are depleted and increased levels of the hormone cortisol begin to break down muscle tissue. Of course, you want to avoid such conditions – the only way to switch from a catabolic to an anabolic state is to consume a fast-digesting post-workout meal as soon as you can after leaving the gym."

workout you should take one or two scoops of protein to maximize both fat loss and muscle gains. Unlike post-workout nutrition when mixing the protein with milk and a simple sugar is probably the best strategy (see next section), your pre-workout nutrition should consist mainly of a fast-absorbing protein – and whey is the clear frontrunner in this category.

POST-WORKOUT

No doubt most readers have heard the old saying, "You don't grow in the gym but outside of it." The reason is that after an intense training session, your muscle glycogen levels are depleted and increased levels of the hormone cortisol begin to break down muscle tissue. Of course, you want to avoid such conditions – the only way to switch from a catabolic to an anabolic state is to consume a fast-digesting post-workout meal as soon as you can after leaving the gym.

Photo by Alex Ardenti
Model Rick Figoni

"In addition to the actual components of your post-workout meal, the other crucial aspect is timing. The body's muscle cells are most sensitive to insulin for the first 45 minutes after exercise. By consuming carbohydrates and protein within this time window, you'll stimulate many more anabolic processes than if you were to take in the nutrients much later. "

Your post-workout meal should consist of two primary nutrient groups: protein and carbohydrates. You may think protein alone would do the trick, but studies have found that there is a better insulin response (and hence the creation of an improved anabolic environment) when carbs and protein are mixed together. This information is not new – food scientists discovered almost 40 years ago that high-protein foods combined with carbohydrates raised blood-insulin levels more than other combinations. Researchers at the University of Texas compared the effects of carbohydrate-protein supplements on blood insulin levels after intense exercise. The carb-protein group produced the greatest insulin response followed by the carb-drink group and then the protein-only group. Surprisingly, subjects who consumed only protein supplements produced an insulin response that was just one-eighth of what was experienced by those who took in a combination of carbs and protein.

Another study carried out by the University of Texas Medical Branch (Galveston) compared the post-training effects of carbohydrates, amino acids and a mixture of amino acids and carbohydrates. They found that protein synthesis was greatest among the amino acid-carbohydrate group; the least synthesis took place in the carbs-only group. In fact, the carbohydrate-amino group demonstrated 38 percent more efficacy than the amino-alone group and 100 percent more than the carbohydrate group.

Your post-workout drink should also include glutamine and creatine. Both compounds are powerful anabolic and anti-catabolic supplements – adding 5 grams of each to your shake will optimize your body's recovery potential.

In addition to the actual components of your post-workout meal, the other crucial aspect is timing. The body's muscle cells are most sensitive to insulin for the first 45 minutes after exercise. By consuming carbohydrates and protein within this time window, you'll stimulate many more anabolic processes than if you were to take in the nutrients much later. One study carried out at Vanderbilt University (Nashville, Tennessee) confirms this. The researchers gave two groups of exercisers a carbohydrate-protein supplement after they performed 60 minutes of exercise. One group received the drink immediately after working out, and the other group waited three hours before consuming the drink. Protein synthesis was found to be almost three times higher in the first group compared to the second group. In addition, subjects who consumed their protein immediately following training had a significant increase in overall net-protein balance (protein synthesis minus protein degradation), whereas those who took it later actually had a net loss.

With regards to body composition, a study published in the *Journal of Physiology* showed that subjects receiving a carbohydrate-protein supplement immediately after exercising had an eight-percent increase in muscle size and a 15-percent increase in strength levels. Subjects who were given the supplement after a two-hour post-workout period showed no increase in either size or strength. Animal studies on rats have found similar results including a six-percent increase in muscle mass and a 24-percent decrease in abdominal fat when a protein supplement was given right after exercise.

The best ratio seems to be 75 to 100 grams of high-glycemic carbs and 30 to 50 grams of protein. You need the carbs as a means to replenish muscle glycogen and reduce the effects of rising cortisol levels that occur post-workout; a quick-digesting source of protein is necessary to provide the amino acids required to begin repairing those taxed muscles. The surge of carbohydrates and amino acids in the body will promote an insulin spike from the pancreas, which in turn shuttles nutrients into the muscle cells.

POST-WORKOUT MEAL TIMING

The optimal time frame for consuming a meal after you train is called the "nutrient window," and for good reason. From the moment you complete your last set, until just shy of an hour later, your body is literally begging for nutrients. Now, this doesn't mean you have to drop the dumbells or hop off the treadmill and start eating the next second, but you typically want to try to get this meal into your body within that first hour. If possible, consuming it within 30 minutes would be even better.

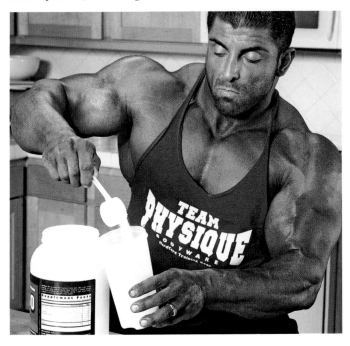

Photo by Robert Reiff
Model King Kamali

LEFT: When mixing your post-workout shake, research has shown that the best ratio is 75 to 100 grams of high-GI carbs and 30 to 50 grams of protein.

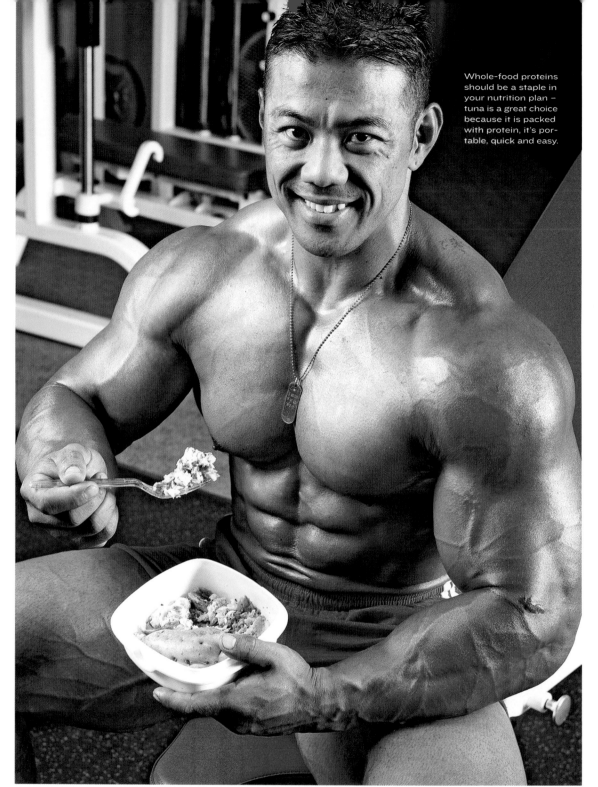

With regards to protein sources, you have two main options – whole foods and supplements. Your best choices for whole-food protein are egg whites, chicken breast and tuna. As animal sources they contain a complete amino-acid profile (as opposed to most plant sources, which are deficient in one or more of the essential amino acids) and are low in fat. While great proteins, they do have one draw-

Photo by Ralph DeHaan
Model Ray Arde

back – they digest rather slowly. By the time the protein is digested and finally ready to be used by your body, a considerable amount of time may have already passed. This is why the ideal source of protein to take in after your workout is a supplement derived from whey protein – it's the fastest-digesting protein there is. And the fact that it's taken in liquid form (powder mixed with water or milk) makes it even quicker for the body to digest.

The primary reason for including carbs as part of your meal immediately after you work out is to restore your muscle glycogen levels. If your post-workout meal doesn't contain a sufficient amount of carbs, your body may end up breaking down muscle tissue for this same purpose. Carbs also create an insulin spike, which helps to more quickly transport other nutrients, including amino acids, into your muscle cells.

Most of the studies on post-workout nutrition have shown that about 1 to 2 grams of carbohydrates per kilogram of bodyweight works best. Keep in mind, however, that the amount you ingest should also be reflective of your training intensity and volume. If you only do two to three sets to failure, you definitely won't tax your body's energy reserves nearly as much as if you complete 15 sets. The specific studies we're referring to used 1 to 1.5 grams of carbohydrates per kilogram of bodyweight for individuals who performed about eight sets to failure. Your specific intake of this nutrient will thus need to be adjusted based on your own training volume.

You also need to remember that all carbohydrates are not created equal. The type you should be ingesting post-workout is either liquid or powdered form. The reason is simple – faster absorption. The quicker you can get glucose into your bloodstream and muscles, the less protein is destroyed and the more glycogen stored. The glycemic index of the carbohydrates you take in should also be relatively high. Therefore, a combination of fruit juice and maltodextrin would be a great option. Maltodextrin is derived from starch and is rapidly absorbed; when combined with fruit juice, you reap the benefits from an excellent source of high-glycemic carbohydrates. Try to stick to juices that are rich in glucose as these will be absorbed most rapidly. Another great feature of juices and simple sugars is that they can satisfy even the worst sweet tooth, seeing as this is the one time of the day when you can get away with sweets in your diet. Even individuals trying to maximize fat loss can drink high-glycemic carbs after a workout because there is very little chance they'll be stored as fat.

Reference

1) A pre-exercise lactalbumen-enriched whey protein meal preserves lipid oxidation and decreases adiposity in rats. *Am J Physiology, Endocrinology and Metabolism.* 283, E565–E572 (2002).

> "The primary reason for including carbs as part of your meal immediately after you work out is to restore your muscle glycogen levels. If your post-workout meal doesn't contain a sufficient amount of carbs, your body may end up breaking down muscle tissue for this same purpose. Carbs also create an insulin spike, which helps to more quickly transport other nutrients, including amino acids, into your muscle cells."

ONE, TWO, THREE, FOUR – CALORIE COUNTING

One of the most fundamental aspects to building a great physique is tracking your caloric intake. On one hand you're trying to consume enough high-quality nutrients to build new muscle tissue, restock energy reserves and enhance your overall recovery system; at the same time, however, you don't want to take in too many calories and end up counteracting all your efforts in the gym.

If you're serious about competitive bodybuilding, you need to be proficient at keeping track of the calories you consume daily. You should also have a solid grasp of what those calories consist of. There's a whole world of difference between 200 grams of protein and 200 grams of saturated fat. And let's not forget that individual genetics will be a huge factor in determining how each calorie will be used by your body.

THE GREAT ENERGY DIVIDE

There are three primary ways that the human body expends energy: basal metabolism (called basal metabolic rate or BMR), physical activity (PA) and the thermogenic effect of food (TEF). If we add all three components together, we get total energy expenditure, or TEE. When combined, the trio comprise the energy needed for physical movement, the body's ability to maintain its normal functions (breathing, heartbeat, body temperature, etc.), and cell tissue repair. Every calorie ingested will be used for one of these essential functions. Once the body gets all the calories needed to carry out the various processes, however, any extra ones will be stored. No matter how healthy your diet is, you'll gain weight if you take in more calories than what your body requires to sustain and maintain BMR, PA and TEF. And logically, you'll lose weight if you take in too few calories.

CALORIE MATHEMATICS

Most bodybuilders are probably aware of the nutrient groups (protein, fats, carbs, etc.) and their respective calorie contents. For those not familiar with the conversion of nutrient amounts (usually measured in grams) into calories, the following table will give you an idea:

> "There are three primary ways that the human body expends energy: basal metabolism (called basal metabolic rate or BMR), physical activity (PA) and the thermogenic effect of food (TEF). If we add all three components together, we get total energy expenditure, or TEE."

432

Grams into Calories

1 gram of protein = 4 calories
1 gram of carbohydrates = 4 calories
1 gram of fat = 9 calories
1 gram of alcohol = 7 calories

Based on those numbers, a 200-pound bodybuilder who eats 200 grams of protein per day (remember, the recommended amount is approximately one gram of protein per pound of bodyweight) would have to ingest 800 calories from protein daily. Likewise, 200 grams of carbohydrates translates to 800 calories (because one gram is equal to four calories). Have a look at the fat conversion, though – nine calories to each gram means consuming 200 grams of fat would tack on 1,800 calories to your diet! Despite the benefits of certain healthy fats, you still need to pay close attention to how much of this high-calorie nutrient you're ingesting on a daily basis.

Now that you have a better understanding of the gram-calorie relationship for each of the major nutrient groups, let's take a closer look at energy expenditure. In order to accurately adjust your eating for maximum output, you need to know how calories are utilized. We'll begin this discussion with the component that has the highest demand for calories – basal metabolic rate.

433

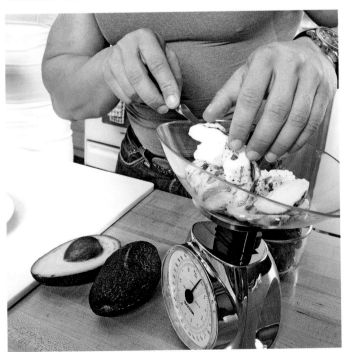

Photo by Robert Reiff

LEFT: As a bodybuilder, your daily caloric intake is crucial. You need to know how much of each nutrient you're getting to ensure optimal health.

"The thermogenic effect of food is the energy it takes to digest, transport, store, absorb and metabolize the foods you eat. Although nowhere near as high as BMR and PA, TEF can burn an extra 10 to 12 percent of the calories you ingest. The process takes place in the first couple of hours after you eat and is influenced by the types of nutrients consumed."

BMR

BMR is the number of calories expended or utilized during a 24-hour period of absolute rest. In other words, if you were to wake up in the morning and not move for the entire day, your body would still need calories for basic, life-sustaining tasks such as breathing, heart function, cell repair and general body regulation. Though you may think otherwise, basal metabolism requires far more overall calories than even high-intensity exercise – 60 to 70 percent of your total daily expenditure.

A person's BMR is controlled by a number of factors including individual genetics, weight and ratio of muscle mass to fat. The last determinant is why bodybuilders and other muscular athletes can ingest so many calories and not get fat – the extra calories are being burned to support the muscle mass (growth, repair and energy resupply).

BMR Calculation

Calculating your BMR is more art than science, and over the years numerous formulas have been developed for this purpose. One of the most commonly used is the Harris-Benedict principle. This equation uses the variables of height, weight, age and gender to calculate specific basal metabolic rate (BMR). While still somewhat approximate, this method is more accurate than calculating calorie needs based on total bodyweight alone.

Harris-Benedict Formula for Men

Formula: BMR = 66 + (13.7 x weight in kilos) + (5 x height in centimeters) - (6.8 x age in years)

Note: 1 inch = 2.54 cm and 1 kilogram = 2.2 lbs.

Example

You are a 28-year-old male who is 5′9″ (180 cm) tall. Your weight is 200 pounds (91 kg).

Apply the Harris-Benedict formula: 66 + (13.7 x 91) + (5 x 180) - (6.8 x 28) ==> Your BMR is 2,022 calories.

PA – PHYSICAL ACTIVITY

Although it utilizes fewer overall calories than BMR, physical activity is probably the most important energy-neeeds factor given that you have more control over your actions. PA is the sum total of all the energy used during a 24-hour period via every form of physical activity you engage in. By "every" we mean everything from cardio and weightlifting to walking and picking up a book or even brushing your teeth. PA accounts for approximately 20 to 30 percent of total energy output.

TEF – THERMOGENIC EFFECT OF FOOD

The thermogenic effect of food is the energy it takes to digest, transport, store, absorb and metabolize the foods you eat. Although nowhere near as high as BMR and PA, TEF can burn an extra 10 to 12 percent of the calories you ingest. The process takes place in the first couple of hours after you eat and is influenced by the types of nutrients consumed. Sources high in protein and complex carbohydrates have a higher TEF than fat calories.

CALCULATING TOTAL CALORIC NEEDS

Now that you have a grasp on the relationship between ingested calories and energy, it's time to calculate your specific total daily caloric needs. Although not foolproof, the following method will give you a relatively accurate estimation.

Start by multiplying your BMR by the appropriate activity factor, as follows:

• You are sedentary (little or no exercise)
   Calculation = BMR x 1.2
• You are slightly active (light exercise/sports 1–3 days per week)
   Calculation = BMR x 1.375
• You are moderately active (moderate exercise/sports 3–5 days per week)
   Calculation = BMR x 1.55
• You are very active = BMR x 1.725 (intense exercise/sports 6–7 days per week)
   Calculation = BMR x 1.725
• You are extremely active (very high-intensity, daily exercise/sports and physical job or twice-a-day training)
   Calculation = BMR x 1.9

Example

You are an extremely active male, so you multiply your BMR of 2,022 (used from previous example) by 1.9, which equals 3,842.4 calories. This means you need approximately 3,842 calories to maintain your weight. The key word here is "maintain." If you're trying to lose bodyfat for a bodybuilding contest, you'll need to cut about 400 to 500 calories per day from this figure (500 calories per day for seven days equals 3,500 calories, or one pound). Conversely, if you're engaged in off-season training and/or trying to gain muscle mass, you'll need to add a few extra calories to this total. It's difficult, however, to provide an exact number, as everyone's body and digestive systems are different. Some bodybuilders may need an extra 500 calories per day to grow, while others might get by on an additional 100 to 200. A few genetically fortunate individuals may even grow by sticking to their maintenance number.

435

PACKING ON SIZE – THE BASICS

For many professional bodybuilders, gaining muscle mass isn't a very difficult task. Heck, a lot of guys almost seem like they grow just by thinking about a barbell. Their main focus is instead on dropping bodyfat and ripping up for a contest. Likewise, the average person usually has no problem pushing the scale's needle up on a regular basis. Of course individuals, both male and female, who eat poorly or don't exercise regularly, tend to put the majority of gained weight around their hips, quads and stomach.

There is, however, a small minority of people who actually want to gain muscular bodyweight. They sometimes slave for years trying to add an extra ounce or two to their frames, but may still fall short. It seems no matter what they do, their bodies simply refuse to grow. In bodybuilding, these individuals are known as hardgainers.

And some people struggle with weight for other emotional reasons. For these individuals, food doesn't hold the same type of obsession as it does with the chronically obese or even the moderately overweight. While many people overeat in response to stressful situations or circumstances, and hence gain weight, underweight people with disordered eating behaviors sometimes tend to avoid food because of their fear of gaining weight. These patterns of thinking cause individuals with this condition to remain skinny or lose even more weight off of their already slight frames. Compounding the problem is that such individuals often dwell on their condition to the point that they give up and accept their skinny frames as being set for life.

Well for those readers who fall into the category of "skinny," "underweight," or "hardgainer," don't give up. With a few simple, basic tricks, you too can change your appearance. We can't promise that you'll achieve a Mr. Olympia physique – most professional bodybuilders who've won that title have been dealt a full deck of playing cards with regards to genetics and training success. Provided you are willing to work hard and follow the advice in this chapter, however, you can reasonably expect to develop a body that will cause your friends to sit up and notice. More important, you'll do wonders for your self-esteem and confidence. Just as an obese person has to make

> "There is, however, a small minority of people who actually want to gain muscular bodyweight. They sometimes slave for years trying to add an extra ounce or two to their frames, but may still fall short. It seems no matter what they do, their bodies simply refuse to grow. In bodybuilding, these individuals are known as hardgainers."

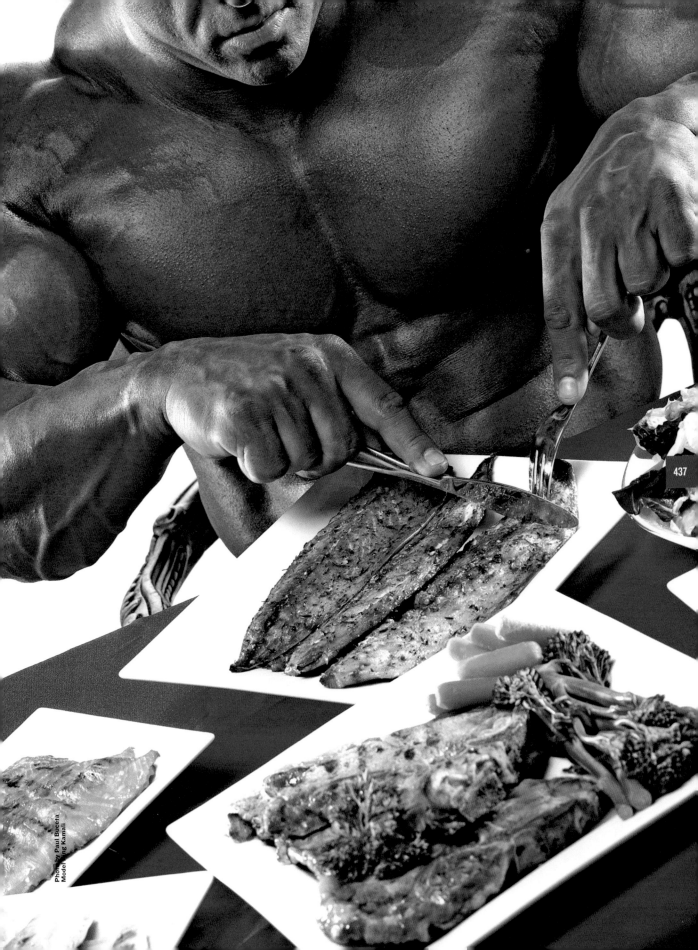

437

Photo by Paul Buceta
Model Ing Kamali

specific diet and exercise changes to get the weight off, so too must underweight individuals modify their lifestyles to put quality weight on – and keep it on.

NO MAGIC PILL

Despite what supplement manufacturers may advertise, there simply isn't a magic pill or powder that will put muscular weight on your frame. Yes, supplements can and will play a role, but the products alone won't accomplish your physique goals for you. Your first step is to map out a healthy eating plan to follow. If you aren't consuming the minimum requirement of fats, carbohydrates and protein, along with the recommended amounts of important vitamins and minerals, all the weight-gain powders in the world won't offer much benefit.

For the building blocks of a solid diet, look no further than protein, starches, fruits and vegetables. It may sound simple, but the combination of these nutrients is effective. For breakfast, you don't have to get much more complicated than having a couple of eggs, a scoop of cottage cheese, and some instant breakfast powder or protein powder mixed with milk. If you find you have a big appetite in the morning, add in a bowl of oatmeal, bran cereal, shredded wheat or a whole-wheat bagel (you can use one tablespoon of margarine made with canola oil or natural peanut butter as a spread). Finally, include a piece of fruit – fresh varieties are better as they contain more nutrients. In no particular order, you can consider trying grapefruit, a banana, any type of berries or a few slices of melon.

The breakfast philosophy generally applies at lunchtime as well. For protein, you can't go wrong with tuna, chicken breast, turkey breast, lean ham, roast beef and low-fat cheese. Complex carbs can be obtained from brown rice, a whole-wheat pita or bread, or whole-grain crackers. A nice fresh garden salad will provide your vegetable needs. Drizzle some olive or flaxseed oil over your greens for both taste and to get a good amount of EFAs. If you want to add more protein and key minerals like calcium to your lunch, include a glass of skim or one-percent milk.

Your supper meal should include a meat, fish, chicken or egg dish. Get your starches from potatoes (sweet potato is a great choice), brown rice or whole-wheat pasta. It's also a good idea to include peas, corn or beans for the fiber content. And another small garden salad would be beneficial to make sure you meet your daily needs of vegetables.

With the three basic meals taken care of, now it's time to start building the rest of your daily eating schedule. One of the most important for bodybuilders is a nighttime snack. A nutritious option at this time is a peanut butter (natural) and jelly sandwich on whole-wheat bread with a glass of milk and a banana.

Give this basic meal plan a try for a couple of weeks before making any other adjustments. By following it, you will have a chance to get accustomed to the increased calories and evening snack (assuming you weren't already eating one before). Often it only takes a slight tweak to your eating habits to shock the body into growth. If you find you still aren't gaining muscular weight, don't despair. You'll simply move on to the next area for change: modifying your daily exercise activities.

With the exception of those genetically blessed individuals (or pharmacologically enhanced), most people can't perform an excessive amount of physical activities outside of training and still maximize their bodybuilding gains. You've only got so many calories to work with and all that extra exercise will only burn them. Your next step is to start focusing on the bodybuilding workouts that will benefit you the most. By this we mean basic, compound power movements, not single-muscle isolation exercises. Your main goal is to stimulate the most muscle mass as possible. The following exercises are considered the best for achieving maximal muscle stimulation:

Squats
Deadlifts
Bench Presses
Barbell Rows

If you've never worked out before or have been draining your body on a six-day split routine, we suggest you start off by working out just three days per week. Take a day's rest between each workout – two days is even better if it fits with your schedule. Do only three sets of eight to 12 reps per exercise. Follow this approach for three weeks and then start piling the weight on the bar – enough poundage so you're limited to getting just four to six reps per set. As soon as rep seven or eight becomes possible, add more weight to the bar.

Further to the amount of muscle you are targeting, another benefit of doing these basic exercises is the increase in appetite they'll ignite. Your muscles will be screaming for nutrients and your late-night snack should be enough to start your body on the road to large gains. For most hardgainers, these adjustments will likely be as far as you'll need to go. But there are, however, a few unfortunate individuals whose bodies will still refuse to cooperate. If this is the case, you'll need to experiment with adding even more calories.

The logical and healthy way to incorporate more calories would be to include another snack or two in your daily diet. The best times to do so are mid-morning and mid-afternoon. Another option you should consider is taking in a meal-replacement or protein drink on a daily basis. Busy schedules and even lack of hunger make it difficult at times to prepare and eat food, but a liquid protein or weight-gainer drink can be ready in minutes and is easy to drink.

> "There simply isn't a magic pill or powder that will put muscular weight on your frame. Yes, supplements can and will play a role, but the products alone won't accomplish your physique goals for you. Your first step is to map out a healthy eating plan to follow. If you aren't consuming the minimum requirement of fats, carbohydrates and protein, along with the recommended amounts of important vitamins and minerals, all the weight-gain powders in the world won't offer much benefit."

439

But what about those readers who still have trouble gaining weight on three meals and three snacks per day? Should you give up? Definitely not. If you're really serious about putting on some quality muscle mass, you can add another snack in the middle of the night. While not ideal, try setting your alarm clock for three or four in the morning. Have a supplement drink right beside your bed. You'd be amazed at what an extra few hundred quality calories will do for a hardgainer's recovery abilities during the sleep cycle.

BEEF-UP SNACKS

The following recipes are examples of some easy-to-make, tasty snacks that you can add to your diet to increase your nutrient and calorie totals. Keep in mind that some of these are very calorie dense, and thus probably shouldn't be eaten by anyone trying to lose weight or get cut for a contest. But for our skinny, ectomorph readers – dig in!

Two-Handed Sandwich

2 slices whole-grain bread (toasted if you like)
3 oz. sliced turkey or chicken
1 oz. Swiss cheese
½ avocado, sliced
2 tbsp. mayonnaise
Lettuce, tomato, pickles (optional)
Enjoy with a glass of milk or juice (fruit or vegetable).

Tuna Burrito

1 12-inch whole-wheat tortilla
½ cup tuna
¼ cup cheese, shredded
½ avocado, sliced
Enjoy with a glass of milk or juice (fruit or vegetable).

Yogurt Sundae

2 cups nonfat/low-fat yogurt
1 banana, sliced
½ cup nuts, chopped
Top with chocolate sauce (if you really want to add extra calories)!

Super-Salad

2 cups iceberg lettuce, spinach, tomatoes
Top with ½ cup diced peaches, ¼ cup sunflower seeds, ½ cup peanuts, 2 tbsp. raisins. Add olive oil, flax oil or Italian dressing.

Quick Snack

    6–8 graham crackers

    2–3 tbsp. natural peanut butter

Enjoy with a glass of milk or juice (fruit or vegetable).

Open-Faced Sandwich

    2 slices whole-wheat bread

    2–3 tbsp. natural peanut butter

    1 apple, peeled and diced

    2–3 tbsp. raisins

Mini Pizzas

    1–2 English muffins, toasted

Top with spaghetti sauce, shredded cheese, sliced olives and other diced vegetables. You can also add Canadian bacon and ham.

BELOW: There are countless options for fast, tasty muscle-building snacks and meals, like a tuna burrito, for example.

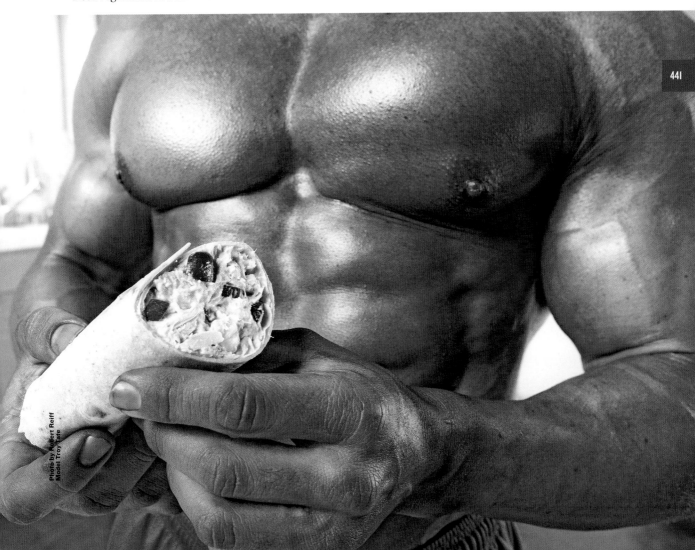

Photo by Robert Reiff
Model Troy Tate

MUSCLEMAG INTERNATIONAL'S SURGE EATING

> "One of the most effective eating strategies to come along in recent years is called 'Surge.' Thanks to Steven Stiefel and *Muscle-Mag International,* you can use surge eating to break through any weight plateaus and boost your muscle mass to the next level."

For many aspiring bodybuilders, the greatest challenge is adding bodyweight in the form of lean muscle tissue and not bodyfat. The old approach was to eat everything in sight during the off-season, gain 40 or 50 pounds and then burn the excess fat during the pre-contest phase. Many bodybuilders, however, have abandoned this practice. For one, all of that extra weight is primarily fat, not muscle. In addition, gaining weight rapidly tends to produce unsightly stretch marks on the skin. Finally, as most doctors will tell you, the human body – particularly the heart – doesn't take too kindly to massive, short-term fluctuations in bodyweight.

Your goal should instead be to follow an intelligent nutrition plan that supplies all the right nutrients to promote muscle tissue growth and repair, while keeping bodyfat gains to a minimum.

One of the most effective eating strategies to come along in recent years is called "Surge." Thanks to Steven Stiefel and *MuscleMag International,* you can use surge eating to break through any weight plateaus and boost your muscle mass to the next level.

Before implementing the principles of surge eating, you should first try to understand why your gains have slowed or halted in the first place. Many young or inexperienced bodybuilders fall into two general categories in this regard. The first includes ectomorphs who are hardgainers and have trouble adding muscle mass because of either their high metabolic rates or tendencies to under-eat. The second group is comprised of those who have a good deal of muscle mass but tend to carry a lot of extra bodyfat because of either overeating or poor eating habits.

The surge approach is ideal for both groups of individuals. This method is also perfect for those who simply want to complement their off-season strength and size weight-training program. Many bodybuilders have gained 10-plus pounds of quality muscle mass while following surge eating principles.

SURGING BASICS

Despite the great results this strategy may produce, there's nothing complicated about the surge program. You simply double the calories

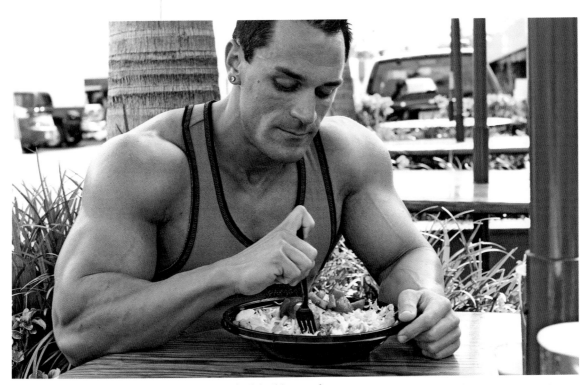

443

you need for maintenance every fifth day. Many bodybuilders tend to add extra calories every day. While some of these surplus calories will no doubt be converted into muscle mass, many will also end up being stored as bodyfat. The advantage of surging is that most of the supplemental calories eaten on day five will go toward promoting the growth of new muscle tissue because your body will use much of the excess calories for heat production. Not only will this create an increased anabolic environment within the body, but since you're only overeating every fifth day, there's also less chance of increasing your bodyfat level.

The key to making the surge program effective is to follow these four steps:

ABOVE: With surge eating, you maintain your regular diet from days one to four and then double your calories on day five.

STEP 1

Calculate your multiplying factor – the amount of calories you burn per pound of bodyweight per day (see Step 2).

STEP 2

Determine the number of calories you should eat each day.

Before looking at the specific nutrients, you need to know how many calories you should be consuming on your four maintenance days and your surge day. For a precise number, refer to the informa-

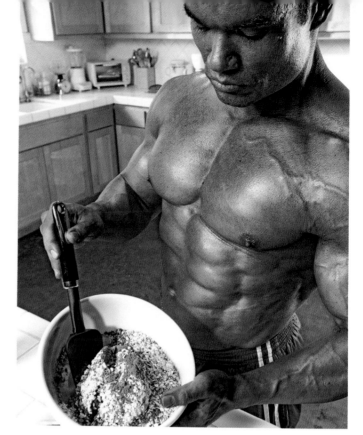

RIGHT: Complex carbs are an integral component to proper nutrition. Focus on sources such as oatmeal, brown rice and whole grains.

tion in Chapter 71. If you want to guesstimate your daily requirement, the average young male bodybuilder burns about 17 calories per pound of bodyweight each day (the multiplying factor). This means that a 150-pound male will expend a little more than 2,500 calories a day (17 x 150 = 2,550). Using the same equation, a 200-pounder would burn 3,400 calories. For underweight ectomorphs or those who engage in other forms of exercise, use a multiplying factor of 20. Conversely, those who are carrying a 15-percent bodyfat or higher should use a multiplying factor of 15.

Now that you know your caloric needs for your four maintenance days, it's just a matter of doubling that amount for your surge every fifth day. The following table outlines the calorie breakdown for the average bodybuilder, a hardgainer or ectomorph and an off-season bodybuilder:

Average Bodybuilder

Day	Bodyweight	Multiplying Factor	Total Calorie Intake
1–4	180	17	3,060
5	180	34	6,120

Hardgainer or Ectomorph (or Highly Active)

Day	Bodyweight	Multiplying Factor	Total Calorie Intake
1–4	160	20	3,200
5	160	40	6,400

Off-Season 220-Pound Bodybuilder

Day	Bodyweight	Multiplying Factor	Total Calorie Intake
1–4	220	15	3,300
5	220	30	6,600

STEP 3

Break down your surge eating into specific nutrient groups.

Although ingesting copious amounts of food on your surge day is your primary goal, you don't want to just scarf down empty calories. You want to ensure that you're fueling your system with only the best recovery and muscle-building nutrients. (The numbers provided in the following suggestions are an example based on a male bodybuilder who weighs 180 pounds.)

Up the Protein

We're sure most readers are doing this already, but the recommendation needs repeating. The primary building material of muscle tissue is protein. You should be consuming around one gram per pound of bodyweight on your maintenance days and even higher on your surge days – try 1.5 grams per pound of bodyweight. For a 180-pounder this works out to 270 grams. The easiest and most effective way is to consume increments of at least 40 grams of protein six to seven times per day.

Get Fat!

Healthy fats are one of the most under-recognized nutrient groups. Besides boosting recovery, they also serve as the building blocks for numerous anabolic compounds including hormones and prostaglandins. On your maintenance days you should be eating at least 20 percent of your calories from healthy fats. Using our example, the 180-pounder should be eating at least 65 grams of fat on days one through four and over 150 grams on surge days. The best sources of healthy fats include salmon, avocados, nuts and seeds, and oils such as olive, canola and flaxseed.

Increase your Starchy Carb Intake

If you overeat on carbs regularly, the excess will cause you to pack on fat, but this nutrient won't cause weight gain if you only consume extra amounts on surge days. Try to limit your carb intake to about 50 percent of your total calories on regular days and up to about 60 percent on surge days. On maintenance days, focus on having slow-digesting carbs including brown rice, yams, oatmeal and whole-grain breads. Every fifth day, switch to more starchy carbs such as bread, pasta, rice and potatoes.

Nutrient Percentages

	Protein	Carbs	Healthy Fats	Other Fats
Regular Days	30%	50%	10%	10%
Surge Days	15–25%	50–60%	15%	5–10%

> "Healthy fats are one of the most under-recognized nutrient groups. Besides boosting recovery, they also serve as the building blocks for numerous anabolic compounds including hormones and prostaglandins. The best sources of healthy fats include salmon, avocados, nuts and seeds, and oils such as olive, canola and flaxseed."

445

STEP 4

Apply the nutrient percentages to your food choices.

Now that you know the breakdown of nutrients percentage-wise, it's time to translate these numbers into actual foods. The sample meal plan that follows is specific to a bodybuilder who eats about 3,000 calories on regular days and 6,000 on surge days. You will need to individually tailor the proportions to suit your own bodyweight, and you'll also need to pay close attention to your physique.

Sample Meal Plan

Food	Regular-Day Amount	Surge-Day Amount
Breakfast		
Eggs	4	6
Turkey bacon	3 slices	4 slices
Oatmeal	1 cup	2 cups
Fruit	1 piece	1 piece
Mid-Morning Snack		
Whole-grain bread	2 slices	4 slices
Chicken breast	6 oz.	8 oz.
Avocado	½, medium	1
Cheese	1 oz.	2 oz.
Lunch		
Salmon	9 oz.	12 oz.
Broccoli	1 cup	1 cup
Brown rice/pasta	1 cup (rice)	12 oz. pasta
Salad	1 cup	1 cup
Olive oil	1 tbsp.	2 tbsp.
Pre-Workout Shake		
Protein powder	1 scoop	2 scoops
Complex carbs	25 g	50 g
Post-Workout Shake		
Protein powder	1 scoop	2 scoops
Sugar	25 g	50 g
Dinner		
Steak	9 oz.	12 oz.
Baked yam	1 medium	1 large
Asparagus	1 serving	1 serving
Dessert	–	1 portion

Bedtime Snack

Deli meat, lean	4 oz.	4 oz.
Whole-grain bread	–	2 slices
Almonds	–	2 oz.

FINAL COMMENTS

After you've consumed double the calories on your surge day, you may find that you're not very hungry on the subsequent day. You need to be aware of this, however, as it becomes possible that you may under-eat every sixth day. Pay close attention to the total number of calories that you do eat. You don't want to derail your progress by not getting in enough calories on each first day of your maintenance cycle.

If you still find you're not adding weight, reduce your training volume to no more than four one-hour workouts per week. Also try a surge eating cycle that's spread out over seven days. In this case you'd surge on days five and seven, and then eat to maintain on days one to four and day six.

If, on the other hand, you start gaining too much bodyfat, cut your maintenance multiplying factor back by two (i.e., from 17 to 15, 20 to 18, etc.). Then use this modified number to recalculate your daily caloric needs. You should also try adding in three 30-minute cardio sessions to your program per week.

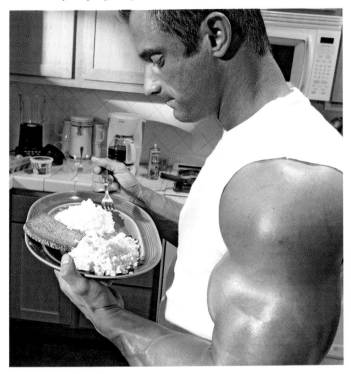

Photo by Robert Reiff
Model Dan Decker

LEFT: When using the surge eating program, be conscious of how you feel the day after your surge day. You may not be as hungry, but you still need to consume your maintenance number of calories.

447

BODYBUILDING'S TOP POWER FOODS

448

Chicken breast, tuna, sweet patatoes ... most serious bodybuilders know the importance of these three sta-ples in a healthy diet. Each supplies either high-value protein to build new muscle tissue or complex carbs to power those high-intensity workouts. Body-building nutrition is much more vast, though, and numerous other foods are just as integral for building quality muscle mass.

If you examine the nutrient profile of the top bodybuilding foods, you'll see that no single source is the "best" all-around food. Some rank highest in protein but low or moderate in carbs. Or, certain items are considered super-carb foods but contain little or no protein. And let's not forget about foods rich with good fats, minerals and/or vitamins. For optimum bodybuilding success, all of the major nutrient groups must be consumed regularly in the proper amounts and proportions.

The following sources should serve as the foundation of your bodybuilding nutrition plan. These foods aren't ranked in any particular order – remember, there isn't a No. 1 – certain choices are just front-runners. We've also included a number of substitutes for each so you can add variety to your diet and stimulate your tastebuds in different ways, or in case you can't obtain the first source for whatever reason. Try to eat a minimum of one serving of each item we've included in the following list on a regular basis – if not daily, you should consume these foods at least a few times weekly.

> "If you examine the nutrient profile of the top bodybuilding foods, you'll see that no single source is the 'best' all-around food. Some rank highest in protein but low or moderate in carbs. Or, certain items are considered super-carb foods but contain little or no protein. And let's not forget about foods rich with good fats, minerals and/or vitamins."

SALMON

Despite the best intentions of *MuscleMag International* and other bodybuilding publications to provide information about the benefits of EFAs, omegas and the like, most bodybuilders still don't obtain enough good fats in their diets. Salmon is a great one-two punch food. It's very high in healthy fats

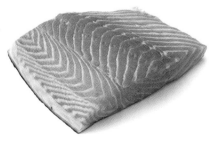

and is also rich in protein. You should aim to include at least two or three servings of salmon or some other fatty fish in your diet every week. Fats from this source provide numerous benefits to your heart, along with the raw materials for hormones, skin, hair and cell membranes.

Alternatives: Trout, mackerel, herring, sardines

BLACK BEANS

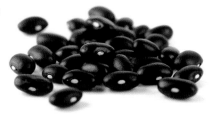

One of the most neglected nutrients in the North American diet is fiber. Bodybuilders are guilty of this shortcoming as well. Consuming enough fiber in your diet is crucial to keep the digestive system working efficiently and even potentially prevent certain forms of cancer. Each half-cup of black beans provides 15 grams of fiber and 20 grams of protein.

Alternatives: Pinto beans, kidney beans, lima beans

FRESH FRUIT

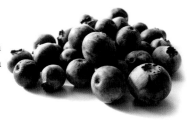

Fruit sometimes gets a bad rap by nutrition experts in bodybuilding because of the sugar content, but it really shouldn't. With the exception of the last couple of months before a bodybuilding contest, all serious trainers should generally be including three or four servings of fruit in their daily diets. While it's true that fruit contains sugar, including the simple sugar fructose, these foods are also loaded with fiber, vitamins and minerals. One of the best choices nutritionally is berries – and the darker the better (think blackberries, blueberries, raspberries). If possible, keep your intake of fruit juices to a minimum as they are generally very calorie dense and lack the fiber whole fruit provides.

Alternatives: Frozen fruit, canned fruit in water (not syrup).

SWEET POTATOES

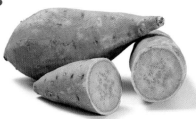

A power food list would not be complete without including the good old sweet potatoes. This vegetable has been one of the staple foods consumed by bodybuilders for decades, and for good reason. Unlike starchy carbs such as pasta and white bread,

449

the complex carbs in sweet potatoes take longer to digest in your system and don't cause the same degree of insulin spiking. Yams are also loaded with fiber.

Alternatives: Whole-grain bread, brown rice, oatmeal

LEAN RED MEAT

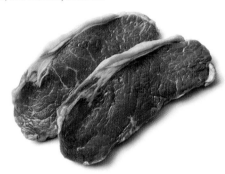

Two of the most important nutrients for packing on serious muscle mass are protein and saturated fats. Yes, you read that correctly – saturated fats. This form of fat (in proper amounts) gets converted by the body into testosterone, which as you know is one of the body's most powerful anabolic hormones. As we've discussed, the more testosterone flowing through your body, the greater your muscle-building potential. Foods that contain saturated fats also decelerate your digestion rate, meaning a slower but steadier delivery of nutrients to your muscles. Red meat is also one of the best sources of protein for gaining muscle mass. Unlike other fast-absorbing proteins such as whey, red meat takes a few hours to digest, thus ensuring a prolonged supply of amino acids to facilitate muscle growth and repair.

So why lean red meat if saturated fat is good? Well, this type of fat is a double-edged sword. On one hand it has the positive benefits we've just discussed. But saturated fat consists of triglycerides, which are major components of LDL or "bad" cholesterol and thus contribute to heart disease. You want to find the happy medium – you want some of this fat in your diet but not a lot. Lean red meat will provide you with just enough to maximize testosterone production and muscle tissue repair, without increasing your risk of developing heart disease. By way of comparison, a cut of prime rib has about 80 grams of fat (23 of which is saturated); a lean cut of sirloin contains just 13 grams of fat, five of which is saturated (the sirloin also has less than half the calories at 407 versus 935 in the prime rib).

Alternatives: Whole eggs, chicken or turkey legs

WHOLE EGGS

Despite the bad rap eggs have received over the years for their cholesterol and fat content, they still remain a top choice among bodybuilders. A single egg (yolk and white) provides 6 grams of protein – top-grade protein we might add.

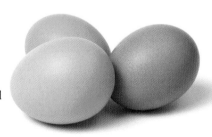

In fact, egg protein is so pure that it's often used as the benchmark to rank other sources of this nutrient. Eggs are also loaded with the fat-soluble vitamins A, D and E, and most of the B-vitamins.

The negative reputation that eggs sometimes receive is unfounded – though this food is somewhat high in fat, most of it is polyunsaturated. And as for the cholesterol relationship, numerous studies now confirm that people who are generally healthy otherwise and eat a couple of eggs per day do not have any higher blood cholesterol levels than those who don't include eggs in their diets. What many people don't realize is that most of the fat contained in the yolk actually helps lower cholesterol levels.

For those who still feel skeptical about eating whole eggs regularly, simply eliminate some of the yolks when you make omelets or scrambled eggs.

Alternatives: Deep-sea fish, lean red meat

> "Your mom was right – you don't get any dessert until you eat your vegetables! Many kids (and even some adults) turn their noses up at the very sight of broccoli. From a health standpoint, this aversion is too bad as broccoli is one of the best power foods out there."

BROCCOLI

Your mom was right – you don't get any dessert until you eat your vegetables! Many kids (and even some adults) turn their noses up at the very sight of broccoli. From a health standpoint, this aversion is too bad, since broccoli is one of the best power foods out there. This green, crunchy vegetable and its close cousins have two major benefits: they are nutrient dense and low in calories. Broccoli is also one of the

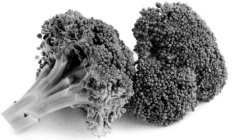

most supreme vegetables because of its excellent nutrient profile and high amount of dietary fiber. Just remember not to steam or boil this source. Both of these cooking methods leech out most of the nutrients and you end up pouring the best part of the vegetable down the drain. Frying is an acceptable way to cook broccoli, but you should use only small amounts of olive or canola oil when doing so to limit the fat content.

Alternatives: Spinach, asparagus

CHICKEN BREAST

While this barnyard bird may look a bit odd, chickens have given iron pumpers two outstanding foods – eggs and lean protein. Chicken meat – especially the breast – is one of the best sources of protein available. One medium-sized

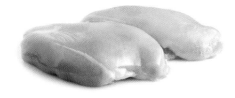

chicken breast contains nearly 40 grams of protein and 180 calories. And with less than 2.5 grams of fat, few other protein foods can match chicken from a health perspective.

Alternatives: Lean turkey breast, goose breast

OATMEAL

Oatmeal is another "mom-recommended" food that should be regularly stocked on your kitchen shelves. Besides being high in fiber, oats are a good source of many nutrients including vitamin E, zinc, selenium, copper, iron, manganese and magnesium. Oats are also an excellent source of complex carbohydrates. The best variety of oatmeal is unprocessed steel-cut oats, which provide 4 grams of fiber per serving – the only downside is they

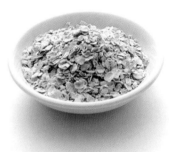

take longer to prepare. Instant oats are cut finer so they cook faster, but that manufacturing process strips away some of the fiber content so you only end up getting approximately 2 to 3 grams per serving. If you're really pressed for time, however, microwave-ready oatmeal is still a good source of whole grains. For example, Quaker Take Heart Instant Oatmeal is fortified with 6 grams of fiber, omega-3 fats, and vitamins C, E and B-vitamins.

Alternatives: Yams, brown rice, brown pasta

"Chicken breasts, tuna, sweet potatoes ... most serious bodybuilders know the importance of these staples in a healthy diet. Bodybuilding nutrition is much more vast, though, and numerous other foods are just as integral for building quality muscle mass."

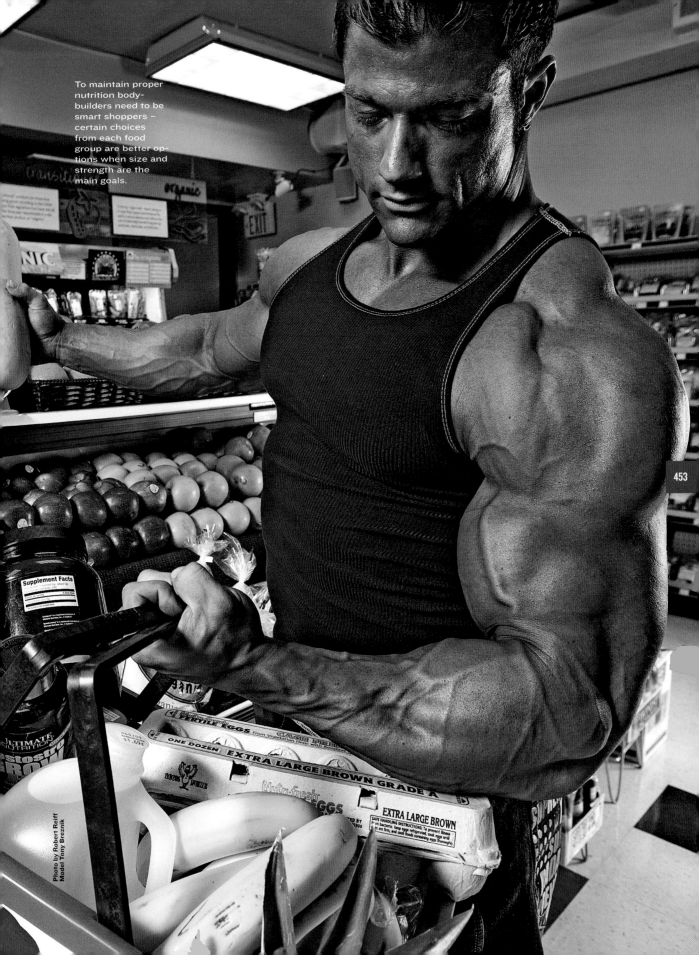

To maintain proper nutrition body-builders need to be smart shoppers – certain choices from each food group are better options when size and strength are the main goals.

453

BODYBUILDING'S TOP POWER SUPPLEMENTS

454

Now that we've looked at some of the best foods for enhancing muscular growth and overall health, it's time to cover the other half of the nutrition equation: the best supplements to add to your gym bag or pantry shelves. Note that all of the supplements we'll discuss have been addressed earlier in the book. This chapter in effect is a "best-of" guide to what's currently out there, based on both anecdotal and scientific evidence. One of the most efficient ways to judge a supplement's merits is to see how long it has been on the market. Supplements that arrive with explosive fanfare and then disappear after a year or two likely do so for a reason. Conversely, specific products like protein have withstood the test of time among athletes because they do in fact work. Similarly, creatine is entering its second decade of use and seems to have become a mainstay among bodybuilders.

Now, be warned that taking copious amounts of the following substances is not a substitute for serious training and sound nutrition. No amount of creatine or glutamine will help you if you sit on your ass all day eating chips and chocolate bars. But provided you follow an intelligent training routine and eat healthy, these supplements will help you more quickly reach your muscle-building goals.

The following forms of supplements are our recommendations (in no particular order).

PROTEIN POWDER

Protein powder has been a staple in bodybuilding diets since the 1940s. And admittedly, while we said this list isn't ranked in any way, few could argue that protein should place at or near the top of your supplement arsenal. Protein is the body's primary building material and if you don't get enough of this key nutrient in your diet, you won't make

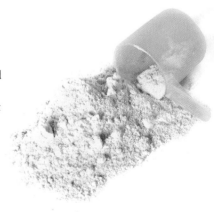

the size and strength gains you desire. Although the "best" amount to consume is still debated, the consensus is that bodybuilders need 1 to 2 grams per pound of bodyweight each day. If you use the median (1.5 grams), a 200-pound individual would need about 300 grams per day. With a can of the old standby – tuna – which supplies about 30 grams, that means you'd need 10 tins to meet your daily protein requirements. Even if you included whole-food protein sources, that's a lot of preparing and chewing. Protein powders are a simple alternative because they're easy to mix and quick to drink. As we discussed earlier in the book, there are four general categories of protein: whey, casein, egg, and soy. Whey and casein are the purest. Whey is rapidly absorbed and thus makes a great pre- and post-workout supplement. Casein is better used just before bed since it absorbs much more slowly and will ensure a steady stream of amino acids in your system over the course of the night. Egg proteins are nearly as pure as whey and casein and make good substitutes. Keep in mind, however, that whey is just as cheap and mixes more easily, so it might be a better option than egg supplements. Soy, while being less pure, offers the health benefits of lowering cholesterol and boosting your immune system. If you're having trouble deciding which type is right for you, do like many bodybuilders and combine both whey and soy in a three-to-one ratio.

> "One of the most efficient ways to judge a supplement's merits is to see how long it has been on the market. Supplements that arrive with explosive fanfare and then disappear after a year or two likely do so for a reason. Conversely, specific products like protein have withstood the test of time among athletes because they do in fact work."

CREATINE

Since its first introduction over 15 years ago, creatine has vaulted to and stayed at the top of supplement best-seller lists. Unlike many muscle-building products that have come and gone over the years, creatine has solid anecdotal and scientific evidence to back it up. As of this publication, hundreds of university-based studies have been done to investigate

creatine for both safety and performance-boosting effects. What they've found is that creatine works in a number of ways. For starters, it increases the body's ATP-regenerating abilities. ATP is the body's primary short-term energy source and the more of it you have, the harder you can train. This organic acid also causes the muscles to hold water, and while most of it is lost after supplement use is stopped, the five to 10 pounds of increased bodyweight is greatly welcomed by those who have been stuck at the same weight for months, if not years. Finally, there is some evidence to suggest that creatine is anabolic in nature. This means it stimulates protein synthesis and hence the growth of new muscle tissue.

> "From energy production and oxygen transport to protein synthesis and hormone production, vitamins and minerals are absolutely vital. You may think you're getting enough from the foods in your diet, but unless you buy only organic and eat all your fruits and veggies raw, you're likely not."

L-GLUTAMINE

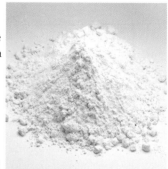

While protein supplements supply the full amino-acid profile, there are a few aminos that should be taken in higher dosages. Glutamine is one such example because it is what's called a "conditionally" essential amino acid. Under certain conditions, the body can't manufacture enough of it and one of these states just happens to be exercise-induced stress. Glutamine helps keep the body in positive nitrogen balance – the environment necessary for maximizing protein synthesis. This amino acid is also central to boosting the immune system. When athletes border on, or slip into, an overtrained state they often catch just about every cold that's going around because their immune systems are weakened. Glutamine supplementation is an easy way to help offset this.

MULTIVITAMIN/MINERAL

In the company of other powerful supplements like creatine and protein powder, multivitamins and minerals may seem pretty basic, but they are in fact key components of muscle-building success. Every metabolic reaction that takes place in your body requires the presence of vitamins and/or minerals. From energy production and oxygen transport to protein synthesis and hormone production, vitamins and minerals are absolutely vital. You may think you're getting enough from the foods in your diet, but 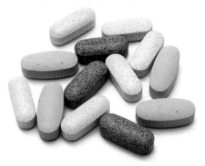 unless you buy only organic and eat all your fruits and veggies raw, you're likely not. There are also environmental factors to consider, such as air pollution, which negatively affect vitamin and mineral absorption in the body. Taking a multivitamin/mineral tablet is an inexpensive way to cover all your bases and protect yourself from all of these health threats. And at about $10 for a month's supply, these pills are also among the cheapest.

ESSENTIAL FATTY ACIDS

Just about every bodybuilder knows that protein is needed for muscle growth and repair, but so is fat – the healthy kind. While the vast majority of bodybuilders of the '50s and early '60s didn't use steroids, they did focus on eating a lot of muscle-building foods such as whole milk, eggs, red meat and nuts. All these sources are loaded with healthy fats. Modern bodybuilders on the other hand try to keep their fat intake to a bare minimum and favor eating such low-fat or fat-free foods as egg whites, chicken breasts, sweet potatoes and oatmeal. While this approach is good practice for avoiding unhealthy fats, it also elim-

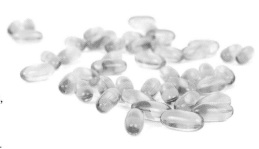

inates the fats that are beneficial for promoting muscle development. An easy way to ensure you're getting an adequate amount of these fats is to include flaxseed oil, fish oil and seal oil (each of which also come in capsule form).

MEAL-REPLACEMENT POWDERS – MRPS

Although these products overlap somewhat with protein powders, meal-replacement powders (MRPs) offer added benefits because they also contain healthy fats, complex carbs, and vitamins and minerals. Like protein powders, MRPs are quick and easy to prepare and drink. Each serving is complete with all the nutrients you need to boost recovery and keep your body and its various systems running efficiently.

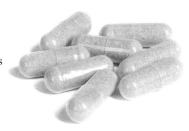

GLUCOSAMINE

Joint pain is probably the last concern on the minds of readers in their teens or early '20s – after all, you're indestructible, right? Don't be so sure. If regular weight training has one negative attribute it's that it can play havoc with your joints down the road. Ask just about any bodybuilder in his 30s or 40s and you'll quickly find out how fragile the human body really is. Most guys in this age group have one or more joints that "talk" to them on a regular basis – shoulders, elbows, knees and the lower back are especially vocal in expressing their displeas-

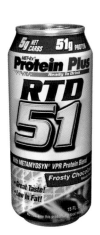

ure with the regular pounding endured over the years. While using good technique on all your exercises and resisting the urge to max out during every single workout is a key factor to preventing injuries, you should also take a quality glucosamine supplement to reduce inflammation, rebuild connective tissue and keep your joints lubricated. When you start including this amino, however, don't expect any overnight miracle cures. It usually takes glucosamine a couple of months to make a noticeable difference. But if your goal is to be lifting pain-free into your 30s, 40s and beyond, glucosamine needs to be a mainstay supplement in your arsenal.

THE ECA STACK

We know we'll get some flack for recommending an ECA stack, but hear us out. Prior to media inflation of the dangers of ephedrine, and the subsequent restriction on the substance, ephedrine (along with caffeine and aspirin) was considered the most effective over-the-counter fat-loss product available. Millions of bodybuilders and other athletes of that generation used it to shed bodyfat and boost performance. It was also the primary ingredient in a vast number of mass-market fat-loss products. When the standard dosage of 25 milligrams of ephedrine was combined with 200 milligrams of caffeine and one aspirin, users had the makings of one powerful fat burner. Virtually everyone who used it shed bodyfat – and you still can. While ephedrine is no longer available in 25-milligram tablets, it is legally available as ephedra, the herbal form, in 8-milligram tablets. By taking three tablets, you would essentially match the same dosage as the old ephedrine tablet. As for safety, unless you have a history of heart disease or stroke, or unless you decide to mega dose, odds are favorable that you won't experience any negative side effects. However, do your own research and make your own informed decision regarding its use.

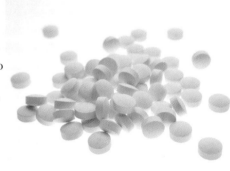

> "When you start including this amino, however, don't expect any overnight miracle cures. It usually takes glucosamine a couple of months to make a noticeable difference. But if your goal is to be lifting pain-free into your 30s, 40s and beyond, glucosamine needs to be a mainstay supplement in your arsenal."

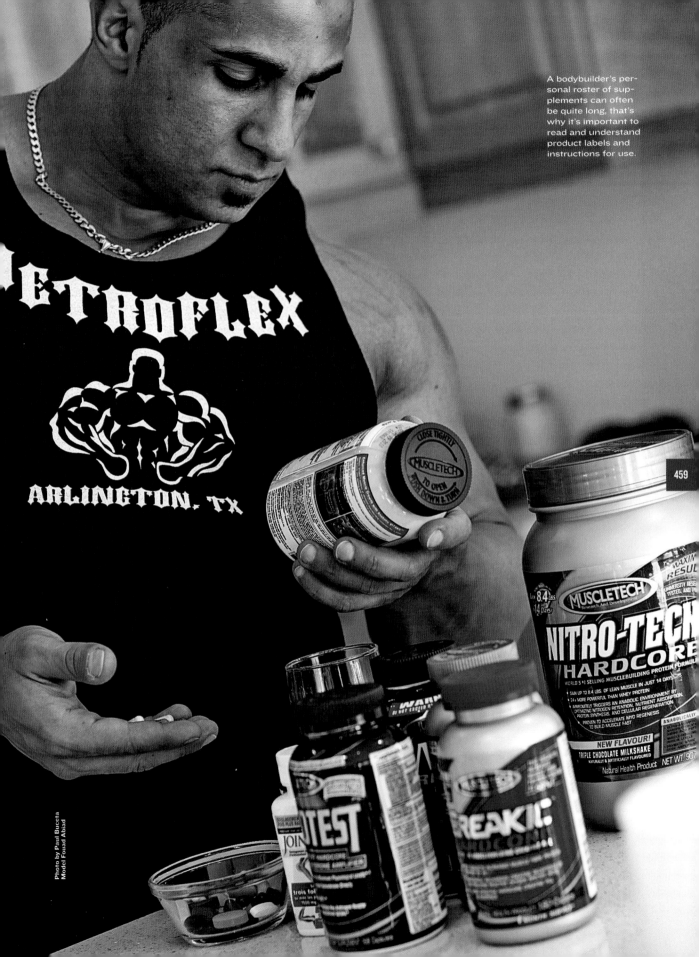

A bodybuilder's personal roster of supplements can often be quite long, that's why it's important to read and understand product labels and instructions for use.

459

THE ANABOLIC WORKOUT

Even though the bulk of the information in this book is geared toward supplements and drugs, there's an entirely separate facet of bodybuilding that focuses on using training as a means to naturally boost the body's various anabolic hormones. You may alternate training styles to optimize strength, size and conditioning, but it's also possible to modify your training to maximize the output of muscle-building hormones such as growth hormone (GH), testosterone and insulin. Of course, when incorporating this approach timing is crucial, and to build muscle, lose fat and increase muscle you'll also need to modify your eating and training habits to ensure you're maximizing your body's internal anabolic environment.

NOT JUST GH

Most of the discussions on using training techniques to stimulate anabolic hormone release have primarily focused on growth hormone, but GH is just one of the major players with regards to muscle hypertrophy. The exercise modifications that boost GH levels also have a dramatic impact on other muscle- and fat-burning hormones like insulin, testosterone and thyroxine.

ANABOLIC POWER!

Before we dive into the details of the routine that will maximize your various anabolic hormone levels, we first need to give you an overview of the exact hormones that are at work when you train. As most readers are probably aware, each hormone has a specific function and associated receptors. At a basic biochemical understanding, the higher the concentration of hormones and the more receptor sites available, the more likely that the hormone will produce its particular actions.

The body's primary muscle-building hormones react to high amounts of stress, so if you're not training with a sufficient degree of intensity, you won't maximize your chances to increase hormone production. For those who love the challenge of training hard, that effort will pay off as hormone levels and the rate of receptor binding will ele-

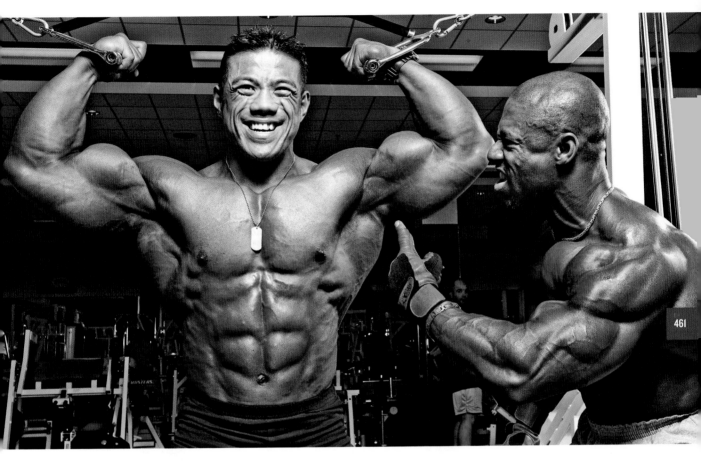

Photo by Kevin Horton
Model Ray Arde and Tricky Jackson

ABOVE: Building a strong, lean, symmetrical physique demands proper training – challenging the body with hard intense workouts will spark muscle-building hormones.

vate with time. Those who've been hitting the iron for years with focus and drive will reap the benefits of incredible hormone production and receptor binding. Hence, tailoring your training is a highly effective method to boost hormone generating and promote binding to the appropriate receptors.

When it comes to building muscle size and strength, the primary helper in the hormone department is testosterone, as it responds directly to high-intensity resistance training. If testosterone is No. 1 in this regard, GH is a close second. Research has shown that moderate-to high-intensity, high-volume exercise involving short rest intervals promotes maximum GH output. Insulin is another hormone that serves numerous purposes in the body. First, it's vital to the process of regulating blood sugar levels, which in turn promotes the uptake of protein for conversion into muscle tissue. Second, during exercise insulin levels decrease, and the hormone itself becomes hypersensitive in response. Therefore, if you consume a high-protein meal along with a simple sugar immediately after your workout, the increased sensitivity of insulin will improve glucose uptake to promote protein synthesis and faster recovery. Also, thyroxine helps to prime your arousal state and also contributes to regulating your metabolic rate.

PUTTING IT ALL TOGETHER

To maximize your hormone output via training adjustments and modifications, a number of factors must be considered:

Workout Volume

Research on the relationship between training intensity and hormone production indicates that the more volume the better – but only up to a certain point. Your workouts must not be so long that your recovery abilities are exceeded. The workout included at the end of this chapter, the "Hormone-Boosting Workout," is designed for beginner and intermediate lifters. Advanced trainers should add 1 or 2 sets to each exercise listed.

Exercise Variety

Although the best exercises for stimulating hormone release are compound movements involving the larger muscle groups (i.e., legs, back, chest), you still need to incorporate exercises for the smaller muscles to keep your physique balanced and in proportion.

BELOW: To produce more GH, testosterone, insulin and thyroxine, workouts must be high volume involving both compound and single-joint moves, using varying reps-and-sets schemes.

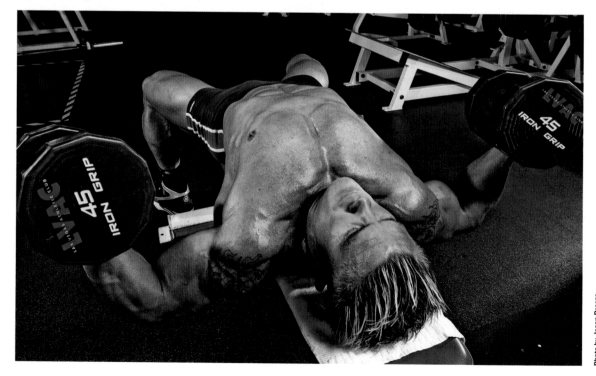

Photo by Jason Breeze
Model Andy Hammond

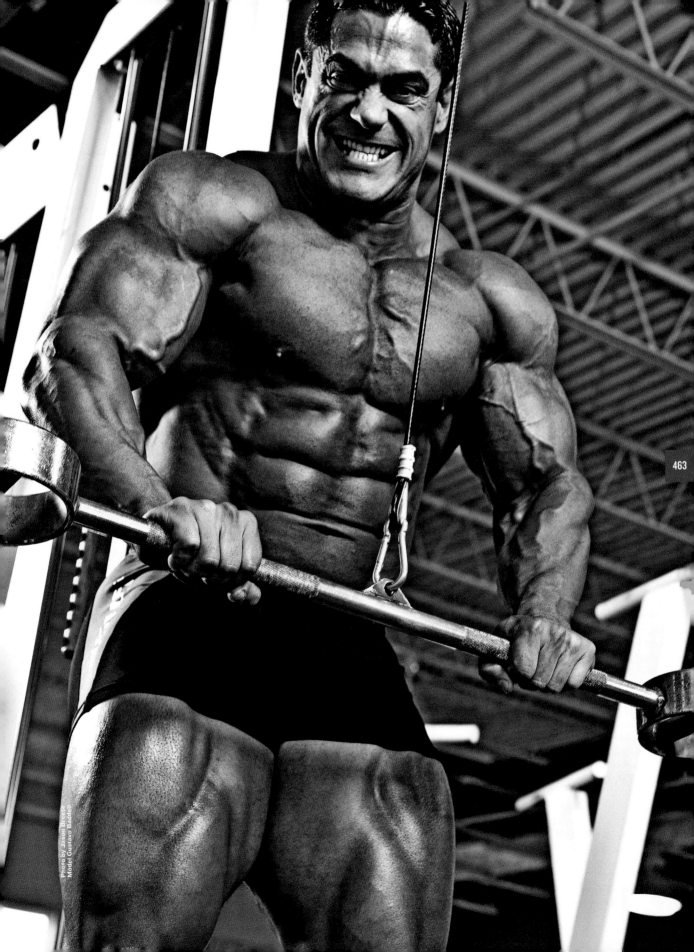

463

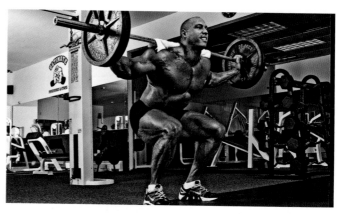

Legs – Once is Enough

Even though you'll be hitting your legs just once per week, trust us, you'll be hitting them hard. So, those few extra days of recovery will be much needed.

Odds and Evens

You'll follow the same workout during weeks 1, 3 and 5, and you'll perform a different training regimen during weeks 2, 4 and 6. The routines vary in a number of ways including exercises, reps, sets and rest schemes. The cycling of reps throughout helps keep your muscles guessing and places stress on different fiber types to prevent stagnation.

During the odd weeks (1, 3 and 5) you'll be using slightly lighter weight for higher reps (10–12), resting 60 to 90 seconds between sets. On the even weeks (2, 4 and 6) you'll use heavier weight for 6–8 reps with upward of two-minute rest periods between sets.

Advanced Techniques

Feel free to incorporate advanced training techniques such as drop sets, rest-pause, forced reps, pre-exhaustion, etc., whenever possible. Doing so will add variety, enable you to push past muscle failure and really force your body to rev up hormone production.

Anabolic Hormone Summary

Hormone	Primary anabolic actions
HGH	Increases fat metabolism and protein synthesis
Thyroxine	Regulates cell growth and overall metabolism
Insulin	Regulates blood glucose levels and protein synthesis
Testosterone	Increases protein synthesis

HORMONE-BOOSTING WORKOUT

This six-week program follows a two-days-on/one-day-off, then two-days-on/two-days-off pattern.

Photo by Jason Breeze
Model Sean Allan

Weeks 1, 3 & 5
Day 1: Chest, Shoulders, Calves

Exercise	Sets	Reps
Wide-Grip Bench Press	3–4	10–12
Incline Dumbell Flye	3–4	10–12
Cable Crossover	3–4	10–12
Smith-Machine Shoulder Press	3–4	10–12
Front Dumbell Raise	3–4	10–12
Bent-Over Raise	3–4	10–12
Standing Calf Raise	3–4	10–12

Day 2: Back, Traps, Abs

Exercise	Sets	Reps
Seated Cable Row	3–4	10–12
Reverse-Grip Pulldown	3–4	10–12
Front Pulldown	3–4	10–12
EZ-Bar Cable Upright Row	3–4	10–12
Dumbell Shrug	3–4	10–12
Crunch	3–4	10–12
Twisting Cable Crunch	3–4	10–12

Day 3: Off

Day 4: Legs

Exercise	Sets	Reps
Squat	3–4	10–12
Leg Press	3–4	10–12
Romanian Deadlift	3–4	10–12
Split Squat	3–4	10–12
Leg Extension	3–4	10–12
Glute/Ham Raise	3–4	10–12
Back Extension	3–4	10–12

Day 5: Arms, Abs

Exercise	Sets	Reps
Parallel Bar Dip	3–4	10–12
Skullcrusher	3–4	10–12
Triceps Pressdown	3–4	10–12
Standing Barbell Curl	3–4	10–12
Barbell Preacher Curl	3–4	10–12
Seated Dumbell Curl	3–4	10–12
Crunch	3–4	10–12
Twisting Cable Crunch	3–4	10–12

Days 6 & 7: Off

"Although the best exercises for stimulating hormone release are compound movements involving the larger muscle groups (i.e., legs, back, chest), you still need to incorporate exercises for the smaller muscles to keep your physique balanced and in proportion."

465

Weeks 2, 4 & 6
Day 1: Chest, Shoulders, Calves

Exercise	Sets	Reps
Incline Bench Press	4–5	6–8
Flat Dumbell Flye	4–5	6–8
Weighted Push-Up	4–5	6–8
Dumbell Press	4–5	6–8
Front Cable Raise	4–5	6–8
Bent-Over Raise	4–5	6–8
Seated Calf Raise	4–5	6–8
Standing Calf Raise	4–5	6–8

Day 2: Back, Traps, Abs

Exercise	Sets	Reps
Weighted Pull-Up	4–5	6–8
Front Pulldown	4–5	6–8
Dumbell Pullover	4–5	6–8
Barbell Shrug	4–5	6–8
Barbell Upright Row	4–5	6–8
Cable Crunch	4–5	6–8
Twisting Crunch	4–5	6–8

Day 3: Off

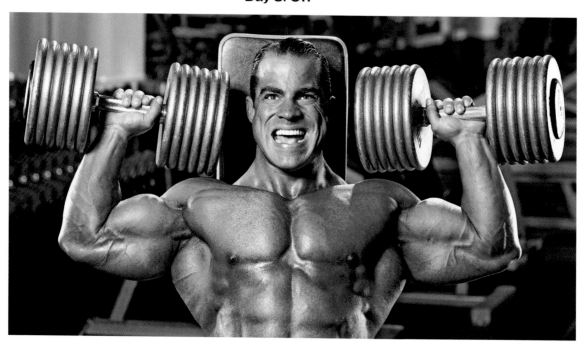

Photo by Robert Reiff
Model Mark Dugdale

Day 4: Legs

Exercise	Sets	Reps
Squat	4–5	6–8
Leg Press	4–5	6–8
Hack Squat	4–5	6–8
Walking Lunge	4–5	6–8
Leg Extension	4–5	6–8
Lying Leg Curl	4–5	6–8
Back Extension	4–5	6–8

Day 5: Arms, Abs

Exercise	Sets	Reps
Weighted Dip	4–5	6–8
Skullcrusher	4–5	6–8
Rope Pushdown	4–5	6–8
EZ-Bar Curl	4–5	6–8
Dumbell Preacher Curl	4–5	6–8
Standing Dumbell Curl	4–5	6–8
Cable Crunch	4–5	6–8
Twisting Crunch	4–5	6–8

Days 6 & 7: Off

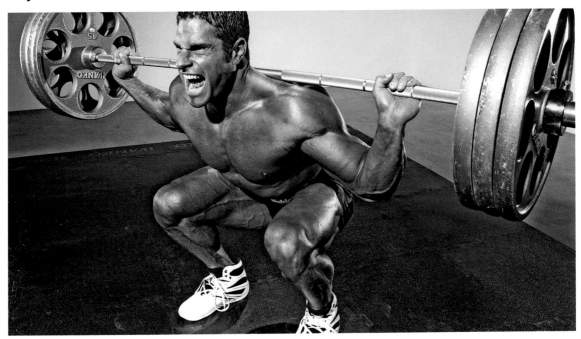

Photo by Robert Reiff
Model David Hoffman

PRE-CONTEST PREPARATIONS WITH THE SUPERSTARS

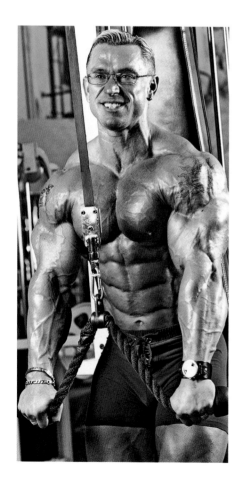

When it comes to "putting it all together" for a competition, the true experts are the top bodybuilding pros. To give you an idea of how our sport's superstars show up on contest day shredded and as big as a house, we present a few samples of their pre-contest training, dieting and supplementing regimens.

LEE PRIEST

Lee Priest has heard it all. Throughout his pro career he's been the target of a rumor mill that has spun wildly out of control. Reports of illness, retirement and physical and professional death, coupled with accusations such as, "He'll never be in shape, he's way too fat," have run rampant about Lee. But as Mark Twain once said, "Reports of my death have been greatly exaggerated."

On December 1, 2001 he weighed a whopping 270 pounds and looked more likely to win a pie-eating contest than a professional bodybuilding show. By March 2, 2002 he had transformed himself to a shredded 199 contest-winning pounds to capture his first pro win, defeating Chris Cormier and Dexter Jackson. Lee routinely gains 60 to 70 pounds after a contest and has always possessed the amazing ability to dial it back in for the next show. Nobody knows more about incredible transformations than Lee Priest. So how does he do it? Read on for the no-frills truths about how this Houdini of contest prep works his magic!

Pre-Contest Training

Lee trains on a four-days-on/one-day-off schedule when preparing for a contest, doing two sessions per day:

	a.m.	p.m.
Day 1:	Back	Cardio
Day 2:	Chest	Delts, cardio
Day 3:	Arms	Cardio
Day 4:	Quads	Hams, cardio
Day 5:	Off	Off

Photo by Ralph DeHaan

Note: Lee trains calves every day and then takes a day off whenever he feels it's necessary. With regards to abs, Lee hasn't trained this bodypart regularly for several years.

Lee does about 20 sets per bodypart and as many as 30 total sets for legs. He usually does free-weight exercises for six to eight reps and machine work in the range of eight to 15 reps. During the final two weeks leading up to a competition Lee opts mostly for machine exercises to minimize the risk of injury.

Anyone who has followed bodybuilding for even a short time knows Lee has one of the best sets of arms in the history of the sport. His training for this bodypart can be summed up fairly easily: supersets for super arms, Superman style. "I get an incredible pump throughout the entire arm by supersetting, and the results speak for themselves," he says. He usually does four exercises with five sets of each, totaling 20 sets for biceps and 20 for triceps, resting one to two minutes after each superset.

Biceps	Sets	Reps
Seated Alternating Dumbell Curl	5	6–8
Incline Alternating Dumbell Curl	5	6–8
Standing Straight-Bar Curl	5	6–8
Incline Side Dumbell Curl	5	6–8

Triceps	Sets	Reps
Pushdown	5	8–15
Rope Cable Extension	5	8–15
Dumbell Kickback	5	8–15
One-Arm Cable Extension	5	8–15

Lee's off-season training differs from his pre-contest approach only in that he trains each bodypart once a week, instead of following the four-days-on/one-day-off schedule. He trains Mondays through Fridays on and takes weekends off.

Monday: Back
Tuesday: Chest
Wednesday: Delts
Thursday: Arms
Friday: Legs
Saturday/Sunday: Off

Cardio

Although his weight training doesn't change much, Lee's cardio goes from zero to 60 in a hurry. Off-season, his total time spent doing cardio is ... zero minutes. Pre-contest, he begins cardio by doing 30 to 40

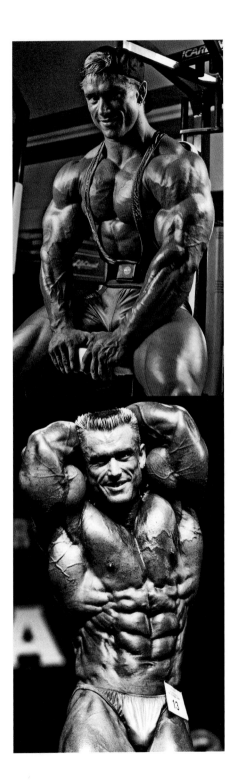

469

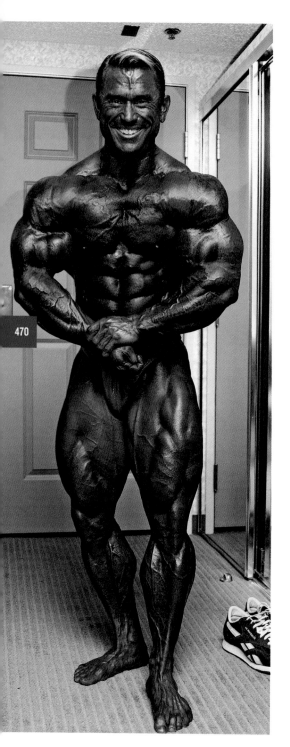

470

minutes a day on the stationary bike for the first two weeks. Then the real fun begins. Lee's regimen bumps up to sessions lasting 40 to 60 minutes, twice a day, seven days a week. He knocks out the first bout on an empty stomach soon after waking in the morning and does the second session following his p.m. workout in the late afternoon.

Pre-Contest Nutrition and Supplementation

Meal 1: (after cardio)
65–80 grams protein powder
¼–½ cup Cream of Rice (dry measurement)

Meal 2:
8–12 oz. New York strip steak (precooked weight)
1–2 cups white rice (cooked measurement)

Meal 3:
9 oz. chicken breast (cooked weight)
½ cup white rice (cooked measurement)
1–2 cups green vegetables

Meal 4:
Same as Meal 1*

Meal 5:
9 oz. chicken breast (cooked weight)
1–2 cups of green vegetables

Meal 6:
65–80 grams protein powder
¼ cup cream of rice (dry measurement)**

*Lee often substitutes 2 cups of egg whites and a half-cup of oats for this meal. However, he has a unique way of cooking it: He mixes the egg whites and oats in a blender and then cooks the mixture in a non-stick frying pan lightly coated with cooking spray. The recipe yields about 12 thin crepes.
**Lee eats the Cream of Rice with this meal only on nights when he feels very hungry.

You may notice that several of Lee's meals include a range for the amounts of rice, protein or cream of rice he eats. In this respect, he applies an instinctive approach to his dieting, listening to his body and checking his condition. "I won my first three bodybuilding shows when I was 13 years old," he says. "I've been doing pre-contest

Photos by Raymond Cassar

diets for quite a few years. I've learned a lot over that time and I trust my experience."

Notes:

– Lee does cardio on an empty stomach and eats his first meal after session No. 1.

– He avoids cheat meals until the contest is over. "I love to eat," he admits, "so in the off-season I allow myself a lot more freedom with food. Once I hit the pre-contest switch, though, all that changes. I don't want to remember how good the fun food tastes in comparison to my diet food. That memory can make returning to a diet very difficult. I'd rather just eat the same food every day and not have to think about it."

– He eats every 2½ to 3 hours and drinks 1½ gallons of water per day.

Pre-Contest Supplement List

– Multivitamin/multimineral
– Vitamin C
– Vitamin E
– CLA
– Coenzyme Q10
– BCAAs
– Fat burner
– Glutamine
– Whey protein powder or egg protein

The Last Week

(This schedule assumes a Friday night prejudging)

Food Intake

During the critical last week before the competition, Lee makes very few changes. "I don't believe in carb depleting and loading or messing with sodium too much," he says. "The day before the show I have some extra carbs, but that's about the only change I make. I always look great a week or two out, so why mess with a plan that works?"

Water Intake

Lee does manipulate his water intake to achieve that dry, grainy look. He makes sure to take in 1 to 1½ gallons of water every day in the final week up to and including Thursday. On the Friday he stops drinking at noon and only sips small amounts of water when he absolutely needs it right up until showtime.

Training and Cardio

In the week leading up to a contest, Lee does his final leg workout on Sunday. He follows his regular upper-body schedule until Thursday,

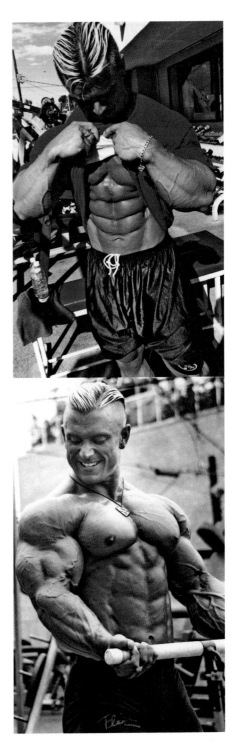

471

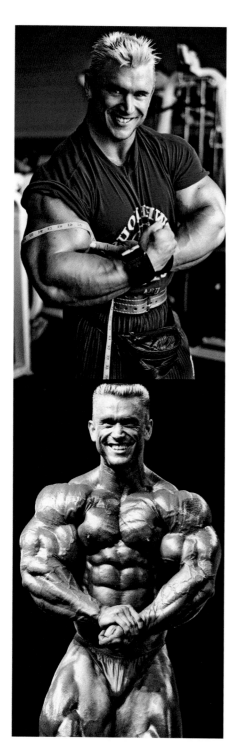

472

in which he trains his entire upper body with about six sets per muscle group. Unlike many athletes, Lee still does two hours of cardio right up to and including the Thursday before a show and an hour of cardio on the Friday. He explains: "If I look great, I don't like to change anything. I think your body gets in a certain rhythm and I don't want to disturb that."

The Finishing Touches
Posing

Lee feels that posing – make that hard posing – brings out more detail and hardness in the muscle, but he doesn't like to practice much at home. "I hate spending a lot of time looking at myself before a show because I always feel I could look better," he explains. "Plus, there's no way I'm going to pose hard enough to make a big difference. My strategy is to set up a lot of photo shoots during the three weeks before. Trust me – after a five- or six-hour shoot I'm sore the next day and I look harder."

Tanning

Lee starts tanning about a month out, hitting the tanning bed every other day. The week of the competition he starts applying Jan Tana coloring on Wednesday – he applies two coats per day on Wednesday, Thursday and Friday, and takes his last pre-contest shower on Friday morning. After the prejudging he showers and applies another coat.

Backstage

Lee pumps up more than just about any other pro. He says: "I get really bored sitting around back there and I like to keep busy. I pump up for about 20 to 30 minutes, doing a combination of push-ups and various movements with bands for my entire upper body. I've always found that the longer I pump up for, the better I look. Plus, it keeps me warm. Once I start getting a pump, I don't want to lose it." Lee also doesn't pose backstage or check himself in the mirror much. "If you're not ready by then," he says, "looking in the mirror isn't going to help. And, if you're not happy with what you see you're probably going to walk onstage depressed, and that's not what you want to project to the judges." Lee opts for Jan Tana posing oil to highlight his hard-earned muscularity onstage.

Flying

He doesn't do anything special to control his water level when flying to a contest. "I've never really had a problem in that regard," he states. "I just eat my normal food on my regular schedule and try to keep my fluids up to offset any dehydration from the flight. In fact, I'm fine to fly in even the day before a contest. My bigger concern

Photos by Jason Mathas and Alex Ardenti

when I arrive is making sure I have everything I need and that the room is in order! Besides, if I arrive too early there isn't anything to do and I start looking at restaurant menus, and that's not good!"

Lee's Tip
After he starts his pre-contest phase, Lee doesn't step on the scale. "The judges don't have scales to help them decide the winner. Weight just doesn't matter."

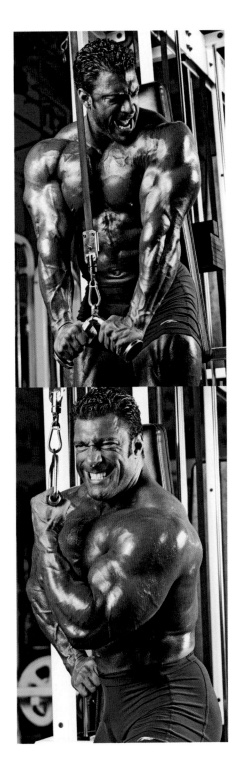

BOB CICHERILLO
Pre-Contest Training
When preparing for a contest, Bob trains six days a week using the following schedule:

Day 1: Chest
Day 2: Back
Day 3: Legs
Day 4: Delts
Day 5: Bi's
Day 6: Tri's
Day 7: Off
Calves: Once per week
Abs: Twice per week

Bob does 12 to 15 total sets of 12 to 15 reps for each bodypart, and keeps his training generally the same year round until a contest approaches. "With the exception of abs, I hit each bodypart once a week year round," he explains. "I eliminate heavy leg work one month out from a show, and during last three weeks I cut the number of sets for every bodypart so I don't overtrain or create a greater risk of injury."

While Bob prides himself on overall symmetry and a classic X-frame physique, he considers his chest to be his best bodypart. Here's the pre-contest routine he uses for chest:

Exercise	Sets	Reps
Flat Hammer-Machine Bench Press	3	12–15
Incline Smith-Machine Press	3	12–15
Incline Dumbell Flye	3	12–15
Pec-Deck	3	12–15
Dip/Cable Crossover	3	12–15

Photos by Alex Ardenti

473

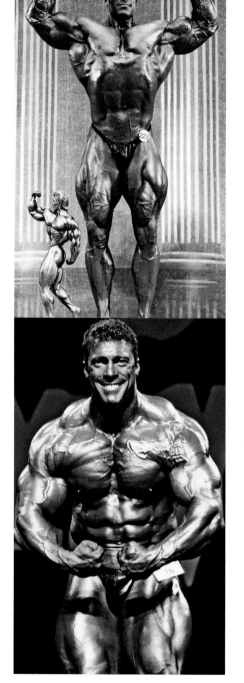

474

Cardio

Bob does not do any cardio in the off-season and doesn't have a pre-set point when he starts. "I generally begin 12 to 14 weeks out," he says, "but you have to be flexible according to your condition at the time. How much you do is always going to depend on how far out of shape you get in the off-season."

Once his cardio commences, Bob starts with one daily session of 20 to 25 minutes on each of his six training days. He then builds up by adding five minutes per session each week. When he reaches 45 to 60 minutes, Bob splits his cardio into two daily sessions. During the last four or five weeks out he does cardio twice a day – an hour each time. Having been criticized in the past for glutes that didn't look hard enough, he prefers the Stepmill and the treadmill. "I can target my glutes on those machines while getting my cardio done," says Bob. "When I do the treadmill, I set it on a high incline, usually 12 percent, and the speed is 3 or 3.1 miles per hour. I don't hold onto the machine either. When I am doing a lot of cardio, I also do some of it on the bike."

Pre-Contest Nutrition and Supplementation

Meal 1:
12 oz. flank steak or 20 egg whites
1 ½ cups oatmeal

Meal 2:
12 oz. chicken
2 cups white rice

Meal 3:
10–12 oz. chicken
10 oz. baked potato

Meal 4:
80 grams protein powder (GNC Pro Performance)
1 cup oatmeal

Meal 5:
12 oz. steak
8–10 oz. baked potato

Meal 6:
80 grams protein powder

Photos by Jim Amentler

Notes:

– Bob weighs his whole-food proteins after cooking and his carbs before cooking.

– He is a big believer in taking a cheat day while dieting. "On my non-training day I eat anything I want while I prepare for a contest. I find the cheat day stimulates my metabolism and provides some psychological relief from the pressures and restrictions of dieting. I really think your body needs and benefits from it."

– He eats every three hours while dieting and usually likes to get two meals in before training. Bob eats his pre-workout meal at least one and a half hours before training and then eats his third meal right after leaving the gym. During the off-season he eats less frequently, consuming only about four meals per day. "My appetite just isn't as big because I'm not doing any cardio," he explains. When it comes to cooking, Bob recommends using a George Foreman Grill for easy food prep and a lot of hot sauce for taste!

Pre-Contest Supplement List

– Whey protein
– L-glutamine
– Glucosamine-chondroitin complex

The Last Week
Food Intake
Sunday through Tuesday

Bob takes in 200 grams of carbs per day and keeps his protein consumption consistent.

Wednesday

He describes his carb intake on this day as "huge." Bob says: "I can't really estimate a number because it varies from show to show depending on how I'm filling up and how I look. But Wednesday is always the highest carb day of the load."

Thursday, Friday, Saturday

To prevent water retention, Bob tapers his carbs as showtime gets closer. In the final 24 hours he leans more toward simple carbs, but not sugar. He instead opts for products like apple-pie filling, dates and dried fruit. On the morning of the competition he eats a 12-ounce steak and 12-ounce potato at 8 a.m. Every hour afterward, he takes in a handful of simple carbs like dried fruit or sugar-free all-fruit jelly. The simple carbs help to add fullness and some hardness, but no drastic changes occur at this state. "If you are worried about carbing up two hours before the show, you should have started earlier," he declares. "Too much at this stage will only bloat and distend the stom-

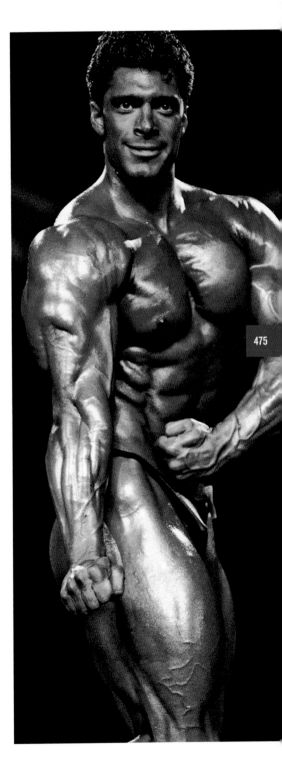

475

Photo by Ralph DeHaan

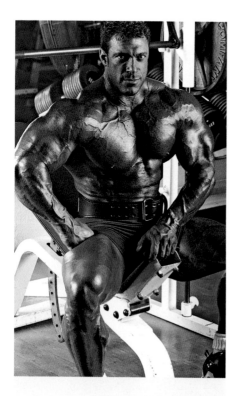

ach when you are trying to keep it as flat as possible. About an hour before the noon prejudging I stop eating, except maybe some chocolate right before I pump up."

Water Intake

Leading up to a contest, Bob drinks about two to three gallons of water every day. This quantity stays constant up to and including the final Thursday. Bob warns, "You have to be very careful not to taper your water too early or you'll go flat and smooth out." On the Friday he takes in about half of what he normally drinks (about one to one and a half gallons). He usually stops his water intake between 6 and 11 p.m. on the Friday night, depending on how he looks.

On contest day he sips small amounts of water. "A lot of guys don't realize that water transports the food and carbs," says Bob. "If you don't drink anything, the food just sits in the stomach, where it does nothing for you."

Training and Cardio

Bob stops doing cardio one week out. He explains: "My metabolism is flying at this point, and when it gets too fast I can't effectively carb up. In the past I would continue with cardio until a few days before the show and my weight would go down as I was carbing up. It was like putting fuel on the fire." Bob does his final leg workout a full two weeks out to allow for his cuts to show through come contest time. As for his upper body, Bob feels very strongly that training after the Tuesday or Wednesday is a big mistake. "If you train past then, you are carb replenishing, not carb loading. You'll end up flat if you train too close to the competition and you'll have a hell of a time backstage when you try to pump up." Here's the schedule Bob adheres to for that last week:

Sunday: Chest, back
Monday: Arms
Tuesday: Delts

The Finishing Touches
Posing

Bob sees posing as a part of his contest preparation, but he has no particular schedule. "At three or four weeks out I start to pose a lot more, but I don't follow any type of regimen. I have done structured posing prep in the past and I really didn't think it made that much of a difference in my conditioning. I like to get my posing routine ready about three to four months in advance. I practice my routine a lot because I want it to be very fluid and smooth onstage, the opposite of my physique!"

Photos by Ralph DeHaan and Alex Ardenti

Tanning

Bob begins using the tanning bed about a month out to get a good base tan. He starts using Pro Tan two days before a competition and puts on four coats. Backstage he uses Pam spray. "Pam gives more sheen than the oils," states Bob. "They tend to blur your appearance, in my opinion."

Flying

Bob doesn't do anything to control his water when he flies to contests. "I just continue following my program as if I weren't flying out anywhere. I always get to the venue three days before the event. Arriving early ensures my body has time to adjust and makes the flying factor largely irrelevant," he says.

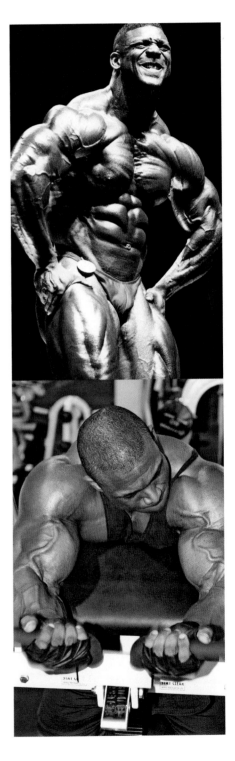

QUINCY TAYLOR
Pre-Contest Training

Quincy trains six days a week when preparing for a contest, but he does not follow a rigid schedule. He tries to train his back, biceps and calves two or three times per week; he feels they are his weak points and thus need to be brought up to par with the rest of his physique. Quincy has a sequence for training his bodyparts, but depending on what his body is telling him, he may postpone the next bodypart he is scheduled to train for a day in order to give his weak areas another session. He takes his rest day either the day before or after he trains quads. In Quincy's training split, abs are listed every day because he does four sets of crunches before every workout as a warm-up. "This is the only ab work I ever do, and I've been doing it this way for years," he says. Here's Quincy's general bodypart rotation that follows a seven-day split:

Day 1: Chest, calves, abs
Day 2: Back, abs
Day 3: Quads, abs
Day 4: Off
Day 5: Biceps, triceps, calves, abs
Day 6: Delts, hamstrings, abs
Day 7: Biceps, calves, abs

Quincy does 14 to 16 working sets per bodypart with the exception of quads, for which he does as many as 20 sets. He generally does eight to 12 reps per set.

Photos by Irvin Gelb and Raymond Cassar

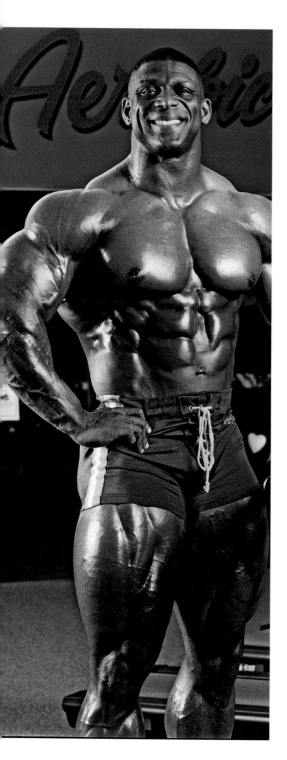

Cardio

During the off-season Quincy does not do any cardio. He starts right into serious cardio when he begins preparing for his contest 16 weeks out; he does two 30-minute sessions per day, the first in the morning on an empty stomach and the second before he goes to bed. At the 12-weeks-out point he increases the length of each session to 45 minutes for a daily total of 90 minutes, which he maintains right into the last week of preparation. Quincy favors three types of cardio equipment: the treadmill, bike and Stepmill. He sets the treadmill to a speed of 3.5 to 4 miles per hour, but does not put it at an incline.

Pre-Contest Nutrition and Supplementation

The following is Quincy's eating regimen when he starts his diet 16 weeks out from the competition.

Meal 1:
4 egg whites
1 egg yolk
8 oz. filet mignon (cooked weight)
1 cup oatmeal (precooked measurement)

Meal 2:
8 oz. filet mignon (cooked weight)
2 cups salad or vegetables

Meal 3:
8 oz. chicken breast (cooked weight)
8 oz. baked potato or yam (cooked weight) – as needed for energy based on how he feels; alternatively, 2 cups salad or vegetables

Meal 4:
8 oz. filet mignon (cooked weight)
2 cups salad or vegetables

Meal 5:
8 oz. filet mignon (cooked weight)
2 cups brown rice
During the day he snacks on cashews if he is hungry. "I probably eat a can of cashews about every two weeks," he says. "My carbs are so low at that point so the added unsaturated fats don't really hurt my condition."

Notes:

– As the weeks go by and he gets leaner, Quincy's hunger level increases and so does his food intake. He ups his meals to six a day,

Photo by Alex Ardenti

adding another serving of steak and vegetables. Some people may wonder why the big man eats most of his carbs with his last meal of the day, before bed. Quincy explains: "If I don't eat carbs with the last meal, I can't sleep. The reason is that simple. If I can't sleep and I don't get the proper rest, I'll never be ready for the show."

– Quincy has a cheat meal, allowing himself whatever he may be craving once per week for the first four weeks of his diet. From the 12-weeks-out point, however, he doesn't deviate from his plan. He eats every two to three hours.

– He drinks two gallons of water every day. "I have to drink a lot," he declares. "In the past I would often get terrible headaches, which I later figured out were caused by dehydration."

– To make his food prep a bit easier, Quincy relies on an outdoor grill. "It's a lot quicker and it makes your food taste better," he says.

Pre-Contest Supplement List
– Multivitamin/multimineral
– Milk thistle
– Vitamin C
– Flaxseed oil (9–10 capsules per day)
– Low-carb protein powder (used when he doesn't feel like eating a whole-food meal)
– Psyllium husk

Quincy feels the psyllium husk supplement is critical to cleanse the body and the colon when he is eating a high quantity of red meat leading up to a show.

The Last Week
Food Intake

Quincy has a rather unusual approach to carb loading in that he makes adjustments to his diet four weeks before the competition. He eats very little carbohydrates when he diets, especially for someone of his size.

When he is four weeks out, Quincy starts eating a medium-sized yam (about 8 ounces, cooked) with every meal. He stops using any protein powder and adds another serving of red meat, often eliminating his chicken meal. He explains: "I'm very close to ready four weeks before the contest. My tendency in the past has been to overdiet, but doing so caused me to come in flat and look softer. When I was in my best shape at the 2001 USAs, I added the carbs a month out and evaluated my hardness. I'm very sensitive to carbs, so if my condition seems to be slipping I cut them back for a few days. I basically work at this adjustment process from the four-weeks-out point right up until the show. I don't carb deplete and load because that approach has always been a crapshoot for me. If I look ready, I don't like to make any drastic changes and risk blowing my chances."

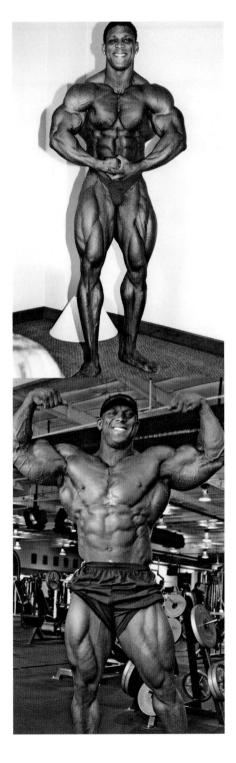

479

Photos by Raymond Cassar

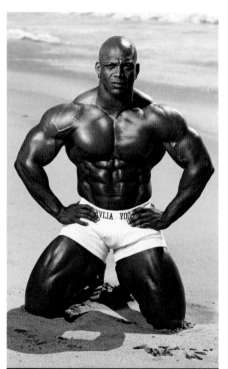

480

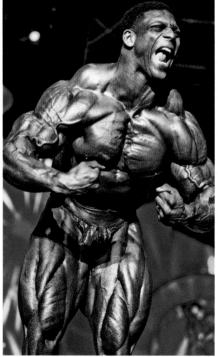

Show Day

In keeping with his "if it ain't broke don't fix it," philosophy, Quincy eats two or three times during the morning – steak and yams or chicken and yams at each meal. He doesn't believe in eating carbs that contain water (e.g., oatmeal, rice) because he is concerned that these foods may cause him to hold water and blur his conditioning onstage.

Water Intake

Unlike many pro competitors, Quincy continues to drink his usual two gallons of water right up to the day before the contest. He does, however, make sure to consume the entire two gallons on Friday by 8 p.m.; he then stops drinking from that point until the prejudging is over. "Every time I cut my water early, I cramp, flatten and look worse. I've come to realize my body needs a lot of fluid and it dries out very quickly," Quincy explains.

Training and Cardio

Quincy stops full leg workouts two weeks out, doing only leg extensions until one week before the contest. At that point he discontinues all leg work. He trains his entire upper body on Monday with three or four lighter sets per bodypart. On Tuesday Quincy repeats this workout in what will probably be his last workout before the show. "On Wednesday I do a lot of posing, but I train only if I really feel I need to."

The Finishing Touches
Posing

Quincy incorporates posing into his contest prep eight weeks out. He practices each of the mandatories five times, holding each one for about 10 seconds. At the four-weeks-out point he does each mandatory pose 10 times. Quincy also prepares and practices his posing routine starting eight weeks before the contest. His posing sessions take place three to five times a week following his afternoon cardio.

"I feel strongly that posing gives you separation and is just as important as all the other aspects of preparation," he states. "You learn how to control and show your muscles, and you condition yourself to pose hard and strong for when you're onstage. By neglecting to practice you do yourself a disservice because you aren't showing the judges the results of all your work."

Tanning

Quincy starts hitting the tanning bed four or five times per week about six weeks before the event. During the last pre-contest week he uses Pro Tan every day, several times per day. "People assume that because I'm black I don't have to do much tanning," he says, "but the stuff just doesn't soak into my skin without a lot of coats."

Photos by Ralph DeHaan and Gary Bartlett

Backstage

Backstage he uses Pam or Muscle Juice. He pumps up by doing two to four sets of push-ups for a total of about 50 reps, followed by four or five sets of biceps curls. He finishes off by hitting each mandatory pose once or twice.

Flying

Quincy tries to consume slightly more water on the plane if he has to take a long flight to the contest. He likes to arrive on the Wednesday before competing to allow his body time to make the proper adjustments and dry out before he has to hit the stage.

SHAWN RAY
Pre-Contest Training

Shawn trains six days a week on a three-days-on/one-day-off schedule when preparing for a contest. Here is the split he uses:

	a.m.	p.m.
Day 1:	Back, calves	Chest
Day 2:	Hams, abs	Quads
Day 3:	Delts, calves	Arms
Day 4:	Off	Off
Day 5:	Repeat Day 1	
Day 6:	Repeat Day 2	
Day 7:	Repeat Day 3	
Day 8:	Off	Off

Cardio

During the off-season, Shawn does not do cardio on a regular schedule. "I'll just do cardio from time to time as the mood strikes me, but not on a structured program." His serious cardio begins 14 weeks out from a contest. He starts with three sessions a week, on Monday, Wednesday and Friday, doing 45 minutes on the treadmill or the Lifecycle®. When using the treadmill, Shawn walks at four miles per hour on a four-percent incline. When he chooses the bike he usually sets it at level three. "I'm not trying to set intensity records when I do cardio. At these settings, I get into a good, even fat-burning range that is challenging but not crazy. I also do all of my cardio between Monday and Friday. I train on the weekend if that's how my three-days-on/one-day-off rotation works out, otherwise I don't do cardio on the weekends."

As the contest gets closer, Shawn makes the following changes to his cardio schedule:

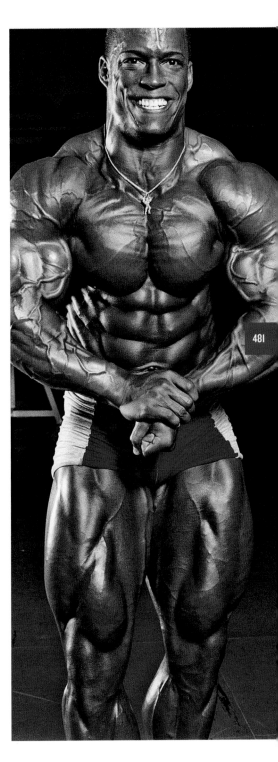

481

Photo by Jim Amentler

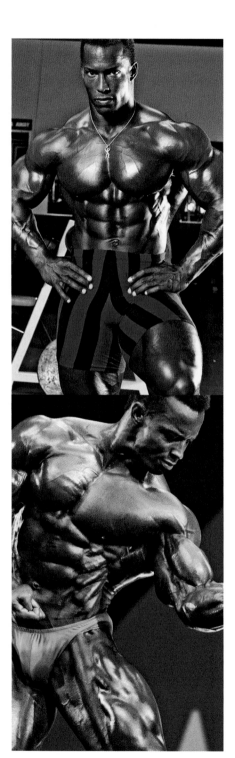

10 weeks out: one session a day, five days a week, 45 minutes each
Eight weeks out: two sessions a day, five days a week, 45 minutes each
Five weeks out: one session a day, four days a week, 45 minutes each
Three weeks out: one session a day, three days a week, 45 minutes each
Last week: no cardio

Shawn does his cardio following his a.m. or p.m. weight training when doing one session a day and after both workouts when double-splitting his cardio. When he is five weeks out, however, he often does the first cardio session at six in the morning. "I can't sleep much once I get to five-weeks-out point, so I'll often knock out the first cardio session, come home, shower and get a meal in, and then go to the gym for my first training session." You'll also notice that Shawn starts to taper his cardio as a competition gets closer. "I believe in being ready early and cutting my cardio as I near a show instead of the opposite like a lot of other bodybuilders do. I see a lot of guys taxing their bodies more and more as the contest approaches, trying to get their conditions right by hurrying the process at the end because they didn't do enough earlier in their prep. These guys usually end up coming in flat or stringy, which is not a winning look."

Pre-Contest Nutrition and Supplementation

Meal 1:
2 New York steaks (approximately 16 oz., precooked measurement)
Broccoli
2 slices watermelon

Meal 2:
12 egg whites
½ cup oatmeal (precooked measurement)

Meal 3:
3 skinless chicken breasts (approximately 10–12 oz., cooked weight)
Asparagus

Meal 4:
3 skinless chicken breasts (approximately 10–12 oz., cooked weight)
Broccoli

Meal 5:
2 New York steaks or lean ground beef (approximately 16 oz., precooked measurement)
½ baked potato
Tossed green salad

Photo by Jim Amentler

Meal 6:

12 egg whites

Pre-Contest Supplement List

– Multivitamin/multimineral
– Lecithin/choline and inositol
– Vitamin B-complex, B-6 and B-12
– Vitamins C, D and E
– Calcium, magnesium and zinc
– Niacin
– Chromium picolinate
– BCAAs

The Last Week

(This schedule assumes a Saturday prejudging)

Food Intake

Wednesday – 10 days out

Shawn uses a seven-day depletion period that starts on the Wednesday prior to the final week (i.e., it takes him to the Tuesday of the last week). During these days, Shawn keeps his protein intake the same as the entire prep period. His carbs change at this point, however, and he takes in a half-cup of oatmeal with his first meal at 6 a.m., half a baked potato with his second meal at 9 a.m. and one cup of cooked rice with his third meal at noon. After this, all of his remaining carbs for the day consist of vegetables and salads. If he feels he needs to deplete further, he eliminates the potato and rice with the 9 a.m. and noon meals for the last few days of the restriction.

Wednesday and Thursday

The carb loading begins. This is the only time Shawn de-emphasizes protein in favor of carbs. "I'm not going to lose any muscle at this point and I have to get sufficient glycogen back into the muscles to get that look onstage like my skin is being pulled tight over my body."

Here's how these days look for Shawn:

Meals 1 and 3:

1 large porterhouse steak and 2 sweet potatoes

Meals 2 and 4:

Oatmeal – very large serving with some type of simple carb such as baby food, banana and/or honey

Meal 5:

2 sweet potatoes

Meal 6:

1 large porterhouse steak and 1 baked potato

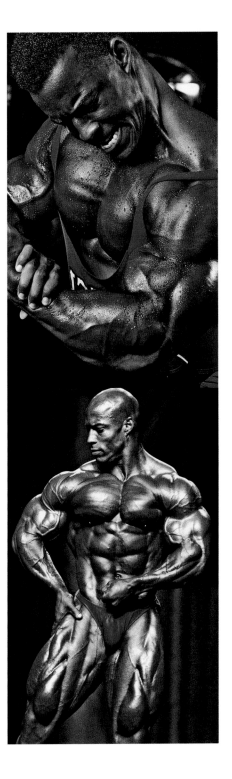

Photo by Irvin Gelb

483

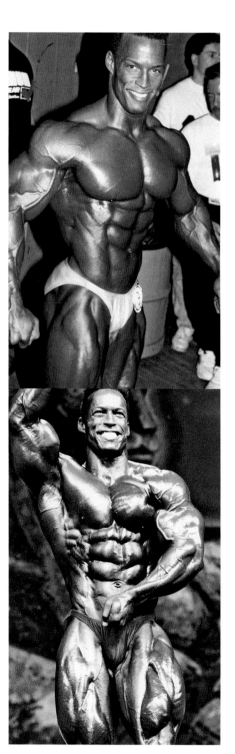

484

Friday

This is perhaps when Shawn's contest prep is most instinctive and when his years of experience come in handy. "Friday is my day to make adjustments based on what I see in the mirror. If I'm looking full I'll raise my protein intake and cut back on my carbs. If I appear flat I'll eat like I did on Wednesday and Thursday."

Saturday

On the day of the show, Shawn's continues to follow his instincts. Unless his condition tells him otherwise, he usually eats two baked potatoes about three hours before the prejudging. "I don't like to eat too much before the prejudging. That's why my midsection is always flat and tight onstage. I'm starving when I'm onstage, but I eat fruit preserves from a jar backstage for a good carb/insulin spike to get through the prejudging and be strong."

Water Intake

On Sunday, Monday, Tuesday and Wednesday, Shawn increases his water intake to approximately five gallons of water a day. "I'm drinking constantly on these days and going to the bathroom all day and all night." On Thursday he cuts it back to about one and a half gallons and makes further cuts on Friday to about half a gallon. On Saturday, Shawn drinks only as he feels it necessary, but isn't afraid to have liquids. "If I still need to carb on Saturday morning, I take some fluid because the carbs won't be fully carried into my system without some water. A lot of guys don't realize this, which is why you see a lot of athletes who come in flat even though they take in a ton of carbs."

Training and Cardio

Shawn stops doing cardio eight days out, doing his last session on Friday. His final leg workout is on the Tuesday before the event, and the rest of his training remains the same as throughout the entire precontest phase.

The Finishing Touches
Posing

Shawn feels posing practice is an important part of his contest prep. At five weeks out he starts posing every training day right after his morning weight workout, followed by a cardio session if he didn't do it in the early morning that day. He does all of the quarter-turns and mandatory poses three times, holding each for 10 seconds. He continues with this method up to and including the day before the contest.

As for his posing routine, the key for Shawn is in choosing the music. "Picking my music is a big part of contest prep for me, maybe the hardest. This is my art on display and I want to find a piece of

Photos by Jim Amentler

music that represents me and my physique. Every song I pose to has special meaning to me. Once I choose the song, the routine more or less just comes to me. In all the times I've competed and done guest posing, that aspect is easy for me. The transitions are critical – they are what really make a great routine. Anyone can get up there and hit mandatories and encourage the audience to clap for them. That is not artistic posing."

"Few bodybuilders ever own a song to the point that when a fan hears the song later on, they immediately think of that athlete. I accomplished that when I posed to Jennifer Holliday's "And I Am Telling You I'm Not Going" from the Broadway musical *Dream Girls*, which I posed to in 1987 when I won the nationals. I'm proud of that."

Tanning

Shawn starts tanning five weeks before the show, lying in the sun four times a week for 30 minutes on each side of his body. If the weather doesn't allow for outdoor tanning, Shawn substitutes at least three sessions in the tanning bed as an alternative. Once he has a good base, Shawn applies two coats of Pro Tan the day before the show, once in the morning and again in the evening.

Backstage

Shawn has always used good old baby oil for his final stage sheen. He pumps up and poses for about 10 minutes backstage. "I'll flex and pose a bit and then do some push-ups, laterals and arm work. Then I'm ready to go. I don't want to pump up too much because I want to be able to really feel the muscles I'm posing onstage, and I want the striations to be very apparent. And I never pump my legs."

Flying

Shawn believes in eating only protein during any flight to a show and drinking as much water as he can. He also tries to arrive at the contest by Wednesday for a Saturday show to offset any effects the flight may have had on his condition.

Photo by Irvin Gelb

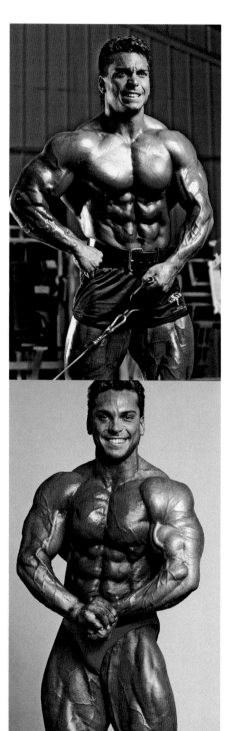

RICH GASPARI
Pre-Contest Training

When preparing for a contest, Rich trained six days a week using the following schedule:

	a.m.	p.m.
Monday:	Chest	Triceps
Tuesday:	Back, lower back	Delts, biceps
Wednesday:	Quads	Hams
Thursday:	Chest	Triceps
Friday:	Back, lower back	Delts, biceps
Saturday:	Quads	Hams
Sunday:	Off	Off

Cardio

You may be surprised to learn that the hardest athlete to step on the Olympia stage in the '80s didn't achieve his condition by living on cardio equipment. "I actually didn't do very much cardio to get ready," says Rich. "I hear about other guys doing two hours of cardio a day. I never did that. But you have to remember, I stayed very lean in the off-season, usually within roughly 20 pounds of my contest weight."

He would begin cardio 10 weeks out from the show, doing three sessions of 30 minutes each. Rich explains: "From there I gauged my time by how quickly I felt my conditioning was coming in. I usually ended up doing no more than four or five sessions of 30 to 40 minutes. I preferred to use the Stepmill or StairMaster because I always felt they burned more calories and hit the glutes and hamstrings better." Rich discontinued all cardio two weeks before a contest.

Pre-Contest Nutrition and Supplementation

Meal 1:
7 egg whites
1 whole egg
1 cup oatmeal
½ banana

Meal 2:
8 oz. turkey breast
½ cup brown rice
Mixed vegetables

Meal 3:
6 oz. salmon
½ cup oatmeal
1 medium apple

Meal 4:
8 oz. fish (halibut, flounder, cod)
3 oz. artichoke pasta
Mixed vegetables

Meal 5:
7 egg whites
1 whole egg

Pre-Contest Supplement List
– Peptide-bond amino acids (throughout the day, with meals)
– BCAAs (before training)
– Multivitamin/multimineral
– Vitamin B-complex
– Vitamin C
– Whey protein
– Digestive enzymes
– Flaxseed oil (2–3 tablespoons a day)

The Last Two Weeks
"My goal was always to be ready for a show two weeks out," says
Rich. "At that point I made a lot of changes aimed at allowing my
body to fill out, get dry and become truly stage ready with my trademark cellophane look."

Food Intake
Rich was never a big believer in the extremes of carb depleting and
loading when he competed. He would instead up his carb intake by
100 to 150 grams per day when he was two weeks out. This increase
usually put him in the range of 450 to 500 grams per day. From there
he would monitor his condition and either keep the carbs constant or
add another 100 to 150 grams if he felt he needed to fill out. He opted
for all complex carbohydrates until the Friday night before the contest, when he would then increase his simple-carb intake with rice
cakes and jelly. Rich also cut his protein in half on Thursday and Friday, usually a drop of about 150 grams, replacing this nutrient with
another 150 grams of carbs.

Water and Sodium Intake
Up to and including the Thursday before a competition, Rich would
continue drinking one to two gallons of spring water. On Friday he
would still drink a gallon of water, but he made sure that by 1 p.m. he
was finished. On Saturday he would sip only small amounts of water.
　　Here's a strategy that Rich would use to get bone dry. He would
brew a box of Weightless Tea into the final gallon of water he con-

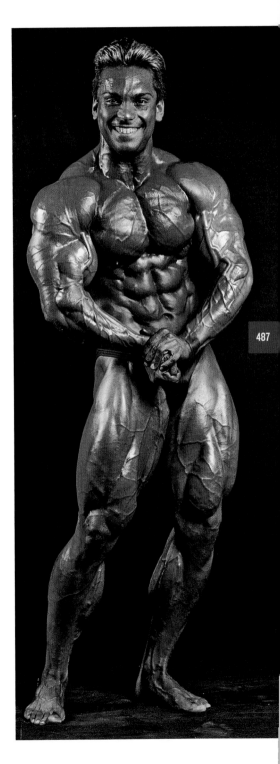

487

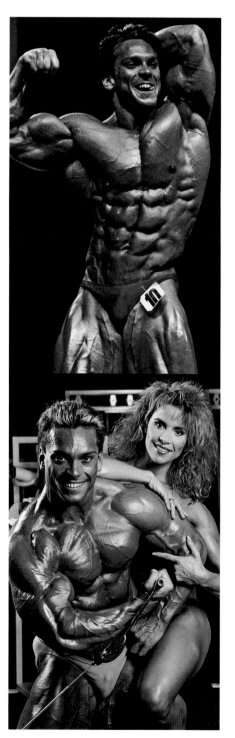

488

sumed on that last Friday. This natural diuretic was all he needed to get rid of any excess fluid that might blur his condition.

As for sodium, he would eliminate eggs from his diet three days out. His sodium level was further reduced as he lowered his overall protein intake over the last two days.

Training and Cardio

Rich would stop all quad training a full two weeks before a contest. Here's the schedule he adhered to for the rest of his body during the last week:

Monday:	Chest, delts, triceps, abs
Tuesday:	Back, biceps, hamstrings
Wednesday:	Full-body workout

The Monday and Tuesday workouts consisted of approximately 10 sets per bodypart, starting with one or two basic exercises followed by isolation and cable movements. The Wednesday session included two exercises per muscle group as a final pump (except for quads).

Rich generally stopped doing all cardio two weeks before a contest, using it during the final phase only if he felt he was spilling over as the day approached. The final Wednesday was the cutoff day that he would allow himself to do a cardio session.

Contest Day

Rich would start the day with a good breakfast consisting of four or five whole eggs, three or four pancakes and syrup. He'd then eat approximately every hour, having small three-ounce servings of chicken with yams, oatmeal or cream of rice. As the prejudging approached, he would switch to simple carbs like rice cakes, jelly and honey.

The Finishing Touches
Posing

If there was a secret to the grainy, crazy conditioning Rich made famous, it was his approach to posing practice. "I think posing was responsible for helping me achieve my conditioning. I practiced it a lot, starting right at the beginning of my contest prep," he explains.

Here's how he did it: at 12 weeks out he would start to choose his music and put his free-posing routine together. Then his posing sessions would officially begin. Three or four times a week, Rich would practice holding all the mandatories and quarter-turns for about five seconds each, ultimately working up to 20 seconds each. He would go through all the poses five or six times and then perform his posing routine three to six times. These sessions would take about an hour and would leave him soaked and tired. At the 10-weeks-out point, he

Photos by Ralph DeHaan and Horton

would do these rehearsals six days a week, after his second training session of each day – that's six hours of posing a week! When he was four weeks out from a show, Rich would often pose twice a day, doing as many as 12 hours of practice over the week.

Tanning

Four weeks before a competition Rich would begin hitting the tanning bed for two or three sessions every day to develop his base tan. From three weeks out he would tan every day until the Wednesday before the show. He would then apply two or three coats of Pro Tan on Thursday and four coats on Friday. "The key to applying your color is making sure you shower after each application to let the excess run off your body. Otherwise, you streak and the tan doesn't look right," he advises.

Backstage

Rich used safflower oil backstage at competitions. "Never use mineral or baby oil as they sit on the skin and don't absorb," he explains. "Once that happens, the lights will reflect off the oil and blur your definition onstage."

To get ready backstage, he would pose and flex a bit before doing push-ups, towel pulls, laterals and dumbell curls. Right before the lineup went onstage, Rich would still be doing push-ups with different hand positions to get a final pump for the judges.

Flying

Rich drank slightly more water when he flew to offset the dehydration from being in an aircraft cabin. To make sure the flight would not affect his condition, he always arranged to arrive in the contest city at least three days before the event. In fact, he even lived and trained in Italy a full month before competing in the 1988 Italian Grand Prix (in which he placed first) to acclimate himself to the new environment!

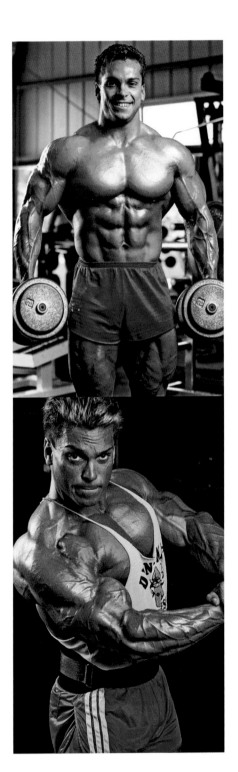

489

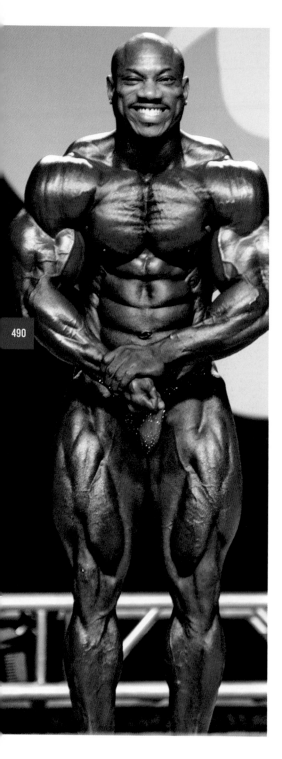

DEXTER JACKSON
Pre-Contest Training

Dexter trains three days a week with the following schedule:

Monday:	Off
Tuesday:	Chest, back, calves
Wednesday:	Off
Thursday:	Legs
Friday:	Delts, arms, calves
Saturday:	Off
Sunday:	Off

Dexter works his entire body over three workouts and hits each body-part once a week as he prepares for a contest. The only exceptions to this regimen are that he trains calves twice per week and never trains his abs. Each bodypart gets no more than 10 working sets of four to eight reps right up until the last week before he competes. "I think a lot of guys make the mistake of going light and doing high reps when they get ready for a show. In my opinion, the best way to be muscularly full and shredded is to diet hard and train heavy. If you change what helped you achieve good muscle fullness in the first place, why would you expect that fullness to stay with you?" he comments.

Dexter doesn't believe he has a "best" bodypart. "I think I'm very balanced, and that has been the key to my success," he says. To give you an idea of how he trains, here's Dexter's formula for building his amazing chest and back.

Chest
Flat barbell bench press 3 x 4–8 reps (after 2–3 warm-up sets)
Incline Smith machine 3 x 4–8
Flat dumbell flye or pec-deck flye 3 x 6–8

Back
Front pull-up 3 x 10–15 or front pulldown 3 x 6–8
Bent-over row 3 x 6–8 or one-arm dumbell row 3 x 6–8

Cardio
Some readers may find it difficult to believe that Dexter never does cardiovascular work. He concentrates on dieting and training harder to bring in the razor-blade detail that few pros have been able to match. There is, however, one exception to his no-cardio rule. He admits: "I did 30 minutes of cardio a day during the first three weeks of my contest prep for the 2003 Arnold Classic. I had to stop though because I was ready for the show at the end of those three weeks!"

Pre-Contest Nutrition and Supplementation

Dexter divides his pre-contest diet into two major phases: Phase one runs from seven to four weeks before a competition. Phase two takes him to the week leading up to a contest.

Phase One

Meal 1:
7 egg whites
5–6 slices of turkey bacon
1 cup grits (cooked measurement)

Meal 2:
MESO-Tech shake (which provides 52 grams of protein, 24 grams of carbs and 3.5 grams of fat)

Meal 3:
6 oz. steak (filet mignon, cooked weight)
3–4 oz. shrimp (cooked weight)
2 cups rice
1 cup mixed vegetables

Meal 4:
MESO-Tech shake (same nutritional value as Meal 2)

Meal 5:
10–12 oz. steak (filet mignon, cooked weight)
1 package Ramen noodles (without seasoning pack)

Meal 6:
10–12 oz. salmon
1 cup rice

Phase Two

During these weeks Dexter drops his carbs, taking in a maximum of 175 grams per day. He also includes more fats in his diet and keeps his carbs very low after 6 p.m. He often varies his carb intake according to how he looks and feels.

Here's a sample of what his diet might look like during this phase:

Meal 1:
7 egg whites
5–6 slices of turkey bacon
1 cup grits (cooked measurement)

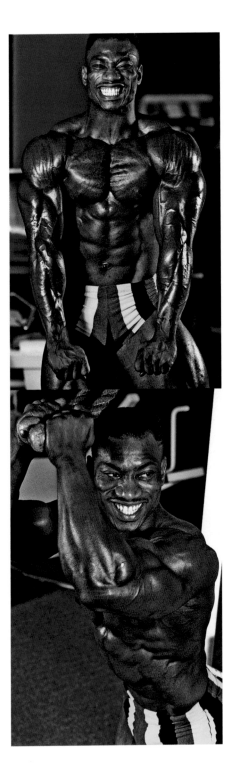

491

Photos by Irvin Gelb

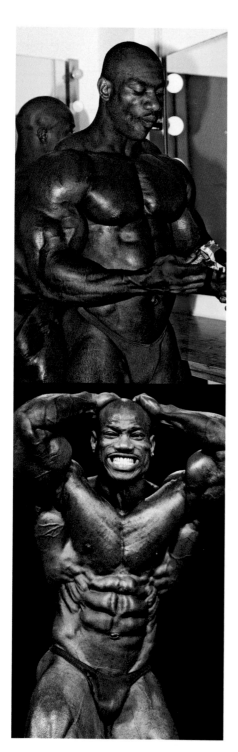

Meal 2:
10–12 oz. steak (filet mignon, cooked weight)
1–2 cups broccoli
1 tbsp. peanut butter

Meal 3:
10–12 oz. salmon
1 cup rice

Meal 4:
MESO-Tech shake (which provides 52 grams of protein, 24 grams of carbs and 3.5 grams of fat)

Meal 5:
10–12 oz. steak (filet mignon, cooked weight)
1–2 cups broccoli

Meal 6:
10 egg whites
5 slices turkey bacon
Chocolate-flavored rice cakes
1 tbsp. peanut butter

Late-Night Snack:
2 fat-free, sugar-free Popsicles
1 serving sugar-free Jell-O
1 handful unsalted peanuts

Dexter eats every two-and-a-half to three hours. He doesn't believe in taking a cheat day or a cheat meal once he begins to prepare for a competition. "If you are ready early, or think you are ahead of schedule, I believe you're better off eating more protein or carbs to stay full. Eating junk food is not a good idea. When you consume a lot of crap, I think your body needs a week to get back to where it was. Cheat days have never made sense to me," he explains.

As for water intake, he just drinks in response to his thirst until he reaches the three-weeks-out point. Then he makes sure to drink a gallon of water every day. Dexter ate a lot more fish when he was preparing for the 2003 Arnold Classic than he has in the past. "I would cook up a large piece of salmon with onions and 'I Can't Believe It's Not Butter!' in a frying pan – great recipe," he comments.

Pre-Contest Supplement List
– Meal-replacement fat burner

Photos by Irvin Gelb

The Last Week

(This schedule assumes a Saturday prejudging)
Dexter stresses that the last week before a contest must focus around instinct and what you see in the mirror. "I know what I need to look like to be shredded," he says. "I'm not a guy who has to have someone else look at me and tell me what to do."

Food Intake
Monday to Thursday

Dexter always checks his weight during the last week. "I know roughly what I need to weigh to be in shape," he says. "So if I weigh a few pounds more, I lower my carbs by eating one less carb meal. If I feel I'm too light or flat, I add a carb meal."

He doesn't use protein powder in the final pre-contest week, but otherwise, he makes no drastic changes at this stage of the game. "I think being ready two weeks out is critical," he reaffirms. "If you are making major moves in the last week, you're in trouble."

Friday

Dexter carbs up on Friday only – he eats one to one-and-a-half pota-toes (white or sweet potatoes) every two hours. He also eats five to six ounces of steak every other meal for protein.

Saturday

Dexter eats the following meal on the day of the show:
6 a.m:
1 cup oatmeal (cooked measurement) with raisins
5–6 oz. steak

If the prejudging is at noon, he does not eat another meal. If the pre-judging is at 2 p.m., he will have a second steak about two hours after the first meal. "I don't eat a lot of carbs the day of the show," he ex-plains. "They can bloat the midsection and do a number on your appearance onstage. I've already carbed up the day before. In my opinion, if you're trying to load the morning of the contest, you didn't prepare right the day before."

Water Intake

Up to and including the Wednesday of the final pre-contest week, Dexter continues drinking one gallon of water per day. On Thursday he reduces his intake to half a gallon. He cuts his water completely on Friday and Saturday before the prejudging.

Training and Cardio

Dexter uses the last few workouts for pumping more than anything

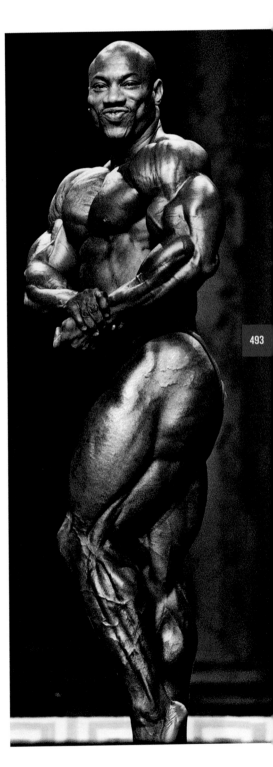

Photo by Irvin Gelb

493

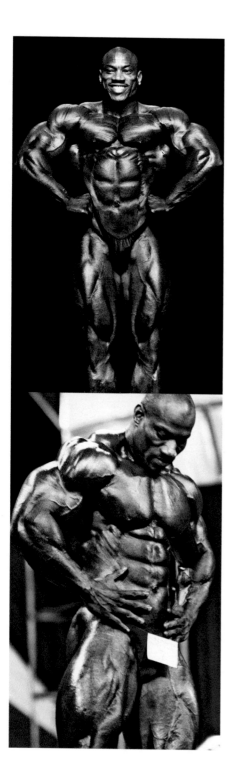

else. He has already done the heavy work, so the last week consists of quick, higher-rep workouts that take about 30 minutes. Here's the schedule he follows during the final week:

Sunday: Legs
Monday: Upper body
Tuesday: Upper body again (depending on how he feels)

The Finishing Touches
Posing

Dexter prepares and starts practicing his posing routine about two weeks before the contest. Several times each week he does every mandatory pose twice. "I don't really feel as though the posing makes much of a difference in my conditioning," he says. "I practice the mandatories for muscle control onstage more than to add detail to my physique."

Tanning

He starts applying Pro Tan on Friday morning, putting on six or seven coats throughout the day and evening. Before going onstage, Dexter uses Pam spray as his posing oil. He pumps up for about 10 or 15 minutes and flexes a lot backstage.

Flying

He does not do anything special to control his water when he flies to contests. "I just keep following my plan. I don't hold water, so that isn't really an issue. I usually arrive at the venue two or three days before the event because that's when we're required to show up for the Olympia and the Arnold. If I had my choice, I'd get there the day before," he says.

Photos by Irvin Gelb

JAY CUTLER
Pre-Contest Training

Jay trains on a two-days-on/one-day-off rotation. He splits each training day into morning and afternoon sessions so he can totally focus on the bodypart being trained. Here's his training split:

	a.m.	p.m.
Day 1	Chest, calves	Biceps
Day 2	Hams	Quads
Day 3	Off	Off
Day 4	Delts	Triceps
Day 5	Back	Traps, back
Day 6	Off	Off

Jay's training style can be described as high volume with high intensity. He flies through approximately 20 to 25 sets per bodypart, resting only 30 to 45 seconds between sets. His back is the only exception to the rule as he does 25 sets in the morning workout and another 25 in the afternoon. Each session takes about 40 minutes, and his reps are usually in the six to 12 range.

Pre-Contest Nutrition

Jay normally begins preparing 16 weeks out if he is starting at his true off-season weight, which varies between 290 and 300 pounds at eight percent bodyfat. During the off-season Jay eats 10 to 12 times per day, taking in a total of approximately 6,000 to 10,000 calories depending on how he feels. He consumes 170 to 220 grams of protein, 900 to 1,300 grams of carbs and minimal fats. His first meal is 10 egg whites, 1 cup of dry oatmeal and a bagel. Meals two through 12 include four or five servings of "Gainers," a protein-carbohydrate powder by ISS Research and another four to six meals that consist of 4 ounces of chicken or top round beefsteak with 2 to 2½ cups of rice.

When his contest prep begins, the major change is his diet. Jay cuts his meals to only six per day, but he still takes in 170 to 220 grams of protein. For carbs he uses a "zigzag" approach whereby he rotates low-, medium- and high-carb days according to how he looks and feels. On a low-carb day he consumes 200 to 300 grams of carbs. Medium is about 700 grams and high is approximately 1,000 grams. He generally eats the high-carb diet only once a week, but Jay will and has used it for as many as seven days in a row close to a show, if necessary. The plan all goes by look and feel – there is no set rotation. Here's what a sample meal plan on a medium-carb day looks like for Jay:

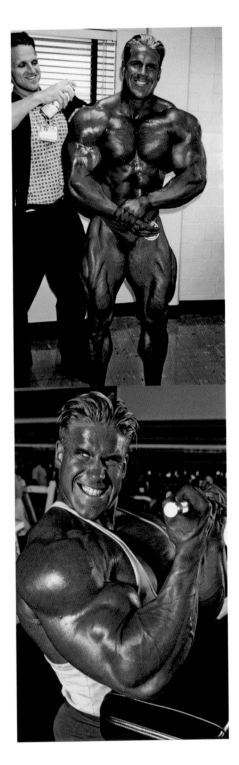

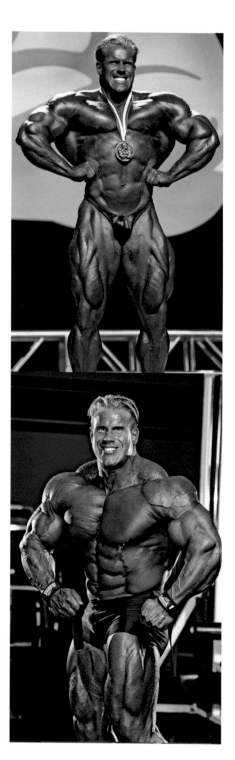

Meal 1:
10 egg whites
1 cup oatmeal (dry weight)

Meal 2: (Post-workout)
35 grams Pro M3 protein (a protein powder by ISS Research)
200 grams carbs from a mixture of rice, rice cakes, banana and Coca-Cola® for the sugar

Meal 3:
5 oz. fish
3 cups broccoli
2 cups rice

Meal 4: (Post-workout)
35 grams Pro M3 protein
175 grams carbs from a mixture of rice, rice cakes, banana and Coca-Cola® for the sugar

Meal 5:
5 oz. fish
3 cups broccoli
1 cup oats (if he feels it's needed)

Meal 6:
40 grams Pro M3 protein

You probably notice immediately that Jay's protein intake is very low for a man of his size. "Protein and carbs have the same number of calories per gram. A lot of guys make choices based on what everyone else is doing and just want to follow the crowd. Being a successful bodybuilder isn't about being a follower. I've done all that. I ate 800 grams of protein and did low carbs and ended up coming down from a very lean 280 pounds to somewhere between 240 and 250. I was losing way too much muscle. One year I came down from 290 to 272 for the Arnold, so my diet is obviously working," he explains. The other feature that stands out in Jay's program is his two post-workout meals that are packed with high-glycemic carbs, including Coca-Cola®. "I drink the Coke for the sugar," he says. "After you train, your body prefers carb sources with a higher sugar content to restore and replenish the glycogen in your liver."

Cardio

Proving again that he isn't afraid to deviate from the norm, Jay generally does only 30 minutes of cardio every other day while preparing for a show. "I've come to the conclusion that bodybuilders aren't meant to do tons of cardio. My sessions are very intense and my heart rate hits 75 percent of my maximum. I favor the treadmill because it calls more muscles into play. I run at about 4.2 miles per hour, which at 290 pounds is pretty fast."

Posing

Jay feels hard posing helps his muscular detail and gives him good muscle control onstage. About six weeks out from the contest, he starts posing every day for about 15 tough minutes. He does each mandatory and each quarter-turn five times, holding each pose for five seconds. Jay's wife Kerry helps out by timing him.

The Last Week

On the Sunday, Monday, Tuesday and Wednesday before a contest, Jay depletes his carbs and trains his entire body, including legs, every day. "I do five sets per bodypart, 15 to 20 reps per set with a light weight. The idea on these days is to get totally depleted, not injured, before filling out. My carbs are basically at zero on those days. Then I carb load and do not train on Thursday, Friday or Saturday morning. I consume four gallons per day up to and including the Wednesday, drop to two gallons on Thursday and then one on Friday."

Lead ... Don't Follow

Jay's philosophies regarding pre-contest cardiovascular work, carbo-hydrate and sugar consumption, and protein intake are very person-alized. He has obviously tapped into what works for him, and in the world of bodybuilding that's what matters. When asked about how he copes when he is tempted to relax and not follow his program on a given day, he said: "Dieting isn't really tough for me because I'm a year-round dieter, but I do have several sources of motivation when I'm getting ready. First are the fans – I realize from my successes and the e-mails I get that there are a lot of great fans out there who rely on me for inspiration. The last thing I want to do is let them down and not be at my best. Next are the several companies that have be-lieved in me enough to sign contracts, and I never wanted to disap-point them either. Getting in great shape is my opportunity to give something back to the people who and companies that have sup-ported me – I can motivate them and show the world they made the right decision. That's all the encouragement I need."

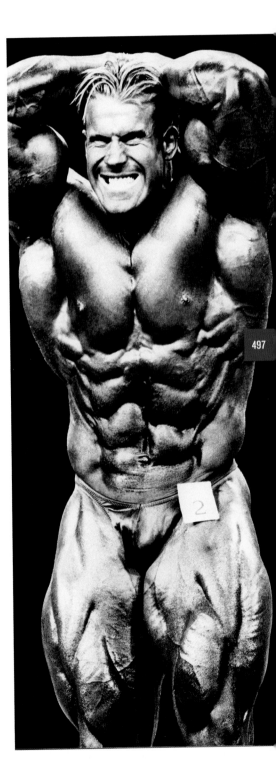

497

QUESTIONS AND ANSWERS

Q. I'd like to try creatine, but I saw on the news that it has killed a few wrestlers. Is this true?

A. Leave it to the media to get their facts wrong. Creatine has been used extensively by athletes for nearly 20 years and no anecdotal reports or controlled studies have yet to show serious side effects. Those wrestlers who died were trying to make a lower weight class and a combination of diuretics and dehydration led them to severely deplete their electrolyte levels. Electrolytes are charged ions that control numerous metabolic functions including heart rate. The creatine had nothing to do with their deaths.

Q. Does whey protein get turned into fat if it's not being used by the body?

A. It's not just protein but any excess calories that will be converted into fat if not burned as an energy source. Fats and carbs, however, will be stored more readily as fat (because fat contains nine calories per gram versus four for protein, and carbohydrates cause a greater release of insulin), but nevertheless, extra protein will get packed around your waist. So, you have to control all of your calories, whether from protein, carbs or fats.

Q. Is there a correct dosage for creatine?

A. There are differing opinions on this topic. Most companies that make creatine powder suggest "loading" with 15 to 20 grams per day for a week, and then switching to a maintenance dose of 5 grams per day. In theory this may make sense, but few studies actually support this approach. Many experts now recommend starting with the maintenance amount from day one. The loading phase, they argue, is just a marketing ploy by manufacturers to convince you to buy and use more of their products.

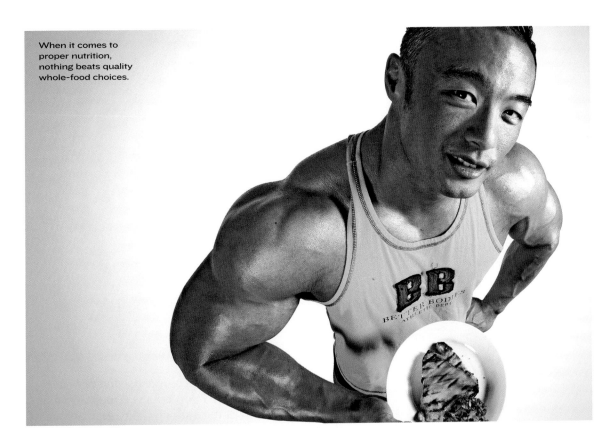

When it comes to proper nutrition, nothing beats quality whole-food choices.

499

Photo by Rich Baker
Model Carl Cheung

Q. I keep seeing the term insulin insensitivity in magazine articles. What does it mean?

A. Insulin insensitivity means that your cells are not as receptive as they should be to this hormone. For those who have this condition, the body doesn't regulate glucose and other sugars as well as it should. The end result is fat accumulation, diabetes and an increased risk of heart disease. Causes of insulin insensitivity include excessive intake of simple sugars, high-fat diets and a sedentary lifestyle. Note that certain nutrients such as chromium, vitamin E, vitamin C, magnesium and omega-3 fatty acids have been found to improve insulin sensitivity.

Q. I just tried one of the newest meal-replacement powders and love it. How many meals should I substitute with the meal-replacement supplement?

A. None! The word supplement means just that: "supplement" not "replacement." No supplement will ever replace a high-quality nutritious meal. Food contains far more nutrients to build your body than even the best of meal-replacement powders. Your goal should be to eat four or five meals a day and then fill in the gaps with a meal replacement.

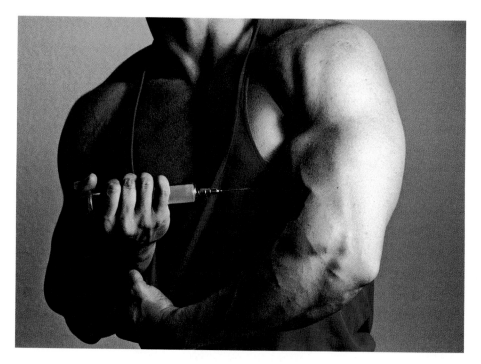

Photo by Alex Ardenti

Q. I keep hearing that steroids cause liver cancer and heart disease. While I don't plan on mega-dosing, I have thought about doing a short, six- to eight-week cycle. Are steroids as dangerous as claimed?

A. While there are risks associated with using just about any drug, the side effects of steroids are blown way out of proportion by the media and many sports organizations. Sports organizations exaggerate the performance-enhancement issue because they're trying to get drugs out of sports. This is a noble cause to be sure, but we question their approach at times. With regards to the media, it's largely sensationalism. Usually they interview doctors and sports officials who are biased against steroids in the first place. Many media outlets rarely check with real experts who have studied the use of steroids among athletes. So generally speaking, steroids are relatively safe if used in low to moderate dosages by those in their 20s or older, while under medical supervision.

Q. When I go into a health-food store I see so many different brands of supplements that promise such wonderful effects. Are all supplements created equal, and are the marketing claims true?

A. The answer to both questions is, no. Given the profits made by the supplement industry – billions of dollars every year – there are some pretty money-hungry characters getting in on the act. And while price is not always an indicator of quality, if you see "Jim's Protein" on sale for $9.99 while most of the competition is averaging $25 or $30, you should know something's up. Odds are that "Jim" is using inferior ingredients in his manufacturing process. Your best bet is to stick with the larger, reputable supplement companies like MuscleTech, Twin Lab, EAS, Optimum Nutrition, etc.

Another rule of thumb is to follow the old saying, "If it sounds too good to be true it probably is." No over-the-counter legal supplement has drug-like effects. Four or five taken together may produce a low to moderate anabolic effect. But don't believe for a second that one natural product has "steroid-like" capabilities.

Q. How important is it to eat right after a workout?

A. Your pre- and post-workout meals are your two most important. Specifically post-workout, from the moment you finish your last set until about an hour later your body is just begging for nutrients – carbs to replenish glucose levels and protein to start repairing muscle tissue. If you don't eat for a few hours after your workout, your body may start using protein tissue (in the form of amino acids) as a fuel source. At the very least you'll make no progress, but if you do this on a regular basis, you run the risk of actually losing muscle size. The best post-workout nutrients are whey protein and simple sugars, as both are absorbed very rapidly.

Q. Is it okay to drink wine and beer occasionally? I keep hearing that it interferes with the benefits of exercise and recovery abilities.

A. The adage of "everything in moderation" certainly applies to alcohol. One or two beers aren't that detrimental in terms of the number of calories. Of course, if you consume a 12-pack of beer every night then yes, it's going to negatively impact your training (and your general health). The same applies for wine. There is even some good evidence to suggest that a couple of glasses of red wine a day can actually improve your cardiovascular health. This is one of the reasons put forward to explain why Europeans have lower incidences of heart disease than North Americans. Keep in mind, however, that it's not just the calories in alcohol you have to consider. Alcohol also tends to slow your metabolism, meaning those on a pre-contest diet might want to give it up entirely until the show is over.

Q. Is it possible to overdose on minerals and trace elements?

A. Both minerals and trace elements are needed by the body in small amounts for metabolic processes such as digestion, hormone

501

"Your pre- and post-workout meals are your two most important. Specifically post-workout, from the moment you finish your last set until about an hour later your body is just begging for nutrients – carbs to replenish glucose levels and protein to start repairing muscle tissue. If you don't eat for a few hours after your workout, your body may start using protein tissue (in the form of amino acids) as a fuel source."

502

> "While virtually every supplement on the market these days is over-hyped, the claims about creatine are closer to the truth. Creatine is one of the few athletic supplements with good scientific evidence showing that it does in fact boost performance. Creatine offers bodybuilders numerous benefits: it increases energy levels by improving ATP regeneration, increases strength and size levels and decreases recovery time between workouts."

synthesis, nerve conduction and heart-beat regulation. If you are consistently eating a well-balanced diet, you probably don't need to consume extra amounts of either in supplement form. As for any dangers, there is a risk with overdosing on certain ones including potassium, sodium and iron. Unless you are deficient in one or more of any mineral or trace element, or you have been advised by a physician, we suggest getting all of your minerals and trace elements from your diet and perhaps a daily multivitamin tablet.

Q. I made the mistake of going on a steroid cycle for six weeks and now I have this swelling around my left nipple. I'm embarrassed to take my shirt off in gym class. I thought by going off the juice it would clear up, but it hasn't. What should I do?

A. Your first step is to go straight to your family doctor. The condition you have is called gynecomastia, which occurs when excess testosterone (in this case from the steroids) is converted into the female hormone estrogen. The high levels of estrogen then stimulate the estrogen receptors in the nipple region, making it swell and creating the appearance of female breasts. You've probably also heard the term "bitch tits" used to describe the condition. For most people it clears up when steroid use is stopped, but for some individuals (like yourself), this isn't the case. We'll be honest – your doctor might give you a lecture about using steroids (and rightly so seeing as you're still school-age), but he or she can prescribe an anti-estrogen. You may be tempted to ignore the condition and hope it goes away, but any time such a mass of tissue is left untreated you run the risk of it turning cancerous. So please take the safer route, suck up the embarrassment and go see your doctor.

Q. I'm not really a fan of eating animal meats. Occasionally I'll eat fish or chicken, but most of my food comes from plant sources. Is it possible to gain muscle strength and size by following a primarily egetarian diet?

A. Absolutely! Some of the greatest bodybuilders in history (multi-Mr. Universe Bill Pearl perhaps being the most well-known) are vegetarians. You just have to be creative and intelligent with your eating, that's all. The reason is that most plant sources are deficient in one or more of the essential amino acids. This means you'll need to consume a wide range of plant foods to obtain all the amino acids. You mentioned you don't eat a lot of animal meats, but what about milk and eggs? Many vegetarians include these animal foods in their diets and both are first-class sources of protein. And unless you're a vegan and completely against the use of any and all animal protein sources, protein powders are another excellent way to add extra high-quality protein to your diet.

Q. It seems every second ad these days is for creatine. Is this supplement really that good or is it just another over-hyped product?

A. While virtually every supplement on the market these days is over-hyped, the claims about creatine are closer to the truth. Creatine is one of the few athletic supplements with good scientific evidence showing that it does in fact boost performance. Creatine offers bodybuilders numerous benefits: it increases energy levels by improving ATP regeneration, increases strength and size levels and decreases recovery time between workouts. Finally, most users report weight gains of eight to 10 pounds while on a creatine cycle. So yes, it's that good and should make a definite improvement to your bodybuilding endeavors.

Q. I'm going to be applying for a job in the near future that has drug testing as part of the interview process. I've done a few steroid cycles over the past year – will the steroids be picked up on the drug test?

A. Unless the company specifically tests for the presence of steroids, you have nothing to worry about. Most companies – especially those involving jobs in the fields of protection and public safety – test for only the more commonly known street drugs such as cocaine, heroin, amphetamines and occasionally marijuana. Steroids won't be detected by such tests, and they won't cause a false positive for the other drugs mentioned.

Q. Now that steroids are illegal I was planning on trying some of the prohormones that are available. Are they as good as steroids?

A. Not even close. Despite the best intentions of researchers and supplement manufacturers, studies showed that none of the popular prohormones came close to duplicating the positive muscle-building effects of anabolic steroids. Prohormones are just compounds that come before steroids. The theory was that the body would be able to convert the compounds to anabolic hormones, and that bodybuilders could get the same results without having to worry about the legal issues. Unfortunately, the conversion rate for most prohormones is extremely low, and some often get converted to estrogen. Finally, even if they did offer some sort of anabolic effect, virtually all prohormones were added to the Anabolic Steroid Control Act in 2004. They're now just as illegal as steroids and essentially warrant the same fines and jail sentences.

> "About the only aspect that simple and complex carbs have in common is their calorie count per gram. In virtually every other respect there's a heap of difference between the two. Complex carbs are also much better for replenishing glycogen stores in the muscles. Simple carbs – or sugars – should only be eaten in small amounts immediately after your workouts."

Q. It seems every time I take my vitamins I get an upset stomach. Is this normal?

A. No, not really. A possible cause could be that you're taking them on an empty stomach. Have you tried having your vitamins with a meal? The problem could also be the time of the day (if you normally take them in the morning, try switching to the evening or vice versa). It may even be something in the particular brand you're using. Consider switching brands to see if another formulation works better. If you've tried all of these options and still get an upset stomach, I'd suggest making an appointment with your doctor.

Q. I'm entering my first competition (which is in a couple of months) and I'm confused about the pre-contest dieting. Some people suggest keeping my carbs high and dropping my protein, while others advise me to lower my carb intake and increase my protein. Do you have any suggestions?

A. Everyone is different, so experimenting is the only sure way to determine exactly what will work best for you. The general consensus, however, is to go with higher protein and lower carb intake. This makes sense for a number of reasons. For one, eating more protein causes a thermogenic effect in the body, raising metabolism and burning more calories. In addition, lowering your carb intake forces the body to switch to fat as a fuel source. Finally, keeping your protein high helps preserve muscle mass.

Q. I was thinking of trying choline and inositol to lose a few pounds. Are these supplements very effective for fat loss?

A. While the medical evidence is sketchy with regards to the fat-burning abilities of choline and inositol, numerous bodybuilders swear by them. Both of these supplements are cheap and relatively safe, so you may want to give them a try. Just don't expect any miraculous loss of fat.

Q. I was thinking of using Synthol because I'm having trouble building my calves. I do three sets of standing calf raises every time I train my legs and nothing's happening.

A. Three sets? Three sets! Don't tire yourself out now. Before you start blaming bad genetics for your mediocre calves take a closer look at your training. How many sets are you doing for your chest and biceps? A hell of a lot more than three, we bet. Try doubling if not tripling your calf training. Don't forget to include seated calf raises to work the lower calves as well. As for Synthol, yes it will make your calves look bigger, but unless it's injected properly, you may end up with a set of lower legs that look more like balloons than calves!

Q. Is there really that big of a difference between simple and complex carbs? They both provide four calories per gram, right?

A. About the only aspect that simple and complex carbs have in common is their calorie count per gram. In virtually every other respect there's a heap of difference between the two. You need lots of complex carbs such as yams, brown rice, whole grains and vegetables

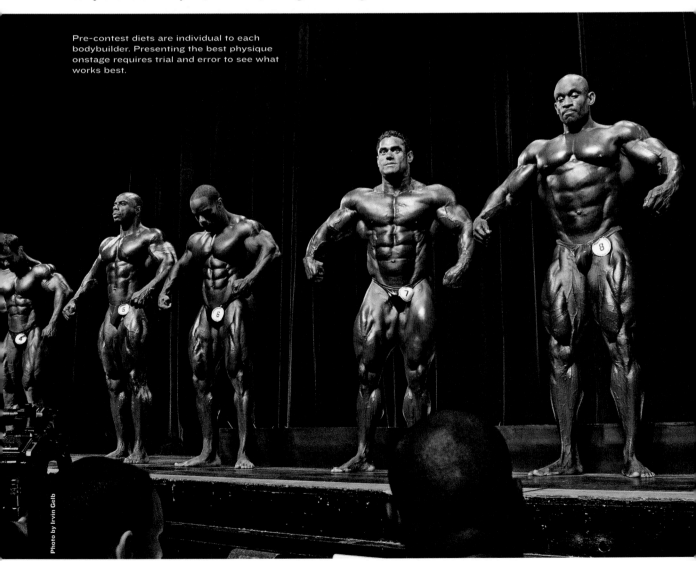

Pre-contest diets are individual to each bodybuilder. Presenting the best physique onstage requires trial and error to see what works best.

Photo by Irvin Gelb

in your diet. Complex carbs are released slowly and don't cause the massive insulin spike that's seen with simple carbs. Complex carbs are also much better for replenishing glycogen stores in the muscles. Simple carbs – or sugars – should only be eaten in small amounts immediately after your workouts. If you consume too much at other times of the day you'll do nothing but enlarge your waistline.

Q. I saw a report on TV the other night that said bodybuilders eat too much protein; they said the RDIs are sufficient for even the most serious trainers and that any more is dangerous. Is this true?

A. If they're talking about the very few bodybuilders who take in 300 or 400 grams per day, then yes, this is probably unnecessary. But I totally disagree with the statement that the RDIs are sufficient for hard trainers. These recommended amounts were calculated based on the lifestyle of sedentary folks and are basically the minimum amounts needed by individuals to survive. Common sense should dictate that a 50-year-old couch potato and a 20-year-old college athlete will have different protein needs. If the 20-year-old is engaged in serious weight training he's going to require much more protein than the channel surfer. With regards to the claims that too much protein is dangerous, unless you have pre-existing health issues such as kidney disease, you have nothing to worry about.

Q. I like the occasional cup of coffee but have been hearing that decaffeinated coffee is actually bad for you. What gives?

A. There is some evidence to suggest that the chemicals and solvents used to remove the caffeine from coffee beans may cause cancer. For example, statistics show that farmers are more at risk for developing certain types of cancers. It's suggested that their increased exposure to pesticides and animal viruses may be the cause. But you should keep things in perspective. If you believe everything you read, then virtually every food chemical is bad for you. You also have to consider what the actual chemical concentrations are that you're being exposed to. Unless you're drinking decaf coffee by the gallon, odds are you're at no greater risk for developing cancer than regular coffee drinkers.

Q. I need to shed about five pounds of water for a bodybuilding contest I'm competing in. I heard that the pro bodybuilders use diuretics and was wondering if I should do the same?

A. The decision whether to use diuretics should not be taken lightly. Yes, diuretics will help you lose water and give you a much

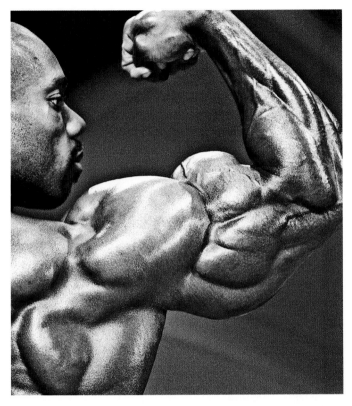

LEFT: Protein builds muscle, and body-builders have a substantially higher muscle mass than the general public. So, it stands to reason that bodybuilders need to have more protein in their diets.

507

Photo by Alex Ardenti
Model Flex Wheeler

harder appearance. But this substance will also cause the body to lose valuable electrolytes, the charged ions that help regulate important biological processes such as muscle contraction, nerve conduction and heart rate. There have been cases of bodybuilders suffering severe muscle cramps and heart attacks during contests from depleting their electrolyte levels so extremely. There have even been a few deaths linked to diuretics. My advice is to stay clear of diuretic drugs and stick with natural herbal diuretics such as dandelion. This type of OTC compound will enable you to shed water without depleting your electrolytes to dangerously low levels.

Q. I think there may be something wrong with my kidneys. Every time I take a B-complex vitamin tablet my urine becomes a yellow color. Is there something seriously wrong with me?

A. You have nothing to worry about. B-complex vitamins, particularly vitamin B-2 (riboflavin), will often change the urine to bright yellow in many people. Other than perhaps using a tablet with a smaller dose to save money literally being pissed down the drain, health-wise you have nothing to worry about.

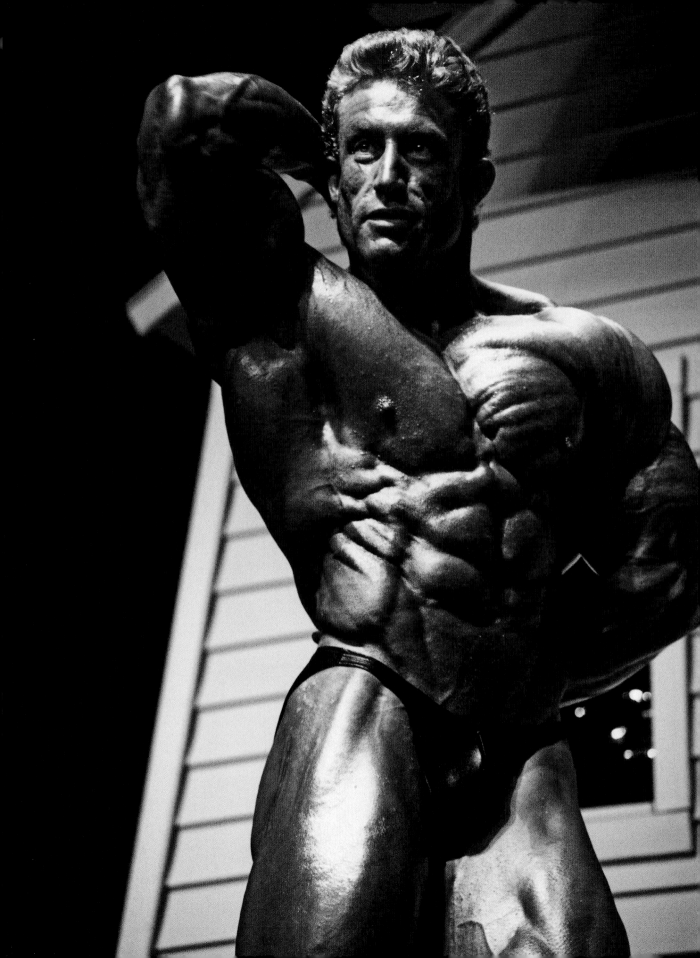

Q. A friend in my class said he put on 10 pounds of muscle using insulin and that I should give it a try. What do you think?

A. In all honesty I think you should get new friends! Insulin is not something to fool around with. It can help you gain muscular bodyweight since it speeds up the transport of amino acids into muscle cells for conversion into protein and new muscle tissue. Unfortunately, insulin also removes glucose (sugar) out of the bloodstream. A number of bodybuilders have died after putting themselves into a diabetic coma after overdosing on insulin. Is it worth risking your life for a few extra pounds of muscle mass? Personally, I think not.

Q. I've been contemplating using steroids but I heard that those with a family history of stroke should not take them. Is this true?

A. There are good reasons that no one should use anabolic steroids, but those with a history of stroke are especially at risk. The primary reason is that steroids cause an increase in blood pressure by causing the body to retain water. And since a stroke is caused when a small blood vessel ruptures in the brain, it's easy to see how steroid users who are genetically prone to this condition could be playing with their lives. My advice for you is to train naturally and stay healthy.

Q. I've been off the juice now for nearly two months and I feel lousy. I've lost nearly 25 pounds and my strength is way down. And worst of all, I haven't had an erection in over a month. What's going on here?

A. What's going on is that your steroid use has shut down your natural testosterone production. While you were on the juice your body assumed that its own testosterone levels were high and thus shut off your testosterone-making machinery (i.e., your testes). But once the steroids cleared your system, the natural production should have kicked back in. Most former users report that within a few weeks to a month they start feeling normal again. In your case, the passing of two months suggests that you may need medical intervention to get your hormonal system straightened out. The doctor will probably give you a few shots of a drug called hCG to stimulate your testes to start generating testosterone again. The condition is fairly simple to treat, but don't try self-administering. Go to your doctor and let a medical practitioner straighten you out.

> "Insulin is not something to fool around with. It can help you gain muscular bodyweight since it speeds up the transport of amino acids into muscle cells for conversion into protein and new muscle tissue. Unfortunately, insulin also removes glucose (sugar) out of the bloodstream. A number of bodybuilders have died after putting themselves into a diabetic coma after overdosing on insulin."

509

Q. My boyfriend has a bit of a temper, but since he started using steroids he's really become agitated and will fly off the handle for the smallest reasons. Will he get worse and develop roid rage or something?

A. Despite what you may hear in the news, most steroid users don't become psychotic killers. Those with short tempers to begin with may become slightly more reactive. Your boyfriend seems to fit this description. And if he's preparing for a contest, his short fuse might be more from the strict diet and extra cardio than the steroids. But as for roid rage, you have nothing to worry about. There's no evidence to back roid rage as a medical condition – roid rage is just a catch phrase invented by a couple of defense lawyers who were trying to get the charges against their clients dropped. The few cases that seemed to gain attention from the media and anti-steroid groups to support the notion of roid rage all involved individuals who had histories of violence before they started using steroids. In addition, most were also using alcohol at the time. Now, by no means are we suggesting that you should put up with an abusive boyfriend. If his behavior continues or gets worse, you should seriously consider getting out of the relationship.

Q. Other than maybe an enlarged midsection or perhaps some bone thickening, are there any other side effects from using growth hormone?

A. While both these potential side effects are cosmetically unpleasant, growth hormone has a few lesser known properties that could endanger your life. For starters, GH can interfere with many of the body's other hormones including insulin. Because insulin controls blood sugar levels, any time you screw with it you run the risk of pushing yourself into a diabetic coma. Growth hormone also has cancer-growing properties, which you don't often hear about. While not conclusive, there is some evidence to suggest that growth hormone can enlarge existing tumors. The question remains the same as with other potentially dangerous drugs: do you want to risk your life for a few extra pounds of muscle mass?

Q. What's the scoop on glucosamine? Does it really cure joint pain?

A. "Cure" is probably too strong of a word. "Helps" is a more fitting description. Glucosamine is a natural sugar-related molecule that has been shown in various studies to promote relief from numerous joint ailments including osteoarthritis. It's also widely used by veterinarians as a treatment for older animals. Bodybuilders and other athletes find this supplement useful for combating the stress and degenerative effects of hard training. It won't cure pre-existing joint problems, but it does provide some degree of preventive medicine.

510

"Despite what you may hear in the news, most steroid users don't become psychotic killers. Those with short tempers to begin with may become slightly more reactive. There's no evidence to back roid rage as a medical condition. The few cases that seemed to gain attention from the media and anti-steroid groups to support the notion of roid rage all involved individuals who had histories of violence before they started using steroids."

Glucosamine also seems to speed up healing following an injury. Unlike true drugs that generally begin to exert their effects in minutes or hours, glucosamine usually takes one to two months before users experience any noticeable benefits.

Q. I saw a report on one of the TV news-magazine shows that said people should be eliminating all fat from their diets. I thought there were certain fats we should be eating. What should I do?

A. Change channels! It's amazing in this day and age that anyone could put together a report that misses the mark entirely. There are specific fats that should be avoided: Saturated fat should be kept to a minimum, and trans and hydrogenated fats should be avoided altogether. While the body does have some ability to break down saturated fat, this form still contributes to heart disease and stroke. As for trans and hydrogenated fats, these are byproducts of the food-processing industry and because they aren't natural, the human body didn't evolve with the necessary enzymes to break them down. These types of fat usually get deposited in and around your organs and on artery walls. The end result is reduced blood flow to the extremities and heart, which can ultimately lead to limb amputation or a heart attack.

511

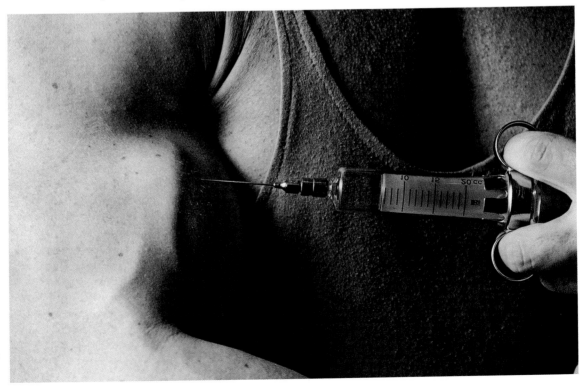

Photo by Alex Ardenti

> "No supplement will ever replace quality whole food when it comes to sound nutrition. Some products actually contain more fat and simple sugar than chocolate bars. Just because a certain bar contains a high amount of protein doesn't mean it won't pack weight around your midsection."

512

The fats that you do need are called unsaturated, and this form can be found in foods like deep sea fish (salmon and herring), flaxseed oil and olive oil.

Q. Is it possible to overdose on vitamins?

A. Theoretically yes, but you'd need to be consuming mega doses over a long period of time. There's no risk of overdosing on the water-soluble vitamins such as vitamins B and C, since any amounts not utilized by the body are simply excreted in the urine. The fat-soluble vitamins such as A, D and E, can reach toxic levels because the body is able to store them, but it would only be dangerous if you were taking many times the recommended dosages. Unless otherwise instructed by a physician, stick to the directions printed on the bottle. For most vitamins the dosage is one or two tablets or capsules a day.

Q. I'm new to bodybuilding and the ads in magazines I've been reading suggest that I need to eat protein bars to gain muscle mass. Are they really that good?

A. It depends on what you mean by "good." Many types taste good – some even taste great. With respect to being necessary for gaining muscle size, however, not a chance. No supplement will ever replace quality whole food when it comes to sound nutrition. Where protein bars do offer an advantage over certain foods is that they're convenient to carry and eat. You only have to tear away the wrapper and away you go. Food often needs to be cooked and prepared in advance and then carried in Tupperware containers. If you find yourself stuck for time and rushing to work or classes, a protein bar can quickly give you 15 to 20 grams of protein or more in a matter of minutes. As a word of caution, make sure you read the labels before you buy a box. Some products actually contain more fat and simple sugar than chocolate bars. Just because a certain bar contains a high amount of protein doesn't mean it won't pack weight around your midsection.

Q. I keep hearing that it's recommended to drink six to eight glasses of water a day. Is this just hype or good advice?

A. We'll be the first to admit there's a lot of hype out there regarding nutrients and supplements, but not in the case of hydration. Water is one of the most – if not *the* most – important of all nutrients. Our bodies require water to function properly. So important is water to our health that the human body has developed conservation-type systems devoted solely to preserving water. At the very minimum you should be drinking six to eight glasses per day – more if you sweat a lot during exercise.

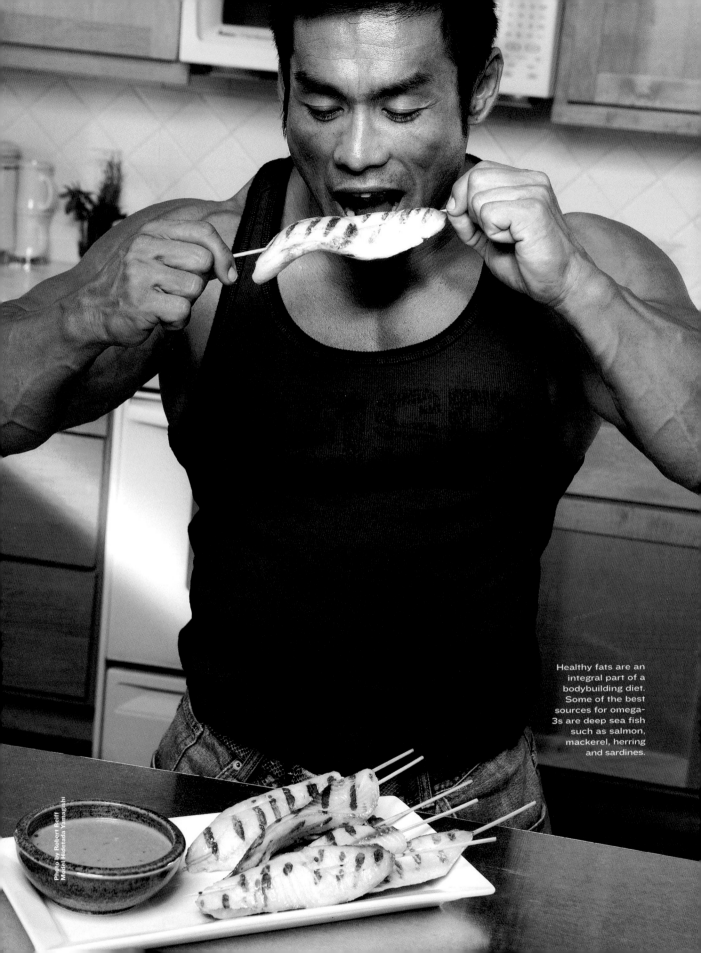

Healthy fats are an integral part of a bodybuilding diet. Some of the best sources for omega-3s are deep sea fish such as salmon, mackerel, herring and sardines.

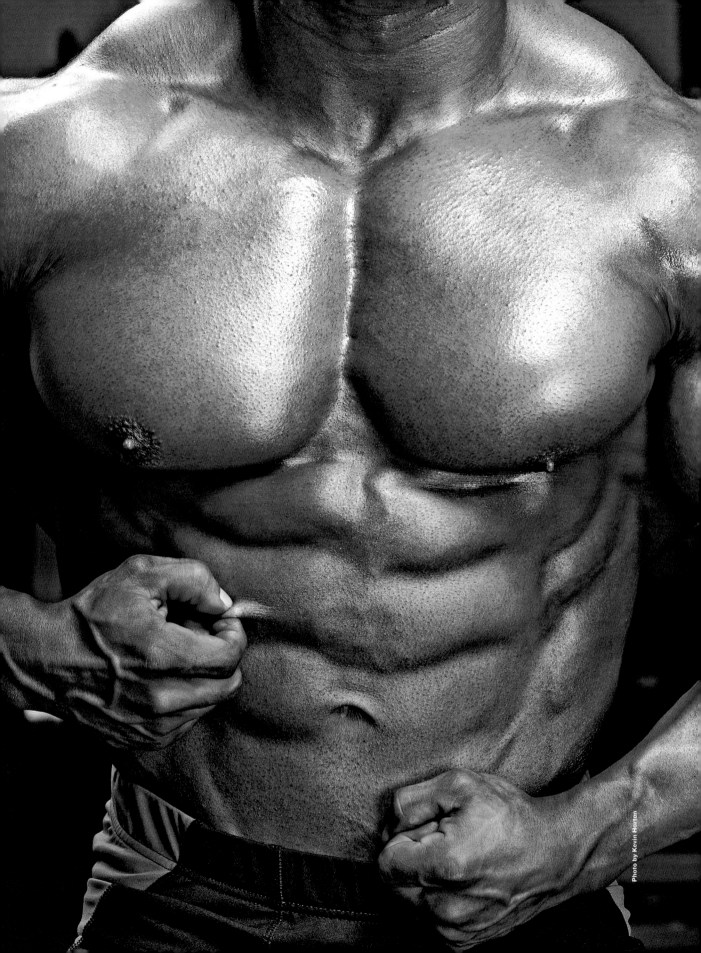

Q. Is it true that you have to eat fat to lose fat? That doesn't seem like it makes sense!

A. This advice may sound crazy, but it's true. By eating certain fats – those categorized as "good" fats – you can actually stimulate the body's fat-burning properties. Some fats such as CLAs actually trick the body into giving up fat deposits to be used as energy. Scientists have yet to discover the exact mechanism for this process, but it is believed that by eating good fats the body realizes it's getting enough fat in the diet and responds by releasing some stored fat. The key to making this work is the type of fat you consume. Saturated and trans fats will only cause you to gain fat. These forms will also increase your risk of heart disease by blocking your arteries with fatty deposits. Try to eliminate them from your diet. You should instead be opting for unsaturated and omega-3 sources of fat.

Q. I've heard that some guys drink alcohol the night before a contest to harden up. Isn't alcohol a no-no for bodybuilders?

A. For the most part you should avoid alcohol. The occasional beer or glass of wine is fine, but moderate to heavy alcohol consumption has no place in a healthy lifestyle. Specifically in regards to consuming alcohol the night before a show, there is some merit to this thinking. Many bodybuilders find that having one or two glasses of wine the night before a contest tends to make their bodies a bit harder and more vascular. It's believed that the body pulls water from under the skin into the blood vessels so the liver can then digest the alcohol. A glass or two of wine will also help you shed a few additional pounds of water because alcohol is a diuretic.

Q. Are there any over-the-counter supplements that actually stimulate fat loss?

A. Most OTC fat-loss products are way over-hyped and are not actually that effective at burning fat. The one that did greatly enhance fat loss was banned – ephedrine, when combined with caffeine and aspirin (popularly called the ECA stack), was probably the most effective OTC fat-loss supplement available. Being a thermogenic compound, it elevated body temperature slightly and made fat deposits more susceptible to being burned as an energy source. The typical ECA stack consisted of 25 milligrams ephedrine, one aspirin tablet and 200 milligrams caffeine (about one cup of coffee). Ephedrine, however, was banned in 2004 after negative publicity surrounding the deaths of a small number of individuals including a couple of athletes. While dehydration or pre-existing heart problems were probably to blame in these cases, all concentrated forms of ephedrine were nevertheless banned. It is still possible to buy the herbal form of ephedrine, which is called Ma Huang.

> "By eating certain fats – those categorized as 'good' fats – you can actually stimulate the body's fat-burning properties. The key to making this work is the type of fat you consume. Saturated and trans fats will only cause you to gain fat. These forms will also increase your risk of heart disease by blocking your arteries with fatty deposits. Try to eliminate them from your diet. You should instead be opting for unsaturated and omega-3 sources of fat."

515

516

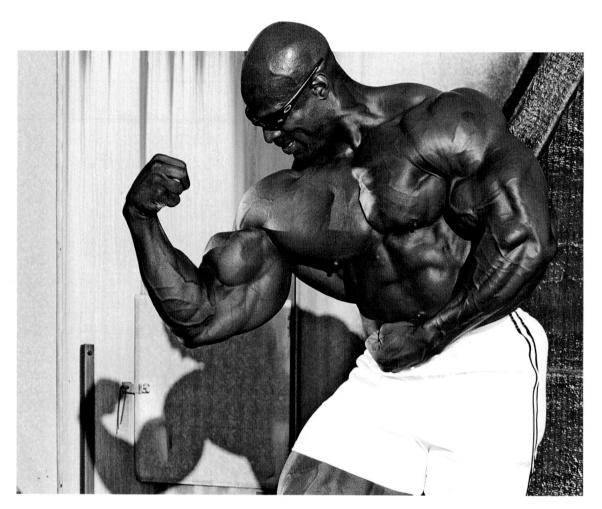

Q. What's the scoop on BCAAs? Are they useful for building muscle?

A. The evidence on BCAAs (branched-chain amino acids) is mixed – some studies show BCAAs can boost recovery abilities while others report no change. Likewise, this supplement has varying degrees of fondness among bodybuilders. In theory, branched-chain amino acids should provide a performance boost since they seem to prevent muscle wasting and counteract the negative effects of catabolic hormones. There is also some evidence to suggest that BCAAs can be burned as a fuel source. This effect would help bodybuilders preparing for a contest since there is a tendency for the body to burn muscle tissue for fuel once bodyfat percentages drop very low. Probably the biggest strike against BCAAs is their cost. A bottle of 100 usually averages $15 to $20. And when you need to take in six to 10 capsules per day, that one bottle will only last you about 10 to 15 days. That same $20 would get you about a month's supply of whey protein – which is also high in branched-chain

Photo by Alex Ardenti
Model Ronnie Coleman

amino acid content. If the cost doesn't deter you, trying them won't hurt, as side effects are rarely reported with use of BCAAs.

Q. I'm on the gear and planning to compete in a bodybuilding contest in a few months. I'm hearing now that the show may be drug tested. Is it possible to beat the test if I go off steroids a few weeks before?

A. It all depends on what form you're taking. Most oral steroids clear your system in a few weeks, so with this type theoretically you could go off, maintain the positive benefits and still pass the test – theoretically. However, because everyone's body is different, there's no way of knowing just how far in advance you'll have to come off the gear to ensure a negative test. Injectable steroids are another matter entirely. Some injectables such as Deca-Durabolin can be detected even 18 months after the last use. It makes no sense to use such substances in preparation for a drug-tested event since any benefits derived from the drug will be lost over the time it takes to clear your system. Most bodybuilders in drug-tested shows use small amounts of injectables and then switch to orals in the last few months before the contest. Guys who use this approach have likely also done their research and thus have a pretty good idea of how close to a drug test they can use the gear and still pass. It's a case of rolling the dice. Keep in mind that the technology for drug tests keeps improving and getting more accurate. For orals, that two weeks required now might become three or four with the next generation of test methods.

Q. Are those electrical stimulator devices any good?

A. It all depends. While no machine – electrical or otherwise – will ever replace good old-fashioned barbells and dumbbells, those electrical stimulation devices (also called electrical muscle stimulation or EMS) do serve a purpose. The machines work by attaching two electrodes at the ends of the muscle and then pass a small electrical current through them. As the muscles contract by electrochemical stimulation (i.e., a nerve impulse triggers a change in the ion concentration in and around the muscle) the EMS machine is essentially acting like the body's own nervous system. Over time, the electrical current can be increased as the muscle gets stronger. EMS machines do have the advantage of muscle stimulation without involving the surrounding structures and tissues. This makes the device great for individuals in rehab for certain injuries. The machine is also relatively cheap when you consider that one $200 unit can stimulate every muscle. You'd need to spend thousands of dollars for a full line of strength-training machines. The downside to EMS machines, however, is that they tend to operate on the all-or-nothing principle. The muscle either contracts or it doesn't. Granted, turning up the juice will pro-

517

"In theory, branched-chain amino acids should provide a performance boost since they seem to prevent muscle wasting and counteract the negative effects of catabolic hormones. There is also some evidence to suggest that BCAAs can be burned as a fuel source. This effect would help bodybuilders preparing for a contest since there is a tendency for the body to burn muscle tissue for fuel once bodyfat percentages drop very low."

518

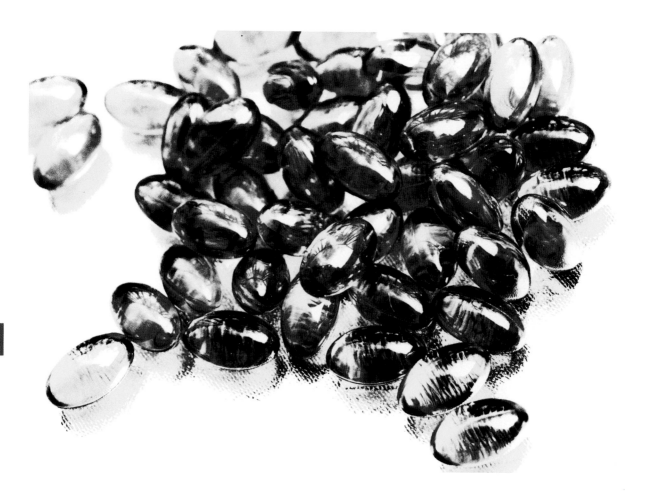

ABOVE: Vitamin E capsules are popular among some bodybuilders to boost energy. While studies don't support this effect, Vitamin E is known to fight off radicals.

duce a stronger contraction, but it's still just one all-out contraction. Conversely, you have much more control over the muscle contraction when using a barbell or dumbbell. You also need to consider that these devices offer no psychological satisfaction – there's just no comparing the feel of working out with barbells, dumbbells and machines with sitting at a table and hooking yourself up to a wire.

Q. I heard that taking vitamin E supplements will increase my energy. Is this true?

A. Unless you're deficient in vitamin E to begin with, supplementing won't make any difference to your energy level. The reason some people tout this vitamin as an energy enhancer is because it plays a role in the manufacturing of red blood cells. But taking extra amounts won't raise your red blood cell count above normal levels. It still wouldn't hurt to take a vitamin E supplement, however. Vitamin E

Photo By Alex Ardenti

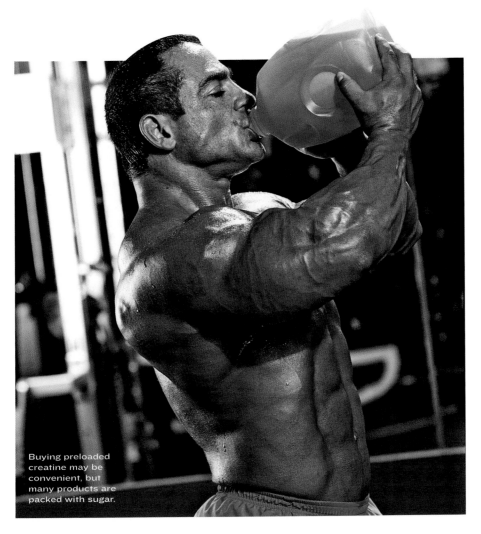

Buying preloaded creatine may be convenient, but many products are packed with sugar.

Photo By Alex Ardenti
Model Mike Ergas

519

is one of the body's primary weapons for combating free radicals, which are charged ions that go around damaging cells and tissues.

Q. Are those preloaded creatine products any better than straight creatine monohydrate?

A. About the only benefit of preloaded creatine is convenience. But even then it only offers a slight advantage. For those not familiar with the term, "preloaded" means the creatine is already mixed with a sugar source. The theory is that by taking creatine with sugar, a larger insulin spike is created. Boosted insulin then increases the transport of creatine into muscle cells. Preloaded products already have the creatine mixed in, so it's just a matter of putting one or two scoops in a glass and mixing it. With pure creatine monohydrate powder, you'd have to add your own sugar. Of course for a couple of dollars you can easily pick up a container of flavored drink mix that would last a few weeks. And how much more inconvenient is it to take one or two spoonfuls and add it to your creatine? Not much. The primary downside to preloaded creatine is cost. You'll end up paying upward of twice the cost for less than half the amount of creatine monohydrate (and much of the container is loaded with sugar). My advice is to buy creatine monohydrate and a container of Kool-Aid or similar drink mix and make your own preload.

Q. I'm having trouble losing fat around my waist. I'm doing 30 minutes of cardio three times per week and the fat still won't disappear. I was thinking about getting liposuction. What do you think?

A. I think you're nuts to be considering liposuction at this stage. Three 30-minute cardio sessions per week is the bare minimum to stimulate fat loss. In fact, this amount might not even be enough to maintain your bodyweight if you have poor eating habits. My first piece of advice is to increase each of your sessions to 45 minutes. I'd also seriously consider adding an extra session or two per week. Finally, take a close look at your diet as there may be room for improvement. With regards to liposuction, I think it should be a last resort, only for those who are grossly overweight despite training and eating properly. For most people, a good exercise program and healthy eating will be more than enough to trim their waistlines.

Q. Does carb depletion/loading make much difference to a competitor's physique on contest day?

A. Assuming you get the timing right, this approach could make a huge difference. Carb depletion/loading is a two-step process. First, you drastically reduce your carb intake and burn most of the glycogen stores in your muscles. Next, you load for a couple of days. The theory is that after a period of depletion, the body will store above-normal levels of glycogen in the muscles. And since every gram of carbs attracts four grams of water, all of that extra glycogen will draw water from under the skin into the muscles. The end result is bigger, fuller muscles and increased vascularity. If the contest is on Saturday, most bodybuilders will deplete on Monday, Tuesday and Wednesday, and then load on Thursday and Friday. But this isn't an exact science – no one knows exactly how his body will respond until he goes through the entire process at least once. Some individuals may need three days to fully carb load, and they end up peaking on Sunday. Conversely, some may peak after just one day and look sharp on Friday but smooth on Saturday. For this reason it's crucial to keep detailed notes. If you hit your condition dead on the first time – great. If not, shift the process ahead or back one or two days the next time and see how your body reacts.

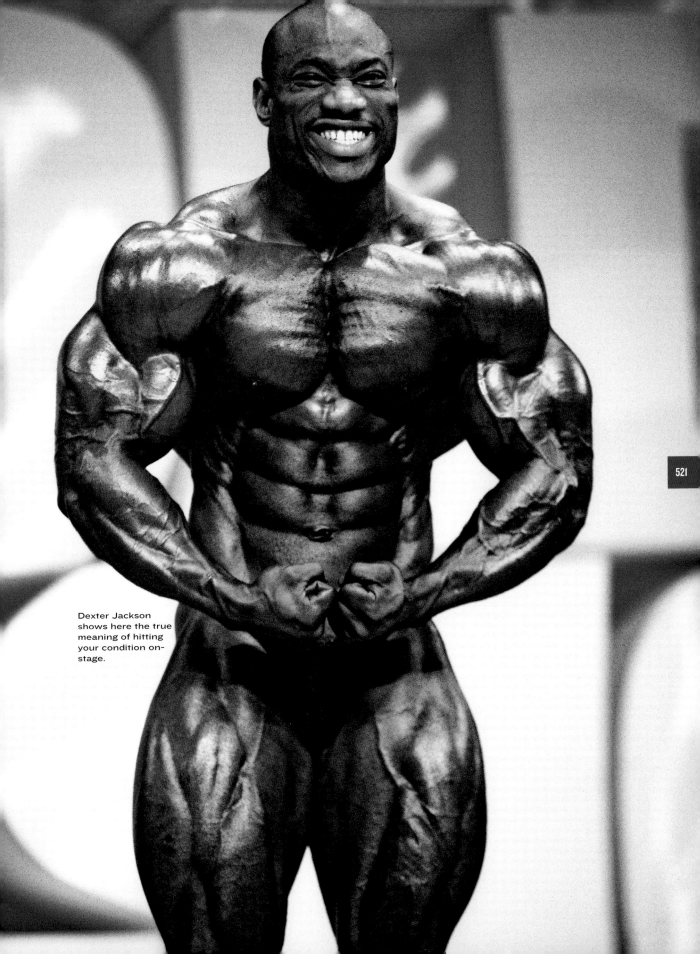

Dexter Jackson shows here the true meaning of hitting your condition on-stage.

521

GLOSSARY

Acromegaly – one of the side effects attributed to excessive amounts of growth hormone. The condition is characterized by a thickening of the ends of bones, particularly the forehead and elbows.

Adaptogens – a group of substances reputed to offer the body varying degrees of protection against internal and external stressors. These compounds were slow to catch on in North America, but were used much earlier by athletes in the former Soviet Union.

Addiction – a condition in which the body becomes so accustomed to a drug that it can no longer function properly without it. Addiction can be physical or psychological in nature, and breaking the condition usually involves a period of withdrawal when the body must readjust to its pre-drug state.

Adenosine triphosphate (ATP) – the body's chief energy source during cellular respiration. During periods of increased energy requirements, ATP is broken down into adenosine diphosphate (ADP) and phosphate (P).

Agonist – a pharmacological term used to describe a drug that stimulates receptors to produce a given biochemical response.

Amino acids – often called the "building blocks of life," amino acids are sub-units that join together in sequences to form protein. Amino acids are named as such because they contain both an acid and an amine chemical side unit.

Anabolic – a chemical reaction that occurs in the body by which smaller sub-units are combined to form larger units (e.g., amino acids are joined together to form long polypeptide chains which in turn join to form strands of protein).

Anabolic steroids – the group of drugs developed to mimic the anabolic effects of the naturally occurring hormone, testosterone. Anabolic steroids are by far the most popular performance-enhancing drugs.

Androgenic – one of the two primary categories of effects produced by such agents as anabolic steroids and testosterone. Androgenic effects include acne, increased facial hair and the development of secondary sex characteristics.

Antagonist – a pharmacological term used to describe a drug that blocks or shuts down a receptor, thus reducing or terminating a given biochemical response.

Anti-catabolic drugs – a class of drugs that halts or slows the wasting effects of catabolic hormones such as cortisol.

Anti-diuretic hormone (ADH) – a hormone produced by the posterior pituitary gland that's responsible for fluid and mineral conservation. Bodybuilders often take ADH blockers to promote water loss in the days leading up to a bodybuilding contest.

Antioxidants – a group of substances reputed to neutralize harmful free radicals produced during cellular respiration.

Arthritis – an inflammation of the tissues surrounding bone joints. There are two types: osteoarthritis, which is produced by the daily wear and tear on connective tissue; and rheumatoid arthritis, which is caused by inflammation of the joint-synovial membranes.

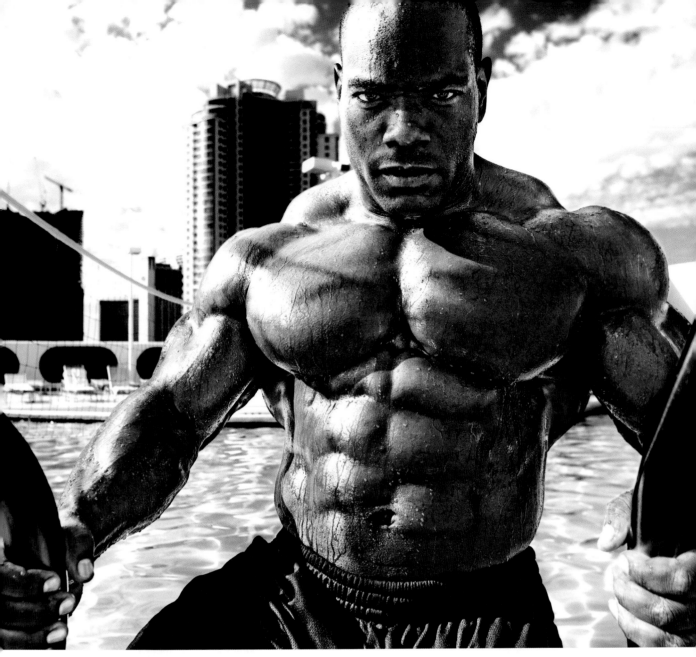

B

Beta agonists – a class of drugs that stimulate the beta adrenoreceptors in the body. Beta agonists are commonly used by bodybuilders as a means to promote fat loss.

Biological value (BV) – the scale of measurement used to determine what percentage of a given nutrient source is utilized by the body. The scale is most frequently applied to protein sources, particularly whey protein.

Blocking agents – the general term used by athletes to describe any class of drugs or substances that prevent a banned substance from being detected in a drug test. In recent years, such agents have declined in popularity since most sports federations have added them to their lists of banned substances.

BMR (Basil Metabolic Rate) – the speed at which the resting body consumes energy (calories).

Buffering agents – any group of substances used to reduce the acidity caused by the buildup of lactic acid during intense exercise.

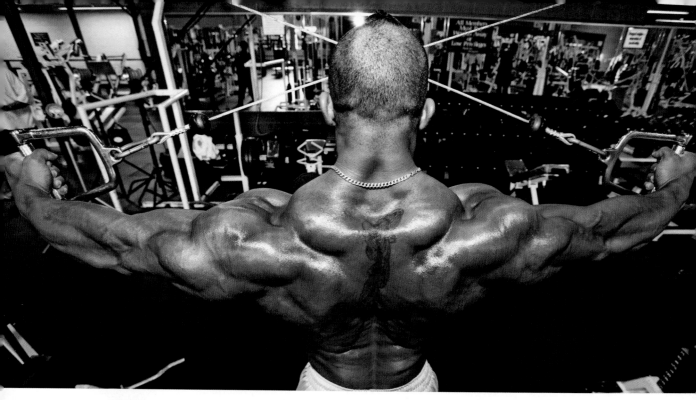

C

Carbohydrate – a molecule composed of carbon, hydrogen and oxygen. It serves as the body's primary short-term fuel source.

Catabolic – chemical reactions in the body in which larger units are broken down into smaller sub-units. For example, muscle tissue may be broken down into protein strands, which in turn may be cleaved into individual amino acids.

Catheterization – an extreme method of passing a drug test whereby the athlete – usually male – injects "clean" urine into his bladder by way of a long, thin hose called a catheter.

Circadian rhythm – daily cycles of bodily function, individual to each human being, commonly called the biological clock.

Cocktailing – the slang term used by athletes to refer to the practice of taking a mixture of performance-enhancing drugs.

Corticosteroids – a class of hormones that are catabolic in nature. Corticosteroids, like adrenalin and cortisol, are released in response to internal and external stressors, one of which is exercise.

D

Cycling – the practice of alternating periods of drug use with periods of abstinence. Cycling is believed to allow the body to readjust to its pre-drug state, thus reducing the risk of developing severe side effects.

Dehydration – the biological state that occurs when the body has insufficient water levels for proper functioning. The human body is over 90 percent water, so athletes must continuously replenish the water lost during intense exercise.

Delivery method – the route of administration of a given drug or supplement. The most common delivery methods are oral (mouth) and injection (needle).

Depressants – a class of drugs that slow the central nervous system. Although not technically performance-enhancing drugs, many athletes use depressants to relax between competitions and training.

Diuretics – a class of drugs used by athletes to decrease water conservation in the body. Bodybuilders use diuretics to increase muscular definition and separation. Unfortunately, further to fluid loss, diuretics also flush life-sustaining electrolytes from the body.

E F

Electrolytes – charged atoms called ions that help regulate the body's various metabolic systems. Athletes regularly consume drinks enriched with electrolytes and important minerals such as potassium, calcium and sodium to replace those lost in sweat.

Electrostimulation – a muscle-stimulation technique involving the use of a low-voltage electrical current. This technique has limited use in physiotherapy, but its merits as an ergogenic aid are questionable.

Epinephrine (also called adrenaline) – this hormone, produced by the adrenal medulla, initiates the "flight or fight" response, preparing the body to deal with a stressful event. Athletes often use the hormone as a thermogenic drug because one of the side effects is fat mobilization.

Ergogenic aids – the umbrella term used to describe any substance that enhances athletic performance. It comes from the Greek *ergo*, to work, and *genesis*, the beginning.

Essential amino acids – a group of nine amino acids that cannot be manufactured by the body and must be consumed in the diet.

Estrogen – one of the two primary sex hormones in the female body (the other being progesterone). In males, excess testosterone is converted to estrogen, which can often lead to the condition of gynecomastia.

Fat – a high-energy molecule that provides the body with long-term fuel reserves. Fat also serves as a precursor for many hormones and offers the body varying degrees of insulation and cushioning.

Feedback control – the process by which the body's hormonal systems monitor and regulate their own levels of circulating hormones.

Free radicals – electrically charged particles that are produced during cellular respiration. It is believed that aging is caused by a buildup of free radicals, leading to a gradual decline in health.

525

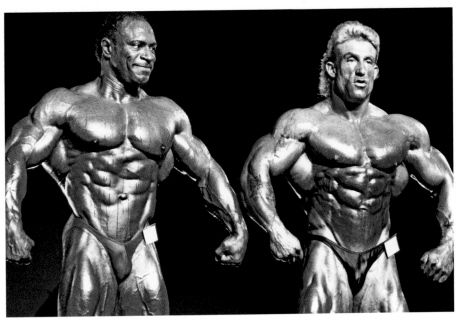

Photo by Robert Kennedy
Models Lee Haney and Dorian Yates

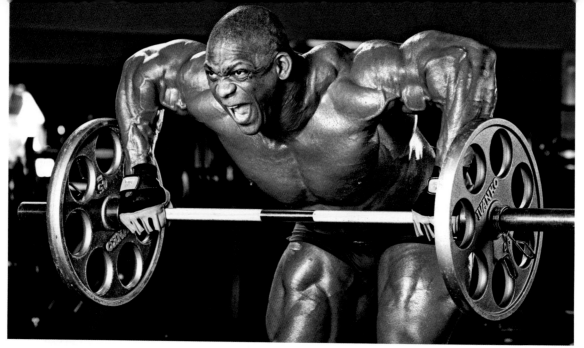

G H I J K

Genetic engineering – the science of manipulating an organism's predetermined genetic code at the DNA level. These processes allow for variations that otherwise would not be possible by natural reproductive means.

Glandulars – a group of supplements derived from the dehydration of animal organs and glands. These substances are reputed to work by stimulating the corresponding organ or gland in humans. As a group, glandulars are generally viewed to be among the most worthless supplements.

Glycogenesis – the biochemical process by which glucose is converted into glycogen.

Glycogenolysis – the biochemical process by which the liver converts stored glycogen back into glucose for use as fuel.

Growth hormone – a peptide hormone secreted by the pituitary gland responsible for the repair and growth of tissues such as bones, muscles and organs. In recent years growth hormone has become one of the most popular agents used by professional bodybuilders.

Gynecomastia – a condition that can occur in males caused by an excess of testosterone or testosterone-derived agent. When it becomes converted (aromatized) to estrogen, the excess estrogen stimulates receptors in the nipple area leading to a swelling that resembles female breasts. The condition is commonly called "bitch tits." In some cases, the condition is severe enough to warrant surgical removal.

Hormone – a chemical messenger released by an endocrine gland that travels to a target organ and produces a given response. Hormones may be steroid or peptide in nature.

Hormonal manipulation – the practice of altering the body's hormonal systems to increase or decrease a given physiological effect. Such manipulations allow athletes to achieve performance levels far beyond those possible through normal means.

Implants – artificial prosthetics, usually silicone, used to increase the size of a given bodypart. In males the calves and chest are the most frequent implant regions, while in females the breasts are the most common site.

Insulin – a hormone produced by the pancreas that controls blood glucose level and amino acids.

Krebs cycle (also called the citric acid cycle) – a complex biochemical pathway that acts as the body's primary method for producing ATP.

526

L
M

Lactic acid – a bodily product given off during aerobic respiration. This acid was once thought to be strictly a waste product, but recent evidence suggests that a version of lactic acid called lactate is used by the liver to replenish glycogen supplies.

Liposuction – a surgical technique in which fat cells are removed by a vacuuming procedure. Originally limited to extremely obese individuals, the surgery has become popular as a cosmetic procedure among the mainstream population.

Masculinization – the general term used to describe the various side effects experienced by female users of anabolic steroids. Common effects include deepening of the voice, facial hair growth and clitoral enlargement.

Meal-Replacement Powders (MRPs) – powdered supplements that can serve as meal substitutes. They contain a full profile and proper amount of recovery and muscle-building nutrients such as protein, complex carbohydrates, vitamins and minerals, and healthy fats.

Medium – in biochemistry, the term used to describe the substance that a given injectable drug is dissolved or suspended in. Most anabolic drugs are suspended in either an oil-based or water-based solution.

Mega-dosing – the practice of taking athletic drugs and supplements in dosages far beyond the recommended or necessary amount to obtain a desired effect.

Metabolic optimizer – the general term used to describe any supplement that boosts an athlete's recovery system. Most metabolic optimizers contain a substance that is reputed to offer some degree of performance enhancement.

Metabolism – the sum total of all biochemical reactions that take place in the human body. Metabolism can be divided into anabolism and catabolism, the balance of which determines whether an individual gains or loses weight.

Mineral – a naturally occurring inorganic element used to support biochemical processes in the body.

Photo by Irvin Gelb
Model Frank McGrath

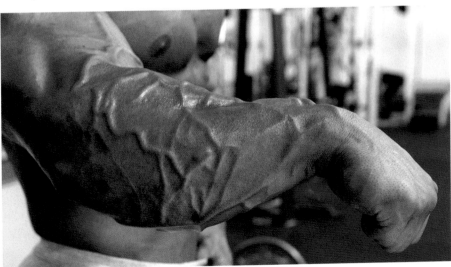

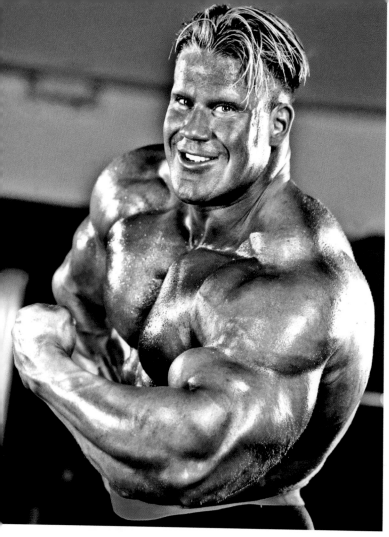

Polypeptide chains join together to form protein strands.

Peptide growth factors – peptide-derived hormone-like substances that promote growth and tissue repair. In athletic circles, insulin-like growth factor-1 (IGF-1) has become one of the most popular agents added to drug stacks.

Placebo effect – a pharmacological term used to describe the effects produced by an inert (inactive) substance. Often called "mind over matter," the placebo effect is used to explain the positive actions of many supplements, which are in many cases nothing more than nutrients. Most medical and scientific studies include a control group (given a placebo) to measure the placebo effect.

Polypharmacology – a term first coined by Dr. Mauro DiPasquale to describe the practice in bodybuilding of simultaneously stacking numerous performance-enhancing drugs.

Positive nitrogen balance – the biochemical state in which nitrogen levels are high enough to allow protein synthesis to occur. This results when more nitrogen is entering the system than is being expended. Positive nitrogen balance is one of the conditions accelerated by anabolic steroids.

Prostaglandins – hormone-like substances manufactured from fatty acids in plasma membranes that control such processes as digestion and cardiovascular function.

Protein – the general term used to describe molecules that are composed of specific sequences of amino acids. The amino acids in protein are the body's primary building material, and while small amounts of this nutrient can be manufactured, most must be consumed in the diet.

N

Neurotransmitters – chemicals released into the clefts between nerve cells that act as transporters to carry nerve signals within the brain.

O

Nostrum – an ancient term used to describe any blend or concoction made by the person who recommends it. Despite the dated origin of this term, it is applicable to modern supplement advertising.

P

Painkillers – a class of drugs used to nullify the sensation of pain. Painkillers range from mild forms (aspirin) to powerful agents (morphine). Some forms can be purchased over the counter, while others require a prescription.

Q

Peptide – a term used to describe any substance that is protein in nature and is composed of sequences of amino acids.

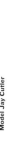

R

Receptor – the point or location on a target cell that serves as the attachment point for a given drug. Receptors are generally specific for only one class of drugs.

Roid rage – the popular name or slang term used to describe the uncontrollable outbursts of anger and violence exhibited by anabolic steroid users. The condition itself has never been proven by the medical community, but the term is continuously exaggerated by mainstream media.

Saturated fatty acids – fat molecules that do not have double bonds between their carbon atoms and are usually solid at room temperature. This form of fat is considered to play a major role in the development of cardiovascular disease.

Shotgunning – another term used to describe the practice of consuming mega doses of multiple athletic drugs. For many athletes the limiting factor on the number and amount of drugs used is cost.

S

Snake oil – a general term used to describe any supplement or concoction that doesn't give the same degree of results as claimed by its advertisers. The origin of this term actually stems from traveling carnivals dating back to the 1800s.

Stacking – the practice of taking two or more performance-enhancing drugs at one time. The actual drugs, combinations and dosages are what compose the stack.

Steroid – the biochemical term used to denote a molecule having three 6-carbon-containing rings and one 5-carbon-containing ring. Steroid molecules form the nucleus of many of the body's hormones.

Steroid replacer – the general term used to describe any naturally occurring substance that supposedly duplicates the effects of anabolic steroids. To date, no steroid replacer has been scientifically proven to be as effective as any anabolic drug.

Stimulants – a class of drugs that increase or excite the central nervous system. Stimulants may be mild (ephedrine) or powerful (amphetamines).

Supplement – any substance that is taken above and beyond the nutrients obtained in the daily diet. Most supplements are simply measured amounts of specific nutrients (usually in pill or tablet form), but a few do enhance physical performance.

Synergism – the biochemical phenomenon in which two or more drugs interact to produce a combined effect that is greater than the individual effects of each drug. In bodybuilding, growth hormone and IGF-1 taken separately produce limited results, but when taken together they produce dramatic increases in size and strength.

T U V W X Y Z

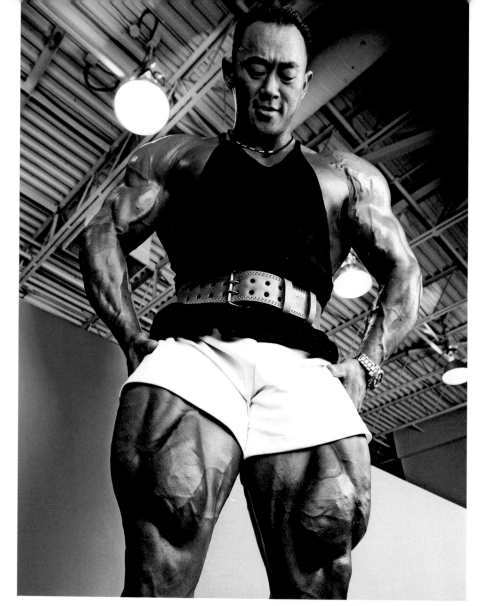

T3 and T4 – the body's two primary thyroid hormones responsible for controlling metabolism. Many competitive bodybuilders take these hormones to speed up fat loss.

Testosterone – the primary male sex hormone. Females also have testosterone, though in much lower concentrations than men, which has led to it being defined as a "male" hormone. Most anabolic steroids are derivatives of testosterone.

Thermogenesis – the process by which stored fat is liberated and mobilized in order to be burned as a fuel source. The most popular bodybuilding thermogenic agents are ephedrine and caffeine.

Thyroid gland – a small gland located in the neck that controls the body's level of calcium and overall metabolic rate. Bodybuilders often add thyroid drugs to their pre-contest drug stacks to increase their body's metabolic rate and speed up fat loss.

Unsaturated fatty acids – a category of fat molecules that have double bonds between their carbon atoms and are usually liquid at room temperature. Generally speaking, as the number of double bonds increase, the fat becomes oilier.

Vitamin – an organic compound used by the body for biochemical functions. Vitamins can be water-soluble or fat-soluble.

Photo by Paul Buceta
Model Jea Jung

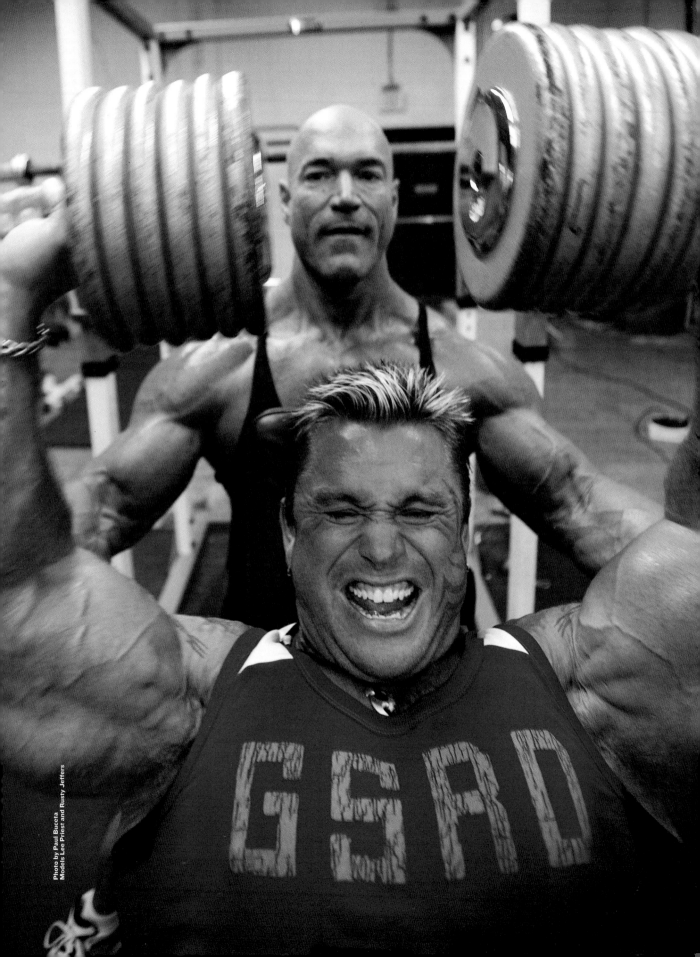

Photo by Paul Buceta
Models Lee Priest and Rusty Jeffers

INDEX

535

tapering off steroids, 100,
  Vitamin C, 342
Morpheus, 238
Morphine, 236-239
morphium, 236
Motrin, 228
Mr. Olympia, 32, 91, 131, 436
Mr. Universe, 46, 502
Multiple Sclerosis (MS), 119
multivitamin, 336, 339, 456
Multivitamin/Mineral, 456
Muscle Builder Power, 19
muscle cells, 190, 204, 284, 307, 310, 340, 359,
  360, 428, 509
muscle contraction, 64, 143, 189, 190, 192, 288,
  338, 352, 354
muscle-building, 110, 116, 120, 167, 169, 188, 252,
  253, 254, 256, 258,
meals, 426-429, 450-451,
  reducing potential, 331
  supplements, 454-460
Muscle Juice, 481
muscle loss, 162
Muscle Media 2000, 20
muscle memory, 107
Muscle Sparing, 284-285
muscle stagnation, 94
muscle tissue, 41, 64, 75, 77, 109, 110, 118, 120, 179,
  204, 205, 218, 248, 269, 272, 273, 284, 285, 340,
  374, 394, 427, 431, 432, 443, 445, 448, 450, 455
Muscle and Fitness, 19, 20, 46, 188, 367
MuscleMag International, 12, 22, 25, 47, 121, 188,
  242, 253, 271, 272, 277, 283, 367, 385, 412
MuscleTech, 20, 264, 501
Muscular Development, 497
myelin sheaths, 192
Myoplex, 264

N

nalbuphine, 234
nandrolone, 371, 373
narcolepsy, 219
narcotics, 90, 234
NASA, 64, 402
nasal spray, 56, 368
National Hockey League, 283
National Institute on Drug Abuse, 88
National Strength and Conditioning
Association's Creatine Symposium, 352
natural testosterone, 103, 509
nausea, 56, 170, 236, 264, 317, 320, 361, 392, 406,
  418, 424
needle, 54, 55, 74, 75, 99, 413
nephron, 139

nervous system, 37, 143, 172, 174, 179, 211, 213, 234,
  236, 239, 283, 340, 391
nervousness, 173
Nescafe, 212
neurotransmitter, 84, 174, 199, 279, 340, 342
neutrophils, 273
New England Journal of Medicine, 32
New York Islanders, 283
NFL-AFL merger, 48
Nicholls, Chad, 256
nitric acid, 360
nitric oxide, 259, 289, 360-361
Nitric Oxide Supplements, 360-361
nitrogen, 64, 242, 248, 251, 269, 272
Nitrogen Balance, 248
No Magic Pill, 438-440
NoDoz, 215
Nolvadex (Tamoxifen Citrate), 111-112
Nolvadex, 106, 111-112
Non-cyclic, 63
noradrenaline, 126, 163, 166
norepinephrine, 118, 157, 166, 179
Not Just GH, 460
NPU (Net Protein Utilization) 261
NSAIDs, 228-229
Nubain, 227, 234-235
nucleic acid, 391
nucleoside, 188
nutrient, 18, 30-32, 36, 192, 194, 242, 244, 245,
  253, 292, 294, 299, 303, 311, 341, 347, 348, 414,
  428, 431, 432, 438, 445, 448, 449, 450, 451, 457,
  499, 501, 512
nutrient window, 429
Nutrition, 30, 31, 32, 60, 95, 100, 101, 248, 263,
  393, 442, 448, 512
  Post-workout, 427-429, 431
  Pre-workout, 306, 426-427
Nutrition Research, 187
Nutritional Journal, 256
Nuts, 192, 445, 457

O

O-methylation, 236
Oatmeal, 452
obesity, 118, 202, 206
off-season, 60, 62, 333
Oils, 312-315
olive oil, 326-327
Olympia, 32, 91, 131, 436, 486, 494
Olympics, 15, 42, 48, 166, 218
  1976 Montreal, 15
  1992 Barcelona, 166, 352
  1996 Atlanta, 352
omega-3, 246, 293, 322, 323, 324, 325, 452, 499

Omega-6, 293, 318, 322, 323
opiate, 236
opium, 236, 238
Optimum Nutrition, 20, 264, 501
oral, 53, 97, 139, 211, 517
Origins, 128
osteoarthritis, 320, 406, 407, 510
Other Routes of Delivery, 56-57
Our Little Secret, 48-49
Over-the-counter (OTC), 22, 27, 178, 179, 182, 216,
  226, 228, 234, 282, 393, 424, 501, 515
Overcoming The Vicious Cycle, 164-165
overeat, 348, 436, 442, 445
oxidation, 253, 344, 391, 426
oxidative phosphorylation, 354, 355
oxygen, 85, 130, 180, 190, 310, 346, 350, 418

P

PA – Physical Activity, 434
painkillers, 224-239
Palmeiro, Rafael, 49
Pam spray, 477, 494
pancreas, 126, 128, 295, 331, 429
Pariza, Dr. Michael, 204
pasta, 294, 296, 445
PDCAAS (Protein Digestibility Corrected
Amino Acid Score), 262
peanut butter, 264-265, 438
Pearl, Bill, 46-47, 48, 502
PER (Protein Efficiency Ratio), 261
Percocet, 227
performance enhancement, 39, 46, 151, 210, 394, 500
  pressures, 51
personality types, 85
pH levels, 288
Phillips, Bill, 19-20, 22-23, 402
phosphatidyl choline (PC), 192
Phosphoenolpyruvate, 186
phosphoglycerides, 192
phosphoric acid, 192
phosphorus, 382
physical activity, 319, 432, 434
phytic acid, 194
phytoestrogens, 259
pituitary gland, 37, 116, 117, 137, 160, 347, 366
placebo effect, 28-29, 379
plateau buster, 121
Platz, Tom, 47
polyphenols, 201, 326, 327, 351
polyunsaturated fats, 292, 293, 318
polyvinyl chloride, 231-232
Pope Clement VIII, 212
pork, 245
Post-steroid Drug Therapy, 105-106